Fitness Programming and Physical Disability

Patricia D. Miller, MA

Editor

A publication for Disabled Sports USA

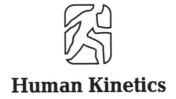
Human Kinetics

Contents

Preface

A new interest in expanding opportunities for all people to develop physical fitness has sparked an increase in exercise research about and programming for people with physical disabilities. Rehabilitation professionals also recognize the importance of physical fitness training for both acute-care and outpatient clientele to correspond with a growing emphasis on recreation and sports in the rehabilitation setting. To meet the demands for professional training created by this expanding interest, we have written *Fitness Programming and Physical Disability* to provide fitness leaders—whether they work in community exercise or rehabilitation programs—with a comprehensive resource for information about the principles and practice of developing fitness programs for people with physical disabilities.

Despite this new awareness and interest in physical fitness for everyone, opportunities for people with disabilities to participate in fitness programs remain quite limited. Physical, attitudinal, and program barriers continue to challenge accessibility. Recent legislation—the 1973 Rehabilitation Act and the 1990 Americans with Disabilities Act (ADA)—has attempted to dismantle some of the barriers our citizens with disabilities continually encounter. Unfortunately, attitudinal barriers and inappropriate stereotypes persist because *programs* are not accessible, which prevents socially integrative experiences from educating everyone about the abilities, needs, and rights of individuals with disabilities. Many instructors are simply unaware that existing programs can be safely and effectively adapted to enable individuals with disabilities to participate— *without* changing the basic quality or nature of the activity.

Fitness Programming and Physical Disability fills the information gap for exercise leaders. This book addresses theoretical and practical details about developing and implementing fitness programs so you can individualize instruction for people with physical disabilities in a group setting. Experts in the fields of exercise science, physical disability, and adapted exercise programming have contributed their knowledge to bring you this comprehensive and practical resource. Because there are so many types and varieties of disabilities, this book attempts only to offer basic information, safety guidelines, and general strategies for adapting exercise classes. The successful program will depend on the skills, knowledge, creativity, and genuine interests of the instructors and directors who shape accessible fitness programs.

Fitness Programming and Physical Disability is divided into four parts, addressing disability, exercise science, program modifications, and program management. Part I provides an introduction to disability: It heightens awareness about facility and program accessibility, suggests preferred behaviors and appropriate language for interacting with people who have disabilities, and reviews general characteristics and exercise implications associated with several of the most common disabilities. This information is particularly worthwhile for the community exercise leader who has limited experience working with people who have physical disabilities or for the rehabilitation professional who needs a review of general exercise implications in the context of health-fitness training for specific disabling conditions.

Part II provides a theoretical base of exercise science that must underlie decisions about adapting exercises and techniques. The principles presented take into consideration how physically disabling conditions might alter the structure and function of the physiologic systems that interact to support aerobic and anaerobic exercise.

We offer guidelines for adapting fitness programs, including modifying principles of conditioning and developing individualized resistance training, stretching, and aerobic dance exercise programs, in Part III. These ideas provide a framework for developing safe, effective, and appropriately modified exercises and routines.

We address practical issues associated with managing accessible fitness programs in Part IV. We include tips for promoting and implementing integrated programs, intervention techniques for medical conditions and emergencies in the exercise setting, and information about wheelchairs and providing assistance to individuals who use them.

Fitness Programming and Physical Disability is not a cookbook with recipes and formulas for program designs but a resource guide to stimulate your interest in taking on new challenges. We hope that after reading this book, you will assume the responsibility you have as an exercise leader for offering fitness training opportunities to people of all abilities who deserve access to the benefits and pleasures of group or individualized exercise programs.

Patricia D. Miller, Editor

Acknowledgments

Many people have contributed to the development of *Fitness Programming and Physical Disability*. It has been a true team effort. I am especially indebted to the chapter authors for their dedication to the project and for the contribution each has made to educate others about the importance of fitness and recreation for individuals with disabilities.

Thanks also to the fitness consultants to *Disabled Sports USA*; all of them have devoted their energy and expertise unselfishly to further the growth of accessible fitness programs through instructor training workshops, and they are largely responsible for expanding my knowledge in this field. I am especially indebted to Kate Baxter, Terry Chase, Pat DiRocco, Nancy Gillette, Kim Hardin, Diane Huss, Karen Jacobs, Kevin Lockette, Greg McMahon, and Kathy Normansell for their support and enlightenment.

I am also indebted to the volunteers who offered their time as models and who appear throughout the book—including Jeff Miller, Nadine Taylor, Herb Talbert, Brenda Levy, and Dave Stradley (to name a few)—and to Dennis Crews, our studio photographer.

I would also like to thank Steve Figoni, Jennifer Heyman, Leanne Monroe, Daniel Kosich, and the reviewers selected by Human Kinetics for their support and advice. Very special thanks to Trudy Orgel and Pearl Paper for their administrative and clerical assistance.

Last but not least, I am indebted to Mary Fowler, Rick Frey, and the staff at Human Kinetics for their talents, support, and patience over the long period involved in producing this book.

Patti Miller

Disabled Sports USA (DS/USA, formerly National Handicapped Sports) wishes to acknowledge the following corporations and organizations for their financial support of DS/USA's Adapted Fitness Instructor (AFI) Program, which was a testing ground for, and contributed greatly to, the development of this manual. They are: **United Airlines, Paralyzed Veterans of America Education and Training Foundation, The Million Dollar Round Table Foundation, U.S. Department of Education**, and the **The Bristol-Myers Squibb Fund**.

DS/USA's deepest appreciation is extended to Patti Miller and the fitness consultants of DS/USA for their dedication and the expertise they devoted to expand accessible fitness programs through instructor training and certification workshops and/or the development of this manual. Special recognition goes to Kate Baxter, Karen Charlton, Terry Chase, Dr. Pat DiRocco, Kim Hardin, Diane Huss, Karen Jacobs, Kevin Lockette, Greg McMahon, Kathy Normansell, and Denise Terry.

DS/USA joins the editor in extending a special thanks to the chapter authors of *Fitness Programming and Physical Disability*, and to Dr. Steve Figoni, Jennifer Heyman, Leanne Monroe, Daniel Kosich, and the reviewers selected by Human Kinetics.

This project would not have been possible without DS/USA's Executive Director, Kirk Bauer, and staff member, Bobbi Avancena, who conceived, funded and directed the original "Fitness Is For Everyone" program and its offshoot, the AFI program. DS/USA is also deeply indebted to its staff, Trudy Orgel and Pearl Paper, for their administrative and clerical assistance.

Human Kinetics has provided invaluable technical support and expertise in bringing this manual to fruition. Thanks to Mary Fowler and Rick Frey and the HK staff. DS/USA is honored to be associated with this outstanding publishing firm.

Disabled Sports USA

Part I

Physical Disability

●

Encouraging your clients to continue with their exercise programs is as important as offering them quality instruction. To do this effectively, you must communicate through your words and actions a respect, concern, and enthusiasm for their participation in your classes. You also must consider the uniqueness of each person, whether you offer group or individual training. This is important for all clients—those with disabilities as well as those without.

Adapting programs for exercisers with physical disabilities may initially seem overwhelming. You may feel uncomfortable interacting with people who have disabilities and worry about speaking or acting appropriately. You also may feel overwhelmed by the many varieties of disabilities and wonder whether you can offer safe and effective instruction. With time, your apprehension will lessen as you learn that people with disabilities are really more like than unlike people without disabilities. You will also find that by experimenting with an individual's movement abilities, referring to the guidelines in this book, and seeking guidance from appropriate health care professionals, you can offer all clients a rewarding exercise program.

Part I offers basic information about physical disability to help you establish a base from which appropriate exercise programs can be developed. Chapter 1 highlights the issues of facility and program accessibility and offers guidelines for communicating and interacting with clients who have physical impairments. Chapter 2 reviews the characteristics, classifications, and general exercise implications of some common physical disabilities. This book builds on that information. Refer to Part I to better understand the ideas in subsequent chapters, which introduce the principles and techniques of adapting exercise programs.

Recommended Readings

Auxter, D., & Pyfer, J. (1993). *Principles and methods of adapted physical education and recreation* (7th ed.). St. Louis: Times Mirror/Mosby College Publishing.

Bleck, E., & Nagel, D. (1982). *Physically handicapped children: A medical atlas for teachers* (2nd ed.). New York: Grune & Stratton.

*Bullock, C.C., McCann, C.A., & Palmer, R.I. (1988). *LIFE Support Manual; LIFE Forms: The LIFE Training Guide;* and *LIFE Resources: The LIFE Resource Manual.* Chapel Hill, NC: Office of Research and Services, Curriculum in Leisure Studies and Recreation Administration, University of North Carolina at Chapel Hill.

*Bullock, C.C, & Palmer, R.I. (1985). *Community reintegration program facilitator's guide.* Chapel Hill, NC: Office of Research and Services, Curriculum in Leisure Studies and Recreation Administration, University of North Carolina at Chapel Hill.

Cobble, N.D., & Maloney, F.P. (1985). Effects of exercise in neuromuscular disease. In F.P. Maloney, J.S. Burks, & S.P. Ringel (Eds.), *Interdisciplinary rehabilitation of multiple sclerosis and neuromuscular disorders* (pp. 228-238). Philadelphia: J.B. Lippincott.

Dunn, J., & Fait, H. (1989). *Special physical education* (4th ed.). Dubuque, IA: Brown.

Gordon, N.F. (1993a). *Arthritis: Your complete exercise guide.* Champaign, IL: Human Kinetics.

Gordon, N.F. (1993b). *Stroke: Your complete exercise guide.* Champaign, IL: Human Kinetics.

Kottke, F.J., & Lehmann, J.F. (Eds.) (1990). *Krusen's handbook of physical medicine and rehabilitation.* Philadelphia: W.B. Saunders.

Lasko-McCarthey, P.M., & Knopf, K.G. (1992). Adapted physical education for adults with disabilities (3rd ed.). Dubuque, IA: Eddie Bowers.

Marieb, E.N. (1991). *Essentials of human anatomy and physiology* (3rd ed.). Redwood City, CA: Benjamin/Cummings.

Sherrill, C. (1993). *Adapted physical activity, recreation, and sport: Cross disciplinary and lifespan* (4th ed.). Dubuque, IA: Brown & Benchmark.

Thomas, C. (1981). *Taber's cyclopedic medical dictionary.* Philadelphia: F.A. Davis.

U.S. Equal Employment Opportunity Commission and the U.S. Department of Justice, Civil Rights Division. (1990). *The Americans with Disabilities Act: Questions and answers.* Washington, DC: Author.

*Note. Copies of the publications by Bullock can be requested by contacting:

Center for Recreation and Disability Studies
Curriculum in Leisure Studies and Recreation
    Administration
CB #8145, 730 Airport Rd., Ste. 204
University of North Carolina at Chapel Hill
Chapel Hill, NC 27599-8145
(919) 962-0534

Chapter 1

Disability Awareness: Considerations for the Exercise Leader

Charles C. Bullock, PhD
Michael J. Mahon, PhD
University of North Carolina at Chapel Hill

All people have the right to choose what kinds of exercise they do, as well as with whom and where they would like to do it. This is both a moral and a legal right. Yet people with disabilities often are denied access to the full range of exercise opportunities that constitute this right. As an exercise leader you are responsible for ensuring that your exercise programs are accessible to all people, whether or not they have disabilities. To accomplish this you must find out as much as possible about the wants and needs of the people in the exercise program.

This chapter aims to increase your awareness of accessibility and barriers to participation, recent federal laws relevant to public accommodations (including exercise facilities), and how appropriate language and actions can communicate positive attitudes about people with disabilities. It concludes with recommendations for interacting with individuals who have physical, cognitive, or visual impairments to enhance their enjoyment of exercise.

It is important to note that general information of the kind we provide should not be used to stereotype the wants, needs, skills, and capabilities of people with disabilities. Finding out how to make a given program accessible to a particular individual is best accomplished by asking him. It is the easiest and most accurate way to get the specific information that you need to provide the most satisfying exercise program possible.

Accessibility and Barriers to Participation

The legal and ethical ideal is that all exercise programs and facilities should be equally accessible to all people. An opportunity is not, in fact, an opportunity for a person with a disability if it is not accessible. As an exercise leader, it is your ethical responsibility to ensure that your programs are accessible to all, despite any legal loopholes that may not require you to comply with certain standards.

Accessibility applies to exercise opportunities in two ways. The most commonly understood kind is physical accessibility, which generally refers to the physical environment within which an activity or program is offered. Stairs, bathroom facilities, and elevators can all be physical barriers that can make it difficult or impossible for people with certain disabilities to participate.

Administrative policies and procedures are also part of the environment within which exercise activities are offered and can be barriers to participation. Such barriers constitute one major problem in fulfilling the mandate that people with disabilities receive equal opportunities for participation. Eliminating such barriers is essential to achieving equal opportunity.

The second kind of accessibility is programmatic—programs and activities must be designed to enable people with a variety of disabilities to participate fully and have rewarding experiences. Program accessibility means that any criteria for participation are applied to all potential participants equally based on skill levels or realistic safety considerations and not on characteristics such as race, sex, religion, national origin, or handicap. Program accessibility can also mean that program leaders and instructors understand the needs of people with disabilities and that they are skilled in modifying the existing program to meet these needs.

Everyone—not only people with disabilities—encounters some people, things, or conditions that can diminish the enjoyment of an activity, but people with disabilities probably face them more often. These obstacles are potential barriers to participation that can render facilities and programs inaccessible, and they represent challenges to be overcome. Barriers can usually be classified into three broad categories: physical, attitudinal, and resource-related.

Physical Barriers

A physical barrier is a condition of the physical environment that restricts or complicates access, movement, or participation. Physical barriers include more than just architectural barriers, such as stairs, curbs, narrow hallways, or doors that are hard to open; they also include natural physical barriers such as steep hills, thick tree growth, and other frustrating obstacles for many people with impaired mobility.

Attitudinal Barriers

Another class of obstacles to free movement includes the perceptions and consequent attitudes of members of society toward people who are disabled, as well as the perceptions and attitudes of people who are disabled about themselves. Many people who are not disabled believe that people who are disabled should be segregated from the rest of society, especially when it comes to exercise. This attitude is often a convenient excuse to avoid contact with people who are disabled because of fear, discomfort, or an unwillingness to compromise activity to include people with different needs and abilities. Its result is often to discourage people who are disabled explicitly or implicitly from participating in programs with people who are not disabled.

Some people who are disabled may sit at home and not become involved in things they enjoy because of the potential embarrassment and alienation from people who are not disabled due to their performance. People who are disabled may choose isolation to avoid the stares of others. Both of these cases represent attitudinal barriers.

Resource-Related Barriers

Resources that are unavailable but necessary for participation in a particular recreational activity are considered resource-related barriers. Lack of money, transportation, equipment, and moral support are all potential resource-related barriers. For example, a person with a disability who wants to swim for fun and exercise faces a resource-related barrier if there is no swimming pool nearby or if the proper transportation to the nearest pool is unavailable.

Recent Federal Legislation

Over the past several decades, federal laws designed to protect the rights of people with disabilities have aimed at removing barriers that limit opportunities for employment and accessibility of services, facilities, and accommodations.

The Rehabilitation Act

In 1973 the U.S. Congress signed into law section 504 of the Rehabilitation Act, which stated, in part:

> No otherwise qualified handicapped individual in the United States . . . shall, solely by virtue of his handicap, be excluded from the participation in, be denied the benefits of, or be subjected to discrimination under any federal program or activity receiving federal financial assistance.

Section 504 has been one of the most significant pieces of civil rights legislation. In spite of section 504, however, equal opportunity for Americans with disabilities to participate in a wide range of programs, including exercise programs, remained the exception rather than the rule. It became clear that stronger legislation was needed to improve access to public life for citizens with disabilities.

The ADA and Public Accommodations

On July 26, 1990, former President George Bush signed into law the Americans With Disabilities Act (ADA). The ADA was originally introduced to eliminate widespread discrimination against people with disabilities in employment, public accommodations, services, transportation, and communications. The ADA requires employers with 15 or more employees (25 or more employees during the 2 years following enactment to accommodate the needs of medium-sized businesses), labor organizations, industries, employment agencies, public services providers, and state and local governments to make reasonable accommodations to allow people with disabilities an equal opportunity to participate in or benefit from a job, program, service, or activity. The five titles or sections of the ADA cover employment, public service, public accommodations, telecommunications, and miscellaneous. The information that follows concerns only Title III, Public Accommodations, as this section relates to public exercise facilities.

The ADA public accommodations provisions became effective on January 26, 1992. The law defines *public accommodations* as private entities that affect commerce, including restaurants, hotels, fitness centers, theaters, doctors' offices, pharmacies, retail stores, museums, libraries, parks, private schools, and day-care centers. Private clubs and religious organizations are exempt from the ADA's requirements for public accommodations.

Safety

Under the ADA, a public accommodation may exclude someone if you determine that the person poses a direct threat to the health or safety of others. However, the threat must be of a nature that cannot be relieved by appropriate modifications in the public accommodation's policies or procedures or by providing auxiliary aids. You are permitted to establish safety standards based on objective requirements for the operation of your business; however, any safety standard must be based on objective requirements rather than stereotypes or generalizations about the ability of people with disabilities to participate in activities at your facility.

Auxiliary Aids and Services

The ADA requires that public accommodations make auxiliary aids and services available to ensure effective communication with individuals who have hearing or vision impairments. Thus, you may be required to provide qualified interpreters, assistive listening devices, note takers, and written materials for people who are hearing impaired and qualified readers, taped texts, and braille or large print materials for people who are visually impaired.

The ADA does not require you to provide any auxiliary aid that would result in an undue burden or a fundamental alteration in the nature of the goods or services provided. However, you must furnish an alternative auxiliary aid, if available, that would not result in a fundamental alteration or undue burden. (These limitations are derived from existing regulations and are to be determined on a case-by-case basis.) For example, a health spa wouldn't be required to have braille signs and instructions if its employees were available to read to customers with visual impairments. A YMCA wouldn't be required to maintain a sign language interpreter on staff to communicate with customers who are hearing impaired if employees would communicate by pen and note pad when necessary. Evaluate the resources at your facility and establish procedures to employ some means for communication with people who have hearing or visual impairments.

Barrier Removal

The ADA stipulates that facilities that are public accommodations must remove barriers if doing so is "readily achievable," defined as "easily accomplishable and able to be carried out without much difficulty or expense" (ADA, section 303, 1990). Alterations considered readily achievable include providing a ramp over a few steps, installing grab bars where only routine reinforcement of the wall is required, lowering telephones, and similar modest adjustments.

With an existing facility, you must consider how alterations might make it as accessible as possible. For example, if you are relocating a doorway, the new doorway must be wide enough to meet the new-construction standard for accessibility. When you're altering a primary function area, such as the lobby, you must provide an accessible path of travel to the altered area, and you must make the bathrooms, telephones, and drinking fountains serving that area accessible as well.

Other alterations for accessibility are required only to the extent that the added accessibility costs are not disproportionate to the overall cost of the alterations. Elevators are generally not required in facilities under three stories or with fewer than 3,000 square ft per floor unless the building is a shopping center, mall, or professional office of a health care provider.

Discrimination and Legal Action

Failure to adhere to the ADA standards for public accommodations can result in legal action against your facility. The ADA public accommodations provisions permit an individual with a disability to allege discrimination based on a reasonable belief that discrimination is about to occur, even before it does. For example, a person who uses a wheelchair may challenge the planned construction of a new place of public accommodation, such as a shopping mall, that would not be accessible to wheelchair users. Resolution of such challenges prior to the construction of an inaccessible facility enables any necessary remedial measures to be incorporated in the building at the planning stage, when such changes would be relatively inexpensive.

Private individuals may bring lawsuits to obtain court orders to stop discrimination. Individuals may also file complaints with the attorney general, who is authorized to bring lawsuits in cases of general public importance or where a "pattern or practice" of discrimination is alleged. In these cases, the attorney general may seek monetary damages and civil penalties, not to exceed $50,000 for a first violation or $100,000 for any subsequent violation.

Communication, Attitudes, and Preferred Behaviors

Many people are not familiar with the appropriate terminology to use when communicating with or referring to people with disabilities. As an exercise leader, however, you become a role model for others in your facility. The way you refer to and communicate with people with disabilities reflects your attitudes and often shapes the images that others have about someone. By using appropriate terminology and by emphasizing that people with disabilities are people first and not part of a collective group called "the disabled," you can foster positive attitudes about people with disabilities. Appropriate communication techniques can be instrumental in providing welcoming environments.

Word Choices

You must be careful and deliberate about how you refer to people with disabilities. A guiding principle is to refer to the person first, not the disability. Instead of referring to "the disabled," it is more appropriate to say "people with disabilities." Referring to people with disabilities as "the disabled" creates an image of a group of people with many of the same characteristics. Some terms can be dehumanizing and perpetuate negative stereotypes about people with disabilities. Table 1.1 includes a list of phrases that represent positive and negative terminology.

The preferred terms focus attention on the uniqueness and the worth of an individual rather than emphasizing the individual's disabling condition. Avoid the connotation of "dis"-ability. It is not uncommon to hear someone use outdated words that create a negative image, such as *crazy, defective, deformed, retard, lame, cripple, spastic,* and *unfortunate.* It is very important that you model positive behaviors when communicating with people who have a disability—by choosing your words carefully, you can convey positive images about people with disabilities.

Table 1.1 Positive People-First Terminology

Positive terms	Negative terms
A person . . .	
Who is blind	Afflicted with blindness
With a physical disability	Crippled
Who is unable to speak or who is nonverbal	Deaf and dumb
With mental retardation	Retard
With Down Syndrome (a type of mental retardation)	Mongoloid
Who uses a wheelchair	Wheelchair-bound
Who has a hearing impairment	Stricken with deafness

General Preferred Behaviors

As a role model, you can encourage including people with disabilities in your exercise program by practicing the general behaviors listed. (We provide additional recommendations appropriate for specific disabling conditions beginning on p. 12).

❏ Ask if people want assistance rather than assuming they need it. The person with a disability is often the best one to identify the type and extent of assistance needed.
❏ Be careful not to assume that a person with one disability also has others. For example, a person in a wheelchair does not necessarily have a mental handicap, nor is a person who is blind likely to be hard of hearing.
❏ When talking to a person in a wheelchair or a short person, try to sit across from that person at eye level.
❏ Be sensitive to the person's feelings, as you would with any individual. You may discuss the same topics and use the same terminology with people who have disabilities as you would with any other person. For example, do not avoid using *look* or *see* with a person who has a visual impairment. You should not hesitate to say "let's walk or stroll" to a person who uses a wheelchair. People with disabilities are more like people without disabilities than they are different, and they fit into the normative society when normative words are used.
❏ Be patient without being overprotective or overindulgent. A person may not move quickly, but she may want to complete a project or activity independently.

❏ Allow participants with disabilities to take part in all activities you offer to the group. Let people make their own decisions regarding what they can and cannot do. Do not impose limitations upon someone else's capabilities or interests.
❏ Above all, use your imagination. That is the sense, more than any other, that will help you provide accessible programs for all exercise participants.

Guidelines for Specific Disabilities

In addition to using the general recommendations for interacting with people with disabilities, you should follow additional guidelines for interacting with people with specific types of disabilities. Although there are many specific types of physical disabilities, we will provide information about people who fall into three classes of disabling conditions: physical, cognitive, and visual impairments. Guidelines for individuals with mental retardation and hearing impairments are beyond the scope of this text.

Physical Disability

Because of the wide range of causes, definitions, and degrees of severity of physical disabilities, we cannot present a categorical system of reference to people who are physically disabled. Terms referring to physical conditions such as *paraplegia, cerebral palsy,* and *muscular dystrophy* are often used to categorize physical disability, but such terms have little functional meaning because people with the same condition differ greatly in level of ability.

As an exercise leader, it is important to be aware of each person's abilities and the level at which he is capable of functioning. Remember that people with the same physical condition will choose different activities and accomplish the skills associated with that activity to different degrees.

Thousands of people in the United States have some degree of physical disability. Physical disabilities may affect a person's coordination, mobility, balance, agility, strength, endurance, or a combination of these capabilities. Keep in mind that a physical disability may have no bearing on a person's ability to participate in a specific program.

For example, using a cane for assistance in walking may have little or no impact on participation in an aquatic exercise class.

In considering how a potential participant can take part in a particular activity, look at the physical requirements of the activity and the person's abilities—he may be able to take part without adaptations, or some adaptation may be necessary. Be sure to consult your most important resource, the person with the disability, for information about his movement abilities when you develop exercise modifications.

The following recommendations pertain to preferred behaviors for communicating and interacting with people who have physical disabilities:

❑ If a person with a physical disability falls, wait for the person to indicate whether or not help is required. If assistance is required, the person can describe a preferred method of assistance.

❑ Ask people with physical disabilities about special equipment, aids, or techniques they may use to assist them in daily living that may be useful in the exercise environment.

❑ Crutches, walkers, prosthetic devices (artificial limbs), and wheelchairs are often necessary accessories. Do not remove them from the participant's activity area unless requested to do so. Taking away such assistive devices can leave a person stranded.

❑ Do not automatically assume that a person in a wheelchair needs assistance propelling it, but if the person wants assistance, provide it.

❑ Design programs to offer opportunities for success, new experiences, and challenge to all participants.

❑ Minimize environmental barriers that limit functioning. A hard, firm surface will probably be easier than grass or soft dirt for maneuvering a wheelchair. Plan ahead to assess a facility for potential barriers, using a person who is physically disabled or a knowledgeable professional as an evaluator.

Personal Aids and Devices

People with physical disabilities usually depend on personal aids and devices to increase their functional abilities. These aids can range from easily available devices, such as a standard wheelchair, to very personalized, one-of-a-kind devices, such as a form-fitted hand strap to assist in holding a pen. Typically, aids and devices become as personal to the individual as clothes do to other people.

Mobility aids (wheelchairs, crutches, walkers, and braces) are the most visible and easily recognized devices. Aids to body function include prostheses (artificial limbs), ileostomy or colostomy devices (for body waste collection), and breathing assistance devices. In most situations, the individual has mastered the use and care of the aid or device and will not need assistance. If assistance is required, the individual can usually direct the kind and level of help needed. It is not only entirely proper, but also usually essential to ask for guidance when assisting an individual with an aid or device. Be sure to ask a parent or guardian about correct assistance with a device used by a child.

You should also ask if there are any implications for exercise activity associated with the device, like where and when it cannot be used, under what conditions the device might be problematic to the owner or others, special storage considerations, and other concerns.

Wheelchairs

Be aware of proper techniques for handling a wheelchair and assisting with a transfer from the wheelchair to another surface. Refer to chapter 14 for more details about these skills.

Cognitive, Communication, and Behavioral Disturbances

Physical disabilities stemming from injury to the brain (such as stroke, head injury, cerebral palsy, or multiple sclerosis) may also be associated with impaired cognition, communication abilities, memory, judgment, and behavior. Be sensitive to the needs of individuals with these impairments and modify your instructional approach to meet them.

People with impaired cognitive function may have difficulty learning new skills or behaviors. They may learn at a slower rate and may have a limited ability to comprehend abstract ideas.

Communication problems impair the ability to use or understand language. People with severely impaired speech may use a communication board for expression. Do not assume that people with impaired speech also have impaired cognition—such an assumption can be demeaning.

The following guidelines may be appropriate for some people with cognitive, communication, or behavioral problems:

❑ Determine the person's abilities and concentrate on them. Do not underestimate abilities and interests.

❑ Speak to participants, regardless of the severity of their disabilities, with respect and dignity. Do not talk down to anyone, and avoid talking about a person in her presence—these approaches are demeaning.

❑ If a person appears to need help, offer assistance, but wait until the person accepts before giving it. Someone may prefer to perform an activity independently, even if with less skill.

❑ It may be necessary to break down directions into simple steps or basic concepts that can be learned sequentially, especially if short-term memory is impaired. Repeat directions as needed. Demonstrate, where possible, what you expect. Use a variety of teaching methods, including manual guidance and visual aids.

❑ Allow plenty of time for learning and completing a task. Repetition is important to learning. Allow opportunity for participants to independently try new skills.

❑ A person's ability to understand speech is often more developed than his own vocabulary. A speech impairment or lack of speech does not indicate that a person cannot understand language. Allow the individual with impaired speech to speak at her own pace; do not hurry or interrupt the person while he attempts to communicate a thought. It may be necessary to ask someone to repeat a word or phrase until you become familiar with her speaking style. Be patient and allow the individual to complete his own thoughts; avoid attempting to finish phrases for her.

❑ Address people with a receptive communication disorder (difficulty with understanding language) slowly and with short, simple sentences. To ensure that the individual has understood instructions, have her repeat the message.

❑ Some individuals may not have the judgment to foresee dangerous situations or acknowledge personal limits. Be sure to review all safety rules before beginning an activity. Offer private reminders if an individual displays disruptive or inappropriate behavior.

❑ Assign people who tend to overestimate their abilities tasks in an order of increasing complexity and difficulty to prevent them from injuring themselves. Offer frequent, concise feedback and praise. Request that individuals who act impulsively talk themselves through an action.

Visual Impairment

People with visual impairments are able to obtain varying amounts of visual information about their environment. It is important to realize, however, that vision is not the only source of information. People with visual impairments have usually learned to rely on other senses to fill the gap created by their restricted ability to obtain visual information. Smell, touch, hearing, and the perception of movement all become more important sensory channels for people who are visually impaired. Remember this increased reliance on gathering information nonvisually when you plan to make activities accessible to a person with impaired vision.

The only way to know for sure the extent of people's visual disabilities, the methods they use to adapt, and their specific needs in a recreational environment is to ask them—don't make assumptions. One common assumption is that most people who are legally blind can read braille. This is simply not the case. Less than 10% of people with severe visual impairments can read braille. Many people prefer to use audio cassettes.

Chapter 2 provides more information about characteristics of visual impairment. Consider the following recommendations for generally preferred behaviors when interacting with people who have visual impairments.

❑ If someone with a visual impairment seems to need assistance, offer help but do not give it unless the offer is accepted. If it is accepted, ask for an exact explanation of how you can help.

❑ Loss of sight does not affect a person's hearing. Do not shout at the person with a visual impairment. Similarly, visual impairment does not affect a person's mental ability. Talk directly to him, not to others on his behalf.

❑ Do not be afraid to use words such as *see*, *look*, or *blind*. Such words are a part of our everyday vocabulary, and people who are blind also use them.

❑ When you meet a person who is blind, be sure to identify yourself. Remember to let the individual know when you leave, too.

❑ Do not pet a guide dog unless you have the owner's permission. When the dog is in harness, it is on duty. Distracting the dog may place the owner in jeopardy.

❑ Use specific, descriptive language when giving directions, explaining things, or describing a place, an event, or an activity. Using colors, textures, movements, and directional indicators in a description can make it more vivid for someone with a visual impairment.

❑ During activities, orient people with visual impairments to the placement of objects around them that they will be using. People with severe visual impairment often use the military analogy of a clock face to explain position. For example, you could explain that the exercise mats are at 3 o'clock, the instructor is at 9 o'clock, and so on.

❏ Orient the person with a visual impairment to new environments. Describe the size, shape, distances, boundaries, and any obstacles or potential hazards in the environment.

❏ If an individual with a visual impairment accepts your offer of help, ask the person if he would like to take your arm. Brush your forearm against his so the person can grip your arm above the elbow. The grip should be firm enough to maintain while walking without being uncomfortable. Children will use the same grip at the wrist. Some people who are aged or physically disabled may want to walk arm in arm, which offers more support than the grip, and they may wish to travel at a slower pace.

Important: Do not attempt to lead a person who is visually impaired by taking his arm! Instead, relax your arm along your side. The person you are guiding will bend his arm at the elbow and grip your left elbow with his right hand. Be sure to keep your arm close to your body. The person who is visually impaired should travel a half step behind you. Pick a comfortable walking pace for both of you. If the person you are guiding pulls your arm back or tightens her grip, you are probably traveling too fast. Never try to push or steer a person who is visually impaired ahead of you. Try to keep the person aware as conditions or surroundings change—remember to mention curbs, steps, doorways, narrow passages, ramps, and the like. Let the person you are guiding know if the stairs go up or down and when they reach the last step.

❏ When guiding a person who is visually impaired to a seat, simply place her hand on the back of the chair and let her seat herself. Explain what you are doing as you do it.

When approaching a door, say so. Place your hand on the knob and let the person who is blind follow your arm to the door knob. Tell him whether the door opens toward or away from you. Allow the person who is blind to hold the door open for both of you.

Chapter 12 includes additional suggestions for teaching skills to a person with a visual impairment.

Equal Opportunity

For equal opportunity to become a reality in exercise programs, you must provide both physical and program accessibility. You must make every reasonable attempt to enable participants with disabilities to get into the buildings and facilities and, once there, to receive the same benefits, services, and information provided to all other participants.

To achieve accessibility, view people with disabilities the same way as everyone else—they have the same variety of needs, desires, expectations, and abilities as other people and the right to be equally accepted and served. Making programs accessible to people with disabilities has both social and practical benefits. Most importantly, it encourages the assimilation of people with disabilities into the mainstream of society.

It may be possible to make an exercise program accessible through some kind of adaptation—the participant can compensate for a skill or capability deficit, or you can adapt the activity without significantly affecting the other participants' enjoyment and satisfaction. However, the primary reason for making exercise programs fully accessible is the basic right of all people to be judged according to their capabilities, not their disabilities; their right to be included in all aspects of public life; and their right to have fun like everybody else.

The next chapter presents characteristics of common physical disabilities and associated exercise implications. This information will offer guidelines to help you make appropriate decisions about adapting your exercise programs.

Chapter 2

Physical Disabilities: General Characteristics and Exercise Implications

Patrick J. DiRocco, PhD
University of Wisconsin—La Crosse

As a fitness instructor, you may work with people with many types of disabilities. To offer safe and effective exercise programs for these people, you must first develop a basic, general understanding of physical disabilities and their exercise implications.

This chapter describes several of the more common disabilities (see Table 2.1). For each selected disability we will describe the medical pathology, characteristics, classification systems (where applicable), and general exercise implications. We will also include generic recommendations for adapting exercises to develop aerobic and muscular fitness. Although fitness training can have therapeutic benefits, this chapter focuses on exercise training for health and fitness.

We have grouped the disabilities in this chapter according to the site of injury, from the brain to the periphery. Disabilities resulting from injuries at a common level may have similar exercise implications. By using this rough categorization of disabilities according to the site of injury, you will be able to quickly formulate a preliminary approach for working with each individual. To fully develop an appropriate and individualized program, you will need additional information about each person's specific condition and, in some cases, advice from a physician or therapist.

Because it is impossible to present every known physical disability in this text, we discuss only the most common disorders in detail. We include a brief description of several less common disabilities at the conclusion of each category.

Table 2.1 Common Physical Disabilities Classified According to Site of Injury

Site of injury	Nonprogressive	Progressive
Central nervous system		
Brain	Cerebral palsy	Multiple sclerosis
	Head injury	
	Stroke (CVA)	
Spinal cord	Spinal cord injury	Multiple sclerosis
	Spina bifida	
Peripheral nervous system		
Lower motor neurons	Poliomyelitis	
	Guillain-Barré syndrome	
	Myasthenia gravis	
	Spinal cord injury (below cauda equina)	
Peripheral structures		
Joint	Arthritis	
Bone	Amputation	
	Osteogenesis imperfecta	
Muscle	Arthrogryposis	Muscular dystrophy

Nonprogressive Physical Disabilities of the Nervous System

The nervous system regulates all functions associated with human movement. Its two major branches are the central nervous system (CNS) and the peripheral nervous system (PNS). The CNS includes the brain and neurons of the spinal cord, and the PNS comprises the nerves that emerge from the CNS. Figure 2.1 depicts the nervous system's organization.

Cerebral Palsy

Cerebral palsy (CP) is an umbrella term under which several specific types of disorders are classified. Although each of these disorders has different symptoms, they share certain characteristics that define the disorder.

Characteristics

All CP disorders result from a lesion in the upper motor neurons within the brain, which regulate neuromuscular function. The specific site of the lesion determines the nature of the disorder. Ab-

normal muscular behavior results from impaired neurological innervation to affected muscles.

Cerebral palsy (meaning "brain paralysis") can occur before, during, or following birth. It may be caused by a mother's prenatal illness and complications, trauma during birth, or brain injury during infancy. Because the central nervous system is affected before the child has matured physically, development in related areas (motor, speech, growth, and cognitive function) during childhood may be impaired. For this reason, CP is classified as a developmental disability (DD).

As a consequence of CP, primitive reflexes—normally replaced during development by coordinated and integrated motor behaviors—may persist throughout life. Primitive reflexes are elicited by certain body positions or external stimuli that, when invoked, produce reflex postures that limit movement. Table 2.2 presents a summary of primitive reflexes that commonly persist with CP.

Cerebral palsy disorders are noncontagious and nonprogressive. The extent of the disabling lesion never worsens, and as the central nervous system matures, the impairment will stabilize. As yet we have no cure for cerebral palsy; thus, an affected individual has the condition for life.

Treatment of CP is initiated to alleviate symptoms and complications. Bracing limbs may elongate muscles and prevent contractures or may support weak muscles. Physical therapy aims to improve daily functioning, relax muscles, and improve voluntary control of movement and range of motion. Surgery may be used to reposition muscles or elongate tendons.

Classifications

Two systems, neuromotor and topographical, commonly describe CP. CP can be classified further according to whether involvement is mild, moderate, or severe. An additional classification system, functional classification, has been developed to equalize competition in competitive sports. This system uses eight classes of involvement ranging from severe (Class I) to mild (Class VIII).

Neuromotor classification of CP considers the site of lesion in the brain and the associated muscular involvement (see Figure 2.3). This system identifies six specific types of cerebral palsy: spastic, athetoid, ataxia, rigidity, tremors, and mixed.

Spastic CP is the most prevalent type of cerebral palsy (see Figure 2.4)—about 60% to 70% of all people with CP have this type. Spasticity results from a lesion to the pyramidal tract in the motor cortex. The primary symptom is a consistent and

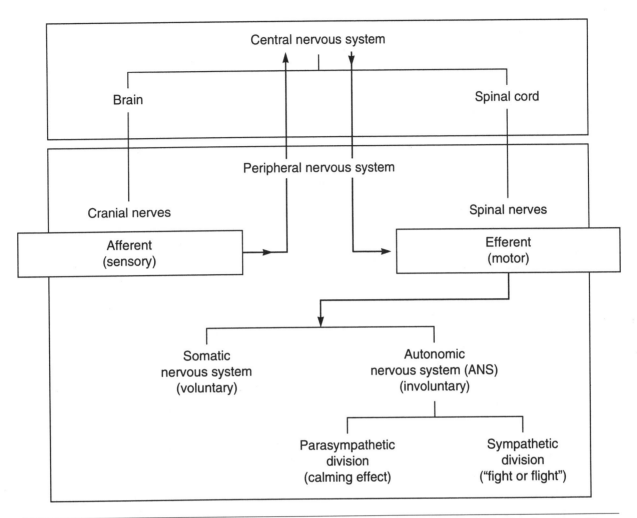

Figure 2.1 The anatomical classification of the nervous system includes the central and peripheral systems. Functional classification further distinguishes the afferent and efferent systems.

INJURY TO THE BRAIN

The central nervous system comprises the brain and spinal cord, which house the upper motor neurons of the nervous system. Injury to the brain can affect movement, cognitive and sensory function, communication, and behavior, depending on the specific area of the brain that has been affected. Figure 2.2 illustrates the major areas of the brain and their primary functions. Some of the more common nonprogressive disabilities resulting from injury to specific or general regions of the brain include cerebral palsy, head injury, and stroke (cerebrovascular accident).

---

increased muscular tone (hypertonicity), which most often affects flexor and internal rotator muscles. Increased tone in adductor and lower extremity extensor muscles may also be seen. Spastic muscles experience a continual state of contraction to some degree (depending upon severity), thereby reducing range of motion at the involved joints. Postural disorders develop in affected body segments.

Hypertonicity, if not properly managed, may lead to contractures that can permanently shorten resting muscle length and cause joint deformities, thereby greatly reducing joint range of motion. The following joints and body parts commonly assume the characteristic contracted state with spastic CP:

Shoulders: flexed, adducted, internally rotated

Forearms: pronated

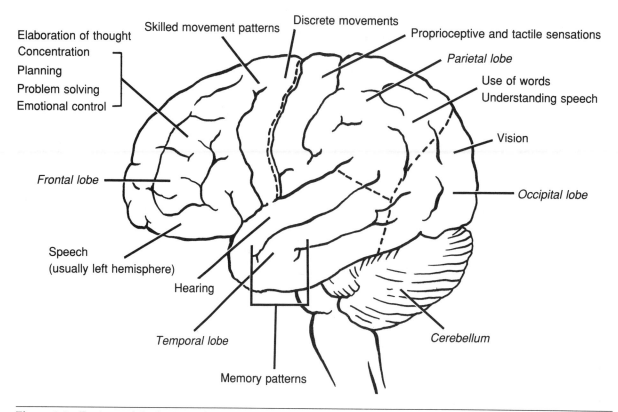

Figure 2.2 Regions of the brain and associated functions.

Elbows, wrists and fingers: flexed

Hips: adducted, internally rotated and flexed

Knees: flexed

Feet: plantar flexed and everted

Spastic CP is also characterized by reflexive contraction of opposing muscle groups in response to voluntary movements, which causes jerky and awkward movement patterns that interfere with intended actions. Spasticity and reflexes are described in more detail in chapter 3, which describes muscle function. Approximately 50% of all individuals with spastic CP also experience seizures, perceptual disorders, or cognitive impairments.

Athetoid CP is the second most prevalent type, accounting for 20% to 30% of people with cerebral palsy. This condition results from a lesion to the extrapyramidal cells in the basal ganglia, and its major symptom is slow, nonrhythmical, random, and involuntary circular or jerky movements. These movement patterns, which tend to persist while the individual is awake, impair hand control, balance, trunk stability, and accuracy of movement. Athetoid movements are often expressed in head, neck and facial muscles as well as limb muscles, and they may also affect postural control.

Stress and emotional arousal may increase abnormal movement patterns.

Athetosis is characterized by fluctuations in muscle tone from hypotonus (decreased muscle tone) to hypertonus. In contrast to spasticity, which is initiated with voluntary actions, athetosis is characterized by a continual state of involuntary movement. Athetosis often accompanies spasticity.

Ataxia affects 5% to 10% of individuals with CP. This condition results from a lesion to the cerebellum and produces several motor impairments, including poor body balance (especially with upright posture); an impaired gait characterized by uncertain, staggering movements; and significant movement incoordination. With ataxia, muscles are hypotonic. People with this type of CP also have an impaired kinesthetic sense, which may cause them to misjudge posture, center of gravity, and body relationships to external objects.

A small percentage of people with CP are affected by rigidity or tremors. Rigidity results in hypertonicity throughout the body, severe postural distortions, and severe mental retardation. Intention tremors are characterized by involuntary and rhythmical movements, usually with the initiation of voluntary movements. Noninten-

Table 2.2 Primitive Reflexes That May Persist With Cerebral Palsy

Stimulus	Reflex response	Instructional considerations
Asymmetrical tonic neck reflex (ATNR)		
Neck rotation	Increased extensor tone in arm in direction of vision	Communicate from position directly in front of person
	Increased flexor tone in opposite arm	Select exercise positions to anticipate reflex actions
Hand grasp reflex		
Stimulus to palm	Finger flexion	
Hyperextension of wrist		
Moro reflex		
Loud noise	Increased tone of body	Avoid surprise
Unstable surface for lying or sitting	Arms and legs involuntarily spread and close	Avoid sudden loud noises
Falling		Select stable exercise positions
Symmetrical tonic neck reflex (STNR)		
Neck flexion	Increased flexor tone of upper body	Maintain awareness of body positions with exercises (e.g., bench press or push-ups) to prevent "locking up" in undesirable postures
	Extensor tone of lower body	
Neck extension	Increased extensor tone of upper body	
	Increased flexor tone of lower body	
Foot grasp reflex		
Pressure on soles of feet	Toe flexion (curling)	May need to exercise in a seated position
Extensor thrust reflex		
Pressure to plantar surface of feet	Increased extensor tone throughout body	Avoid leg movements
		Strap hips, thighs, and lower legs to wheelchair to prevent sliding from chair
		Recommend seated posture of deep hip and knee flexion
Positive supporting reflex		
Stimulation or pressure on plantar surface of foot	Plantar flexion	Avoid leg movements or encourage seated exercise when partially present in ambulatory person

Note. Other primitive reflexes (not listed here) may be associated with more severe movement limitations.

tional tremors involve continuous shaking and trembling.

The rarely seen mixed type of CP involves the presence of two or more types in equal degrees (usually spasticity and athetosis). People with mixed CP are generally severely involved. Although many people with CP are affected by both spasticity and athetosis, they will not be classified as mixed unless neither predominates.

The anatomical approach to CP classification, known as topographical classification, categorizes CP according to the areas of the body it affects. The following terms are used:

Monoplegia: one limb is affected, usually an arm.

Paraplegia: the lower extremities and hip region are affected.

Hemiplegia: limbs on one side of the body are affected.

Triplegia: three limbs are affected, usually both legs and one arm.

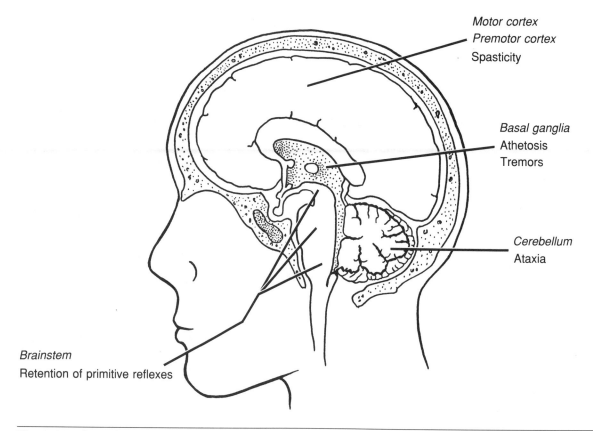

Motor cortex
Premotor cortex
Spasticity

Basal ganglia
Athetosis
Tremors

Cerebellum
Ataxia

Brainstem
Retention of primitive reflexes

Figure 2.3 Sagittal section of the brain showing motor areas that might be affected by cerebral palsy.

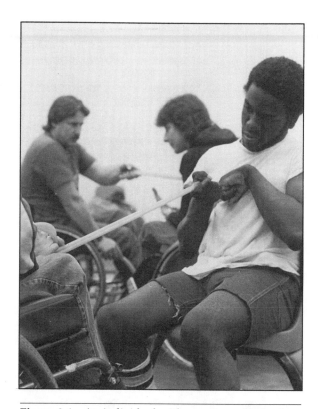

Figure 2.4 An individual with spastic cerebral palsy participates in a resistance training program.

Quadriplegia: all four limbs and the trunk are affected. Neck and facial muscles may also be involved.

Diplegia: all four limbs are affected, the legs more severely than the arms.

Because cerebral palsy results from brain damage, it is not uncommon for individuals with cerebral palsy to have associated disorders. Other conditions most frequently associated with CP are reflex disorders; seizures; and speech, hearing, or visual problems. In about 40% of people with CP, some degree of mental retardation also may be present. When working with individuals with cerebral palsy, it is important to determine whether the person has associated disorders so you can modify instruction appropriately. It is also very important not to assume that speech problems and CP automatically imply mental retardation. Individuals with CP may be of normal or superior intelligence.

Exercise Implications

People with cerebral palsy have impaired movement patterns due to abnormal neural control mechanisms; however, they are capable of movement. You must assess each person's movement capabilities to individualize instruction appropriately. In spite of the impaired neural function, histologically the muscle cells are normal and, therefore, they can adapt to exercise training.

The specific disorder determines what type of modifications you need to make to exercise routines. You can take steps to avoid causing abnormal movements. For example, avoid routines that cause the participant with CP to experience excessive and early fatigue, which will, in turn, cause movement patterns to deteriorate and further limit the duration of participation. Using work-rest intervals is an effective means of delaying fatigue. Avoid exercise in cold environments, when possible, because muscle tone may increase with spasticity under these conditions. Sudden excitement, loss of balance, and fast movements also can activate abnormal movement patterns. You should also minimize actions that elicit primitive reflex responses.

People with spastic CP benefit from a prolonged warm-up of 15 to 20 min that relaxes and warms the muscles before vigorous exercise. The warm-up should include static stretches, held for 40 to 60 s. People with spastic CP will benefit most from large, slow, and rhythmical moves during the warm-up.

People with athetoid CP are typically in constant motion and therefore remain habitually warmed up. These participants should focus more on relaxation and stress reduction, which may enhance movement patterns during subsequent, vigorous exercise.

Stretching regularly should be an integral component of fitness programs for people with spastic CP. Stretching is essential to prevent decreases in functional range of motion and the development of contractures. Holding static stretches, however, may be difficult for individuals with athetosis or ataxia. Keep in mind that full range of motion may not be possible in people with CP. Encourage participants to achieve full functional range of motion during exercise.

Maintaining muscular strength and endurance are very important for people with CP. An effective resistance training program may improve function because spastic muscles, although hypertonic, are not necessarily strong—in fact, extensor muscles that oppose spastic flexors are often weak. People with other types of CP may also benefit from resistance training. Because research about the effects of resistance training with spastic muscles in CP is limited and opinions about its value and safety are varied, recommend an exercise program cautiously. Monitor immediate and delayed post-exercise responses to resistance training to ensure that the program is not causing a decline in function.

Because strength on each side of the body may vary to a large extent and someone with CP may have difficulty coordinating bilateral movements, exercising each side of the body separately may produce better results. If bilateral movements are not a problem, symmetrical actions can be successful, especially during an aerobics workout.

Regular participation in aerobic exercise is as important to the person with CP as to the general population. Consider an individual's impaired balance and coordination, limited joint range of motion, and disposition to early fatigue when designing aerobic exercise routines. Keep movements simple, large, symmetrical, and repetitive for individuals with spastic CP. Repeating movement patterns for an extended period will allow the participant to keep up with the group, even though it may take longer to assume the designated pattern. Participants with spastic CP should avoid continual flexion of spastic muscles due to the potential for increasing spasticity following the workout. People with athetoid CP will benefit from interval or stop-start movement patterns, which facilitate optimal control of large movements. People with CP may regularly use relaxants or anticonvulsant medications that can affect exercise tolerance and performance. A comprehensive preparticipation screening program should highlight the use of these and other pharmacologic agents.

Stroke

Stroke is medically referred to as a cerebrovascular accident (CVA). It results from oxygen deprivation to the brain or hemorrhage due to a burst artery leading to the brain. The immediate symptoms include unconsciousness followed by paralysis. The initial paralysis may or may not be complete.

Following the hospital convalescence period, the person who has had a stroke may commonly have any combination of impairments in motor, cognitive, and sensory function, depending on which areas of the brain have been affected (refer to Figure 2.2). Depression is also common following the initial hospital stay. In many cases the immediate postconvalescence symptoms improve with time. However, complete recovery from all symptoms rarely occurs.

Characteristics

A permanent disability resulting from a CVA includes some degree of muscle weakness (paresis) or paralysis and motor skill loss, often on one side of the body (hemiparesis/hemiplegia). This weakness may require the use of a wheelchair or a cane to assist with locomotion. If the person with this disability is ambulatory, his balance may be impaired. In addition, the hand on one side may be nonfunctioning.

Impaired speech, memory, and vision (on one side) are also common characteristics of a CVA. Some people also experience uncontrollable emotional outbursts (lability) and will have difficulty using or understanding words (aphasia). With expressive aphasia, the person has difficulty expressing thoughts, whereas receptive aphasia involves difficulty in comprehending verbal messages from others.

Classifications

A CVA may be referred to according to which side of the brain is predominantly involved, because injuries affecting either hemisphere are often characterized by common impairments. In general, people with a right CVA have motor dysfunction on the left side (left hemiparesis/hemiplegia). Injury on the right side of the brain also may impair visual-spatial abilities and judgment or cause impulsive behavior. A person with a left CVA will have paresis or paralysis on the right side and may have impaired speech and language. It is important to remember, however, that not all individuals who have had a stroke exhibit characteristics of injury from only the left or right brain, depending on the specific site of the injury. Table 2.3 summarizes functions controlled predominantly by the left and right hemispheres of the brain.

Stroke also may be classified as ischemic or hemorrhagic according to the cause of injury (Gordon, 1993b). Ischemic stroke results when brain cells cease to function due to a lack of oxygen. This may be caused by a build-up of atherosclerotic plaque in arteries of the head or neck, or formation of blood clots that restrict the flow of blood and oxygen. Hemorrhagic stroke occurs when blood accumulates in the brain or brain cavity after an artery leading to the brain bursts. This is caused by an aneurysm, or weak spot, in an artery wall. Neurologic damage tends to be more severe with ischemic stroke, although the survival rate is generally higher.

Exercise Implications

Require anyone who has had a stroke to get physician approval before participating in an exercise program. Because a CVA is a vascular disorder, it is important to monitor exercise heart rates and blood pressure regularly. Advise these participants to keep exercise intensity below 70% of the predicted maximum heart rate. If dizziness, shortness of breath, or chest pains occur, stop the exercise and check blood pressure and heart rate immediately. Report any such occurrences to the person's physician and obtain permission before that person continues participation in the program.

Many people who have had a stroke are on medication. An individual's physician can provide important advice about the expected effects of medications on exercise performance and tolerance. Appendix A summarizes common pharmacologic agents and their effects with exercise.

Participants with hemiparesis and impaired balance exercise more safely from a sitting position. People with mild impairment who prefer to exercise from a standing position should have access to a stable object for support and a chair for rest as needed.

A CVA can cause damage to the memory centers of the brain that impairs memory function. When working with individuals with memory impairment, be prepared to reteach exercises and dance routines. Constantly monitor exercise performance so you can offer assistance as needed. Some individuals with memory impairments may have difficulty identifying objects or tasks from verbal instructions. These people will be most successful when you provide strong visual cues. You may also have to modify your instructional techniques for people with communication disorders. Table 2.4 summarizes teaching strategies for individuals with various behavioral, communication, or memory disorders that may result from a CVA.

When teaching aerobics, you should not necessarily encourage symmetrical movements if someone's attempts to use them decrease the intensity of the effort and thereby reduce the potential for

Table 2.3 General Impairments Characteristic of Left and Right Brain Damage

Right brain damage	Left brain damage
Language comprehension	Speech and use of language
Spatial-perceptual orientation	Arithmetic and calculations
Memory (vision and performance)	Memory (speech and language)
Behavior (may become quick, impulsive, careless)	Behavior (may become slow, cautious, anxious, and disorganized)
Left hemiplegia	Right hemiplegia

Table 2.4 Teaching Strategies for Individuals With Acquired Brain Damage (Stroke or Head Injury)

Deficit	Instructional approach
Language comprehension	Speak slowly
	Offer simple, short, concise instructions
	Provide manual guidance and tactile demonstrations
Memory (from speech)	Repeat instructions frequently
	Offer visual demonstrations or manual guidance
Overcautious, disorganized behavior	Offer frequent feedback
Impulsive behavior, overestimation of abilities	Request that the person talk herself through movements
	Avoid partnering activities
	Sequence movements in small steps of increasing complexity and intensity
	Provide an assistant for exercise that utilizes equipment (especially with resistive weight training)
	Ignore nondisruptive behavior
	Offer private reminders that disruptive behavior is inappropriate
Lability (emotional outbursts)	Ignore nondisruptive incidences

achieving an aerobic training effect. Full, vigorous movement on one side of the body is preferable to limited, symmetrical movement when cardiovascular conditioning is the objective of the exercise session.

Encourage resistance training and stretching for noninvolved limbs. Participants with hemiparesis should use caution and lower intensity with muscular conditioning on the involved side. Resistance training should be avoided if movements cannot be isolated. For this reason, suggest unilateral instead of bilateral exercises during resistance training and stretching. A key objective of the exercise program when spasticity is present on the involved side should be muscle balancing to maintain good posture by strengthening antagonists and stretching spastic muscles. Consult with the participant's therapist for advice about muscular conditioning.

Head Injury

Because head injury can affect large regions of the brain, the symptoms are quite varied and diffuse. In many cases head injury will result in a combination of physical, cognitive, sensory, and behavioral impairments. More than 50% of head injuries occur in people between the ages of 15 and 24 years, and head injuries occur twice as frequently in males as in females.

Brain damage as a result of head injury can be caused by a primary trauma and complicated by secondary responses to that injury. Traumatic injuries produce brain damage in two ways. A closed head injury is caused by an external source that imposes an acceleration, deceleration, or rotational force, or any combination of these forces, on the brain. The inside of the skull is not smooth, so as these forces cause the brain to move within the skull, they result in tearing, shearing, and puncture wounds, as well as bruises, in soft brain tissue. An open brain injury is caused by a penetrating wound. Besides the location, pathway, and depth of the wound, complications from debris and infection also determine the nature and extent of the brain damage.

Brain damage can also occur from a secondary response to an injury or fever (e.g., encephalitis). These responses may be swelling, which causes tissue damage due to increasing intracranial pressure, or severe deprivation of oxygen (ischemia) to a region of the brain.

Characteristics

The general symptoms resulting from brain damage depend upon the region of the brain in which it occurs. Examples of possible impairments include these:

Physical: motor weaknesses, incoordination, impaired balance, and spasticity

Cognitive: impaired short-term memory, perceptual function, and decision making, along with impaired ability to adequately deal with a new setting

Behavioral: emotional outbursts or impulsive behavior and emotional blunting, which involves distorted reactions and a lack of internal motivational responses

Other: aphasia, slurring of speech, and epilepsy

The majority of posttrauma recovery occurs within the first year. Some continued progress may be observed over the next few years. Beyond this time, the individual's impairments will be permanent.

Exercise Implications

Symptoms related to head injury are individual, and therefore we cannot offer any general movement adjustments. When working with people who have had a head injury, you need to become familiar with the full extent of the resulting physical, behavioral, and cognitive impairments. In some cases, the behavioral and cognitive challenges are more serious than the physical impairments.

You may need to modify your exercise program for the impaired balance, poor motor coordination, spasticity, paralysis, and perceptual distortions someone with a head injury may have. We provided specific suggestions for instructional strategies and effective ways to interact with people with aphasia in the previous chapter about disability awareness (see chapter 1, pp. 8-9).

Spinal Cord Injury

Spinal cord injury (SCI) is caused by a lesion to the spinal cord that disrupts control of muscles innervated at and below the level of the injury. Motor function, sensation, or both will be impaired even though muscle tissues remain intact.

SCI is usually caused by a traumatic injury, and the majority of the incidences occur to people in the 15- to 30-year age bracket. Other causes are viral infections or toxic conditions. Trauma may result from severing the cord or from severe bruising that creates swelling and rupturing of the myelin sheath on nerve fibers. The myelin sheath does not repair itself to restore normal nerve function.

Medical treatment for people with SCI proceeds through three stages. The first stage is the acute-care period that begins immediately following the injury and lasts for about 30 to 60 days. During this stage, treatment prevents death. The injury or sickness that caused the SCI is also given treatment, including antibiotics to treat infections. Health care professionals provide such assistance as managing incontinence, preventing pressure sores, and offering nutritional counseling.

Following acute care, people with SCI enter the rehabilitation period, conducted in a rehabilitation unit, for 3 to 6 months to develop the maximum functioning the disability allows. The rehabilitation team provides physical, occupational, and recreation therapy, along with counseling services to assist with vocational pursuits and such issues as family stress, anger, depression, and denial.

When in-patient rehabilitation is completed, the person returns home, hopefully to function within society. Beyond this point, some individuals need additional periodic out-patient medical care for treatment of pressure sores, urinary tract infections, and for dietary counseling.

Characteristics

Two major symptoms of SCI are loss of muscle function, a corresponding loss of sensation, or both. Disrupting innervation to a muscle causes partial or complete paralysis of that muscle, and disrupting innervation to the skin and joint receptors causes a partial or complete loss of sensation to those areas.

The specific symptoms resulting from SCI depend upon the specific location and severity of the injury (see Figure 2.5). Generally, higher level SCI results in greater functional impairment.

Individuals with SCI also may have other associated medical conditions such as

- incontinence due to a loss of innervation to the bladder or bowels;
- pressure sores (decubitus ulcers), which result from poor circulation and skin breakdown in weight bearing areas;
- sporadic limb spasticity and joint contractures;

INJURY TO THE SPINAL CORD AND PERIPHERAL NERVES

The spinal cord and peripheral nerves transmit sensory and motor impulses to and from the brain and periphery. Damage to any of these pathways interrupts the flow of messages and may weaken or prevent movement from the muscle groups they innervate. Injury to spinal cord nerves generally does not affect peripheral reflexes and causes the spastic form of paralysis (with complete injury) or paresis (with incomplete injury). Peripheral nerve injury causes flaccid paralysis or paresis. Injury to these lower motor neurons is character-ized by muscle atrophy and a loss of peripheral reflexes.

Impairment to the nerves of the spinal cord can result from several conditions, including spinal cord injury, spina bifida, or multiple sclerosis. Peripheral nerves are affected with injuries to the spinal column below the T12 level (below the cauda equina) or with poliomyelitis, Guillain-Barré syndrome, and myasthenia gravis.

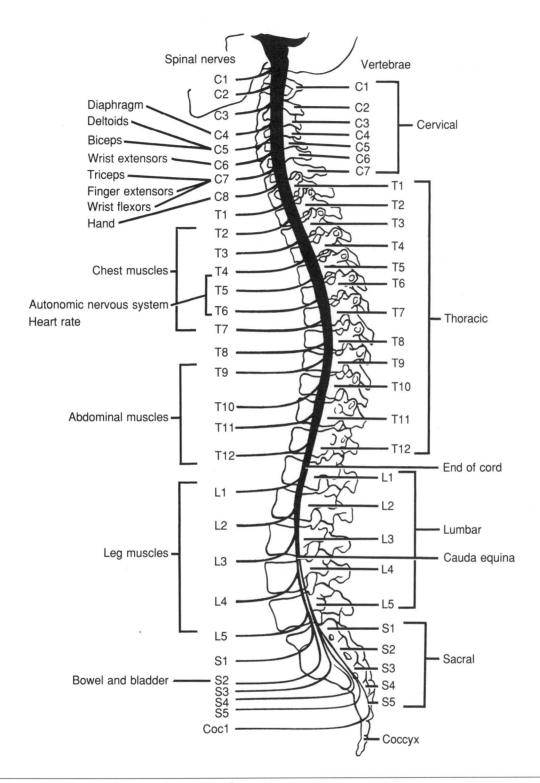

Figure 2.5 The spinal cord and nerve supply.

- residual pain around the injury site;

- urinary tract infections; and

- impaired regulation of heart rate and blood pressure with autonomic nervous system (ANS) dysfunction.

ANS dysfunction accompanying injuries at or above the T1 to T5 level (Mathers, 1985) impairs regulation of body temperature, blood pressure, and heart rate. Heart rates above 100 to 120 beats per minute generally cannot be achieved with this condition, even with intense exercise.

Nerves emerging from the sacral vertebrae regulate bowel and bladder function. Individuals with injury above that level of the spinal cord use a bowel and bladder program to control elimination, which may include use of catheters, laxatives, and regular scheduling of elimination.

Autonomic dysreflexia is a condition associated with impaired autonomic function that can affect individuals with SCI, especially those with high-level injuries. An episode of autonomic dysreflexia requires immediate medical attention to prevent potentially life-threatening complications. Symptoms of autonomic dysreflexia include impaired sweating (which may be absent or uncontrolled), a pounding headache, nasal constriction, goose bumps, and splotching of the skin. Autonomic dysreflexia is commonly caused by distension of the bowel or bladder, infection, spasms, kidney dysfunction, or pressure sores.

Classifications

Spinal cord injuries are classified in three ways. First, the injury is classified according to the spinal root level of the lesion. For example, an injury at the first lumbar level is referred to as L1.

Second, the injury is classified by the type of cord lesion, either complete or incomplete. A complete lesion results in loss of movement (paralysis) or loss of sensation in muscles innervated below the level of the lesion. An incomplete injury causes partial paralysis (paresis), leaving some spinal cord function intact. With incomplete lesions, some movements and sensations are observed in muscles innervated below the level of injury.

The third classification used for SCI describes the body parts that are affected. If functional loss occurs at or below the level of the upper abdominals (T1), the person is classified as having paraplegia. If someone's functional impairment involves all four limbs and the trunk, as occurs with injuries above T1, that person is classified as having quadriplegia. People with quadriplegia, especially with incomplete injuries, have a wide variety of movement characteristics.

Exercise Implications

Because the vast majority of people with spinal cord injury use wheelchairs for mobility, accessibility to gym facilities and locker areas is an important issue. Some people also may need assistance in dressing, showering, and using exercise equipment. Consult chapter 14 for other guidelines relevant to exercise from a wheelchair.

If someone with SCI has impaired trunk balance, check her balance before beginning exercise. En-

courage use of additional support for the trunk if impaired balance limits activity and exercise training potential. When balance is severely impaired, advise the participant to exercise only one side of the body at a time while using the other side for stability.

Many people with quadriplegia have problems with muscular endurance, which has implications for both resistance training and aerobic exercise. For example, they may need to reduce the number of repetitions with resistive exercises and the arm patterns in aerobic dance. Additional recovery time between sets during resistance training or incorporating intervals in aerobics routines may help prevent early fatigue from limiting the workout.

People with quadriplegia also may have impaired gripping ability. Plan in advance to use alternative techniques or modify equipment to accommodate specific needs. Keep in mind, however, that not everyone with quadriplegia has limited gripping ability, depending on the level of the lesion and whether the injury is complete or incomplete.

Although it is important to continually remind all your students to maintain adequate hydration during exercise, it is especially important that people with SCI remain hydrated as an aid to renal function and thermoregulation.

People with SCI commonly develop muscle imbalances due to prolonged sitting and extensive use of the muscles required for wheelchair use. These individuals should be advised to routinely stretch affected muscle groups, including hip flexors, knee flexors, plantar flexors, and anterior shoulder muscles. Be aware that increasing range of motion in some muscles may actually be undesirable because tightness in these areas has functional benefits. For example, overstretched, nonfunctional back muscles can make it more difficult to maintain upright posture. With quadriplegia, simultaneously stretching wrist and finger flexors may lessen tenodesis, which may decrease hand function. (The tenodesis action involves finger flexion in response to wrist extension, which aids gripping.) It is very important that you avoid recommending exercises that may have a negative impact on someone's functional abilities.

Maintaining aerobic fitness is extremely important for people with SCI because it improves their ability to function more independently and decreases the likelihood of developing health problems associated with inactivity. However, because people with an ANS dysfunction have impaired temperature regulation, be prepared to modify or postpone exercise in warm, humid environments. Under these conditions, encourage frequent intake of fluids, have wet towels available for cooling, and incorporate rest periods during the workout to prevent overheating.

People with SCI may use medications to regulate blood pressure and control spasticity, which may decrease exercise training capacity and responses. Be sure to review everyone's medical and health history forms so you can anticipate each person's appropriate exercise responses.

People with incontinence are not necessarily restricted from activity. Because light exercise may stimulate urine production, however, you may wish to remind participants, as sensitively as you can, to empty their bladders before exercise to prevent accidents.

Spina Bifida

Spina bifida refers to a condition in which one or more vertebrae fail to completely fuse on the posterior side during fetal development. The cause, though still unconfirmed, is probably genetic, exacerbated by environmental factors. In many cases the vertebrae remain stable and the condition is not considered serious. The condition becomes serious if the vertebrae become unstable, creating pain and dislocations, or if spinal tissue becomes damaged. Most of the serious spina bifida cases result from damage to spinal tissues.

Characteristics

People with spina bifida have symptoms similar to those of spinal cord injury, depending on the location and extent of nervous tissue damage. The condition weakens or paralyzes affected muscles. Missing or damaged sensory neurons results in a total or partial loss of sensation in the affected muscles. Impaired innervation to the bladder or bowels causes incontinence.

Most people with spina bifida who participate in an exercise class ambulate with the aid of leg braces and crutches, or use a wheelchair. Their hands and arms are generally functional.

Because spina bifida is a congenital disorder, it affects muscle tissue and bone development. Imbalances between opposing muscle groups create postural disorders in the trunk and lower extremities. Bone deformities are often present, and contractures are not uncommon.

Classifications

There are three classifications of spina bifida: occulta, meningocele, and myelomeningocele (see Figure 2.6). The occulta form of spina bifida does not cause neurological damage. In the meningocele form, a sac containing skin, meninges, spinal fluid, and, at times, nervous tissue protrudes from the spinal cord. This type of spina bifida can be corrected shortly after birth, and if there is no spinal tissue damage there may not be any serious disability.

Myelomeningocele is the most serious form of spina bifida—it causes permanent neurologic damage ranging from mild to severe. With this condition, a sac (-cele) containing meninges (membrane covering the spinal cord) and nerve tissue protrudes from the spinal cord (myelo-). The birth process causes some tissue damage. In addition, the spinal cord is not fully developed and fails to completely innervate the affected muscle tissue, both

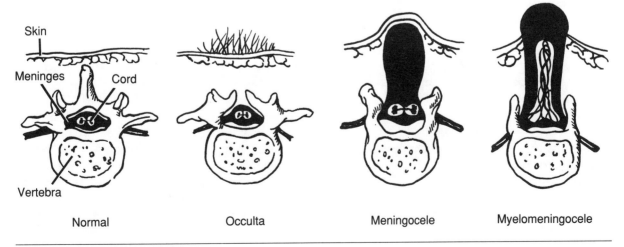

Skin			
Meninges	Cord		
Vertebra			
Normal	Occulta	Meningocele	Myelomeningocele

Figure 2.6 Types of spina bifida.

striated and smooth. Motor and sensory nerves are affected.

In some cases of myelomeningocele, the reabsorption of cerebrospinal fluid in the brain malfunctions, resulting in a condition called hydrocephaly ("water on the brain"). Uncorrected, hydrocephaly can cause mental retardation or death. Hydrocephaly is relieved by surgical placement of a shunt to drain excess fluid from the brain to the venous system.

Exercise Implications

When working with people with spina bifida, determine if any sensory loss is present so you can take appropriate safety measures to prevent injury. When sensation is lacking, the person will not feel abrasions, sharp objects, hot surfaces, and the like. Also check trunk balance from a standing or seated position so you can make any modifications to the position or the exercise program that may be necessary to prevent a loss of balance.

A person's motor and sensory loss cannot be rehabilitated. However, unaffected muscles can benefit from training. People with spina bifida should follow normal training principles. Sometimes their rate of fitness improvement may be slower because the ability to stress the systems being trained is impaired.

In general, exercise modifications for people with spina bifida will be similar to those for people with spinal cord injury and for people who exercise from a wheelchair.

Poliomyelitis

Poliomyelitis (polio) is a nonprogressive neuromuscular condition caused by a virus that enters the body through the alimentary canal. Upon entering the body, the virus settles either in the brain stem or, commonly, in the anterior horn cells of the spinal cord and proceeds to destroy segments of the peripheral neural tracts. The precise location of the lesion determines the type of polio. Lower motor neuron (peripheral) dysfunction is the most common symptom (Frustace, 1988).

Characteristics

Polio is characterized by flaccid paralysis, muscle atrophy, structural deformities, respiratory and circulatory disorders, or a combination of these symptoms. People affected by polio ambulate with the aid of leg braces and crutches or, in more severe cases, use a wheelchair. Poliomyelitis does not affect sensory nerves.

At the onset (acute stage), the disease makes people very sick, causing a great deal of pain and paralysis. After this stage passes the person with polio enters a rehabilitation period (recovery stage) that lasts approximately 8 to 12 months. After this stage, the existing physical impairment generally remains permanent.

Classifications

There are two types of polio. The first type, spinal polio, occurs when the virus attacks anterior horn cells in the spinal cord, which impairs skeletal muscles in the trunk and limbs. The specific muscles affected and the degree of involvement depend upon the location and extent of the lesion. In the second type of polio, bulbar, the virus attacks neurons in the brain stem area. Bulbar polio affects the vital centers of circulation and respiration, and when severe it requires life-sustaining, assistive devices, such as mechanical ventilators. Some individuals have a combination of the two types, which is known as bulbo-spinal polio.

In recent years, a phenomenon known as postpolio syndrome has been identified. In middle age about 25% of people who have had polio develop this syndrome, which is characterized by joint or muscle pain, fatigue and a decrease in workload tolerance, an increase in muscle weakness, and an increase in respiratory weakness (Halstead, 1990). Symptoms most often appear in muscles previously affected by the disease, but they occasionally occur in muscles previously thought to be unaffected by the virus. People affected by postpolio syndrome often find the loss of functional ability psychologically depressing.

Although the actual cause of postpolio syndrome has not been conclusively determined, current medical opinion suggests that this syndrome is a consequence of overuse (Halstead, 1990). Medical authorities suggest that nerve fibers regulating weakened motor units have been overstressed for long periods of time, resulting in muscle or nervous tissue damage and a new loss of function.

Exercise Implications

A general flexibility program is advised for individuals with polio to prevent the development of contractures. Regular stretching also helps relieve muscle tension in the lower back and hip region that affects people who walk with an impaired gait. An aerobic program that places limited stress on joints is recommended for weight management. Swimming in a warm pool is an ideal mode of conditioning for people with a postpolio disability.

When postpolio syndrome has been identified, you should recommend exercises in conjunction with the advice of a physician or therapist. Previously inactive individuals benefit from a baseline fitness assessment and a slowly progressive exercise program. Active participants diagnosed with postpolio syndrome also need a conservative exercise program, possibly limited to gentle stretching and low-intensity conditioning. Recommend resistive work only for muscle groups with no clinically apparent prior involvement (Halstead, 1990), but remember the need for training to achieve muscle balance.

Despite the concerns associated with postpolio syndrome, it is important that all postpolio clients remain involved in some type of physical conditioning program within comfort and safety limits. Keep exercise intensity for both aerobic training and resistance training at a low to moderate level. Although the theory that overuse causes postpolio syndrome and a loss of function has not been conclusively proven, until medical research confirms the actual cause of postpolio syndrome, people who have had polio must exercise with caution.

Monitor the recovery time for clients with postpolio. If it regularly takes more than 24 hr to recover following the workout, lower the intensity level of the workout.

Other PNS Disorders

Guillain-Barré Syndrome, a disease that paralyzes peripheral nerves, is characterized by progressive, ascending numbness and paralysis of the feet, legs, trunk, upper extremities, and finally muscles of the face. Two thirds of those affected by this disorder recover, some completely. People with remaining weakness in limb and respiratory muscles may need to modify their exercise programs as people with postpolio syndrome do, such as by decreasing intensity during aerobic and resistance training.

Myasthenia gravis is a disease that causes abnormal fatigue and muscle weakness. The cause is unclear, although it is believed that the disease affects the transmission of motor nerve impulses. Myasthenia gravis is a nonprogressive disorder, and it often goes into remission for weeks or years. Symptoms do not necessarily worsen with recurrence. Onset of myasthenia gravis may be sudden or gradual. The effects are often seen in weakened back, lower extremity, and intercostal muscles. Fatigue is also a common symptom and affects facial, jaw, and tongue muscles, causing drooping eyelids, vision problems, and difficulty with chewing and speaking.

Exercise training for people with myasthenia gravis should target cardiorespiratory endurance and incorporate resistance training to maintain muscular balance. Because fatigue is a common symptom, exercise must progress slowly in consideration of individual tolerances. Breathing exercises are beneficial for strengthening weakened respiratory muscles.

Progressive Disorders

Progressive disorders involve a loss of function with time due to impairments in the nervous system or skeletal muscles. Functional decreases may be rapid, or they may occur gradually with or without periods of remission. As this type of disease progresses, a person becomes progressively weaker and less capable of ambulating. Maintaining function for as long as possible is critical for people with progressive neuromuscular disabilities.

Multiple Sclerosis

Multiple sclerosis (MS) is a progressive neurological disease that generally causes a continual loss of physical and, at times, some cognitive function. It is considered a disorder of the central nervous system, and it affects myelinated nerve tissue in the brain and spinal cord. Some evidence suggests that MS may affect parts of the peripheral nervous system as well (Chretien, Simard, & Dorion, 1985). The basic pathology is a destruction of the myelin sheath (insulation) surrounding the nerve tissue, which causes a loss of function in the innervated muscles (see Figure 2.7). Both skeletal and smooth (organ) muscle can be affected. Currently there are no cures for multiple sclerosis.

Characteristics

MS is often first manifested during middle age and is characterized by periods of exacerbation (acute illness) and remission. Remission is the period during which the condition stabilizes and function remains at a given level until another loss of function occurs. The rate of progression is highly individualized. Some people maintain function at a high level for long periods of time with minor regressions, whereas others become very debilitated within a 10-year period. For many, however, physical function will decrease to some extent over 3 to 5 years.

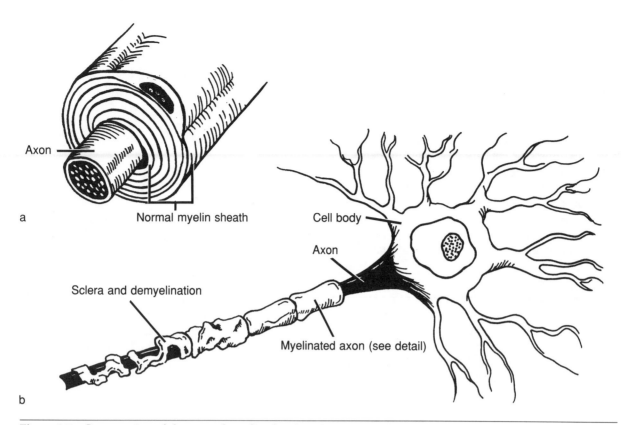

Figure 2.7 Cross section of the normal myelin sheath and nerve axon (a) and the axon of a nerve fiber with normal myelination, sclera, and demyelination with MS (b).

People with MS generally display common symptoms. The primary motor impairments are an increasing loss of muscle function, including partial or complete paralysis; increased ataxia; and, in some cases, spasticity and intention tremors. Some people experience numbness, optic distortions, cognitive impairments, and slurring of speech. Medically, MS may cause incontinence and periodic urinary tract infections. Psychologically, some people have periods of irritation and depression. Commonly, people with MS become progressively weaker, less coordinated, and eventually nonambulatory. Periods of fatigue are also common complaints. If demyelination occurs in nerves regulating the autonomic nervous system, heart rate and blood pressure may not respond normally to exercise.

Despite common impairments associated with MS, the most characteristic symptom of the disease is its unpredictable nature. The location and combination of lesions are very individualized and determine the specific symptoms and course of the disorder for each individual.

Classifications

The following types of MS have been identified to describe the general course of various forms of the disease (Rosenthal & Scheinberg, 1990):

Benign: several attacks (often affecting vision) followed by good recovery and long periods of remission that may last several decades

Exacerbating remitting: periods of exacerbation and good functional recovery for several years followed by a long asymptomatic period for many years with little disability

Relapsing progressive: periods of exacerbation that may, but do not necessarily, alternate with periods of remission; disability accumulates with time

Chronic progressive: slow, progressive decline in function without periods of remission

The most common form of MS is the relapsing progressive type.

Exercise Implications

Multiple sclerosis is a progressive disease that cannot be reversed or halted with therapy and exercise. However, exercise does have an important role to play in the life of the person with MS because it can help him maintain function for a longer period and prevent complications associated with inactivity. Thus, exercise programs, when appropriate, should address all components of physical fitness and include flexibility, strength, and aerobic conditioning.

Because MS progressively weakens the muscles, people with MS can develop contractures, especially in the hip flexors, knee flexors, and plantar flexors, when they become nonambulatory and use wheelchairs. You should develop a daily flexibility routine for each person that can be performed at home, and encourage its use. Emphasize static stretches and avoid ballistic movements with spasticity.

The goal of a resistive strength-training program for people with MS should be to improve and prolong the functionality of muscles that benefit from an exercise program. Because the muscles are very susceptible to fatigue, which will make them less functional for a day or two, limit the intensity and duration of exercises for each muscle group. Heavy resistance training is generally contraindicated.

MS places a great energy demand upon the system, so maintaining aerobic fitness is particularly important. However, people in advanced stages of MS may not be able to obtain an exercise training effect because their muscles may be too weak to provide sufficient stress to benefit the cardiovascular system.

People with MS are often prone to early fatigue with exercise. To delay this effect, a gradual, low-intensity warm-up is essential. Keep in mind that a person with MS may fatigue very quickly when core temperature rises, and warm environments may exacerbate this condition. Hence, exercise in hot and humid conditions is generally contraindicated. If someone chooses to exercise under these conditions, lower the intensity. Remind people with MS of the need for hydration, unless a physician has prescribed diuretics. In this situation, consult the physician or delay training until a cooler environment is available.

Advise people with MS who experience excessive fatigue and a decline in function following exercise against exercising at more than 60% of maximum. More deconditioned participants may require an interval approach to aerobic conditioning, interspersing activity with brief rest periods. If the heart rate response is affected by the disability, use the Rating of Perceived Exertion scale as an alternative measure of exercise intensity (see chapter 5, p. 73).

You should be continually aware of the effect exercise has on daily functioning of participants with MS. A significant decline in function following exercise training indicates that the volume or intensity of the program should be reduced. You might also suggest that your clients with MS plan an additional rest period on days of exercise training to help reduce the effects postexercise fatigue may have on functioning.

Muscular Dystrophy

Muscular dystrophy (MD) refers to a group of chronic diseases that result in the progressive degeneration of skeletal musculature. The age of onset, the rate of progression, and the muscle groups affected vary according to the type of disease. All the various conditions are noncurable and noncontagious.

For the majority of conditions the genetic cause is inherited, although spontaneous genetic mutations are responsible for some cases. All three types of inherited conditions (sex-linked, autosomal dominant, and autosomal recessive) are seen throughout the various conditions. Parents can receive genetic counseling to determine their risk of having other children with MD.

The basic pathology associated with muscular dystrophy appears to be the result of a disturbance in the muscle metabolism. The muscles cannot metabolize necessary substrates, resulting in cell death and tissue degeneration. The actual site within the muscle and mechanism of this disturbance are not known.

Characteristics

The actual muscles affected and rate of progression of muscular dystrophy vary. In some cases, a slow rate of progression precedes a long period in which no further degeneration takes place.

Regardless of the type of MD a person may have, movement restrictions result from the same three factors. Due to a progressive degeneration, affected muscles become increasingly weaker, with weakness ranging from mild to severe. Degeneration in the lower limbs affects balance and ambulation, and degeneration in the upper limbs affects the strength and dexterity of arms and hands. The second factor that causes movement restrictions is a continued loss of muscular endurance, which causes early onset of fatigue with activity. A third factor is postural disorders that result from an imbalance in degeneration of muscle tissue in opposing muscle groups. Most postural disorders appear in the trunk and feet.

People with MD are susceptible to respiratory infections, which can lead to pneumonia, particularly in later stages of the disease. Conditions such as pneumonia and heart failure may reduce the life span of people with MD.

Classifications

Many forms of MD have been identified and labeled. Three of the more common forms of MD are facio-scapulo-humeral, limb girdle, and Duchenne. The facio-scapulo-humeral type is the most common adult form of MD, often not recognized until late adolescence or adulthood. Facioscapulo-humeral MD can arrest during any stage. The disorder involves progressive weakness in shoulder, shoulder girdle, arm, back, and facial muscles. Hip and thigh muscles are less frequently affected.

Limb girdle MD is characterized by slow progressive degeneration of upper and lower extremity muscles beginning after the age of 10 and originating in either shoulder girdle or hip and thigh muscles.

Duchenne MD is the most common (and severe) form with symptoms appearing in children between the ages of 3 and 10. This form progresses steadily, affecting leg, hip, back, shoulder girdle, and respiratory muscles and severely impairing the ability to walk within 10 years. Walking, climbing stairs, and rising from a recumbent position become increasingly difficult. Weakened anterior tibialis muscles cause "foot drop" and frequent falling. Obesity, lower-limb contractures, and extensive atrophy characterize later stages of the disability. Death generally occurs by early adulthood from associated complications.

Exercise Implications

The goals of the exercise program for people with MD should be to maintain muscle function, range of motion, and cardiovascular endurance as long as possible. It is imperative that you be familiar with the medical history of each client with MD. Potential problems common to people with MD are heart complications, fragile bones, or a susceptibility to respiratory infections. Check trunk balance before beginning exercise and recommend the use of a safety belt for trunk support, if indicated.

Encourage stretching as part of a daily exercise routine to maintain range of motion (ROM) and prevent contractures. You also may want to develop an appropriate resistance training program (but only with guidance from the person's physician). In some cases, resistance training may be contraindicated if the physician feels that overloading weakened muscles would accelerate muscle degeneration associated with the disorder.

Exercising to fatigue is not advisable for people with MD because some authorities believe it may hasten the degenerative effects of the disease (Adams, Daniel, McCubbin, & Rullman, 1982). It is essential that you continually monitor all clients with MD to ensure that they adhere to recommended intensity levels.

Other Progressive Disorders

Friedreich's ataxia is a genetic neurological disorder that causes progressive degeneration of sensory nerves in the limbs and trunk. People with Friedreich's ataxia have impaired balance and coordination, tremors, distal limb atrophy, slurred speech, seizures, foot and spinal deformities, cardiac problems, and impaired vision. Fitness training should focus on maintaining muscular strength and endurance, particularly in distal limbs.

Charcot-Marie-Tooth syndrome is caused by demyelination of spinal nerves and anterior horn cells in the spinal cord, causing progressive weakness and atrophy in leg and hand muscles. Hand weakness and gait impairment are common characteristics. Follow strategies and precautions similar to those used with MD regarding exercise intensity during strength training.

Several progressive disorders that are characteristic of middle or advancing age include amyotrophic lateral sclerosis (ALS), Alzheimer's disease, Parkinson's disease, and Huntington's disease. Consult a physician before recommending exercise programs for individuals with these conditions.

Disabilities From Injury Outside the Nervous System

Some disabilities are the result of impairments that affect structures outside the nervous system, such as bone and joint impairments. This category includes amputations and various forms of arthritis. With all these conditions, coordination and reflexes are not affected.

Amputation

Amputation refers to the removal or absence of a limb. An acquired amputation involves the removal of an injured or diseased limb from the body. A congenital amputation, also called a limb deficiency, refers to a limb that is absent at birth or a limb malformed at birth that may subsequently be removed to provide a better fit for a prosthesis (artificial limb). Dysmelia is a congenital amputation resulting in the absence of a complete limb; phocomelia is the absence of the middle segment of a limb with distal portions being attached to the joint, such as hands attached to shoulders and feet attached near the hips.

The most common cause of acquired amputations is a malfunction in the circulatory system that causes a loss of the blood supply to a limb and results in the death of the affected tissue. Other causes include trauma (vehicular accidents, severe burns), cancerous tumors, and serious infections that resist treatment.

Surgical amputation is undertaken to improve a person's health, as in cases of cancer, or to improve an individual's future functioning by removing a severely damaged or deformed limb. Four times more amputations of the lower extremities occur than of the upper extremities.

The remaining segment of an amputated appendage is referred to as the stump or residual limb. A physician uses surgery to construct a stump that will be suitable for a prosthesis. During recuperation following surgery, the stump is monitored to prevent infection. The medical team wraps the stump to control swelling and uses therapy to develop or maintain strength in the remaining muscles of the amputated limb. Within 3 months postsurgery, most people can be fitted for a prosthesis. Shrinkage continues temporarily in the stump and requires periodic fittings to ensure a proper fit. Usually therapists will train people how to use artificial limbs properly.

Classifications

Amputations are categorized according to their location (see Figure 2.8) and are given these labels:

Below knee (BK): the amputation is in the lower leg; the knee joint is intact.

Above knee (AK): the amputation is in the thigh; the hip joint is intact.

Below elbow (BE): the amputation is in the forearm; the elbow joint is intact.

Above elbow (AE): the amputation is in the upper arm; the shoulder joint is intact.

Disarticulation: the amputation is through a joint. (Symes amputation refers to an amputation at the ankle.)

Amputations can also be classified according to cause as acquired or congenital.

Prosthetics

Prosthetic devices are individually constructed by a trained professional, called a prosthetist. The particular design people use depends upon their needs and lifestyles. Due to advances in research

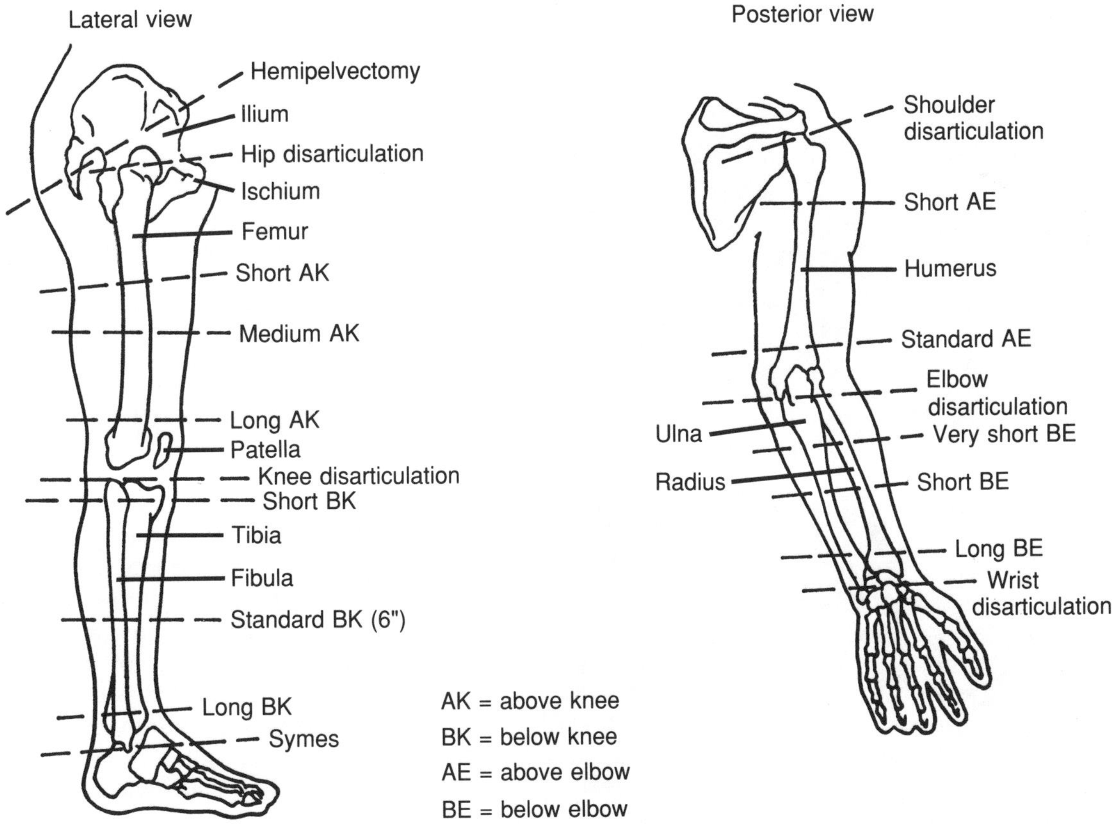

Figure 2.8 Anatomical classification of amputations for the upper and lower extremity.

and modern technology, prostheses now allow for a very active lifestyle (see Figure 2.9).

Except for disarticulation, the lower limb prostheses do not support the weight on the end of the amputated limb. The weight is carried either on the pelvis or the muscles of the thigh for an AK amputation and on the sides of the tibia for a BK amputation. Several methods are used for securing the lower limb prosthesis. People can use a belt that loops around the hips, suction, a lacing corset, or wedges. Except in the case of suction, the person wears a sock over the residual limb to reduce friction.

Lower limb prostheses offer several types of feet, and the person's lifestyle and desires determine the specific type chosen. Some feet are designed to provide a little bounce to the step to make running and other quick movements more natural and allow varying degrees of ankle motion. Other feet are designed to accommodate high-heeled or dress shoes.

There are two types of upper extremity prostheses: one type connected by straps to the opposite shoulder and operated through shoulder girdle movement and a second type activated by sensors placed over muscles. These sensors detect electrical impulses of functional muscles to operate small motors that flex the elbow and operate the terminal device (prosthetic hand).

A good prosthetic fit is essential to permit an active lifestyle. Loose-fitting prostheses decrease stability during movement. Improper prosthetic fit can cause pain and blisters in the stump and further decrease efficiency in walking, which brings on fatigue more quickly.

Other causes of pain from prostheses are ulceration, which results from poor circulation in the stump; infection; and neuroma, which is a nonmalignant tumor that results from an interaction between nervous tissue and scar tissue. Some people also have phantom limb pain—brain messages that give pain from the missing limb. This phenomenon usually diminishes with time.

Exercise Implications

Lower limb amputations present most movement problems. Although lower limb prostheses provide for a lot of movement, they are not as biomechanically efficient as a natural leg and foot. Speed, lateral agility, jumping power, and stair climbing efficiency are generally affected. A lower limb prosthesis decreases gait efficiency, particularly with an AK amputation.

Upper limb amputations primarily affect a person's dexterity. These amputations may also affect locomotion by reducing the counteracting motions of the arms that help reduce upper trunk sway, thereby reducing some of the efficiency and stability of the locomotion pattern. Evaluate each person's movement patterns before exercise to determine if any vigorous movements would create a serious risk of falling. If so, eliminate the pattern or make it less vigorous.

Because ambulation with a prosthesis requires significantly more energy at a given intensity level, many people with an amputation become less active. This reduced activity could lead to stiffness in hip, knee, or elbow joints over time. Some people bring their artificial limbs through the swing phase of their walking gait by elevating the hip during the leg movement, which creates an increased lordotic curve and a potential for low-back pain. This is called hiphiking. Upper body posture may also be affected with development of shortened rhomboids. Postural imbalances can be relieved with regular abdominal and pectoral exercise and with stretching the hips and back.

Removal of a dominant hand or leg can cause awkward movement patterns in the initial months following surgery, challenging movement coordination during activity. This incoordination should dissipate with time as the person becomes skilled at using the nondominant side.

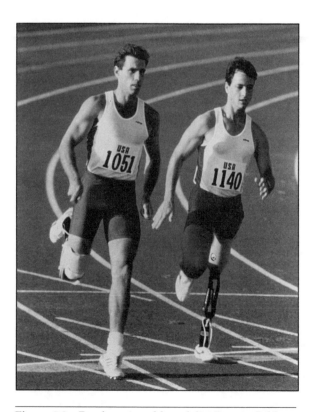

Figure 2.9 Paralympic gold medalist Dennis Oehler trains with Todd Schaffhauser. Photo courtesy of Flex Foot, Inc.

Keep the design features of AK prosthetics in mind when exercise calls for standing postures. Some prostheses require that the knee be kept straight to prevent buckling. Be aware of individual prosthetic knee dynamics so you can offer proper guidance to prevent loss of balance. If the leg prosthesis is designed for use with heeled shoes, wearing sport shoes may create an imbalance. The participant may use lifts in both shoes to compensate for differences. Consult with the individual's prosthetist or therapist to determine the proper choice in this situation.

Sometimes the person with an amputation may wish to remove the prosthesis during exercise if it restricts movement or causes rubbing, shearing, and abrasions. The choice for use or removal of a prosthesis belongs to the wearer. Be aware, however, of the impact of the decision on exercise performance and comfort. People more frequently choose to remove an upper limb prosthesis. Removal of a lower limb prosthesis radically alters balance and causes significant stress to the unimpaired leg, necessitating exercising from a seated position. Also, forewarn the person with an amputation that because exercise can cause slight swelling of the skin and the stump, prosthesis fit may be affected after exercise. Swelling can present challenges if the prosthesis has been removed. A perspiration-soaked stump sock should be replaced with a dry one to prevent rubbing.

During resistance training, the prosthesis can be removed if it provides greater resistance than stump muscles can tolerate. As strength increases, the prosthesis can be used to add resistance. Additional cuff weights can be added to the residual limb to further increase resistance. Resistance should never be applied to the prosthesis itself.

Because of the increased energy demands placed upon a person with an amputation, encourage regular aerobic activity. If a client has an acquired amputation due to circulatory problems, however, you may need to reduce exercise intensity because of associated health concerns. Consult with the individual's physician before making recommendations. In addition to aerobic dance exercise, bicycling and swimming may be effective means for maintaining aerobic fitness.

Arthritis

Arthritis (joint inflammation) refers to various conditions that create pain and inflammation within joints affected by the specific disorder (see Figure 2.10). Arthritis is often referred to as everybody's disease because almost everyone is affected either directly or indirectly. The annual cost to the nation's economy in the treatment of arthritis is in the billions of dollars.

Common Forms

Of about 100 different arthritic conditions, the most common types are rheumatoid arthritis and degenerative joint disease consequent to aging (osteoarthritis). Other forms of arthritis may result from infections, joint trauma and stress, rheumatic fever, and gout. In this manual, we will discuss rheumatoid arthritis, osteoarthritis, ankylosing spondylitis, and juvenile rheumatoid arthritis.

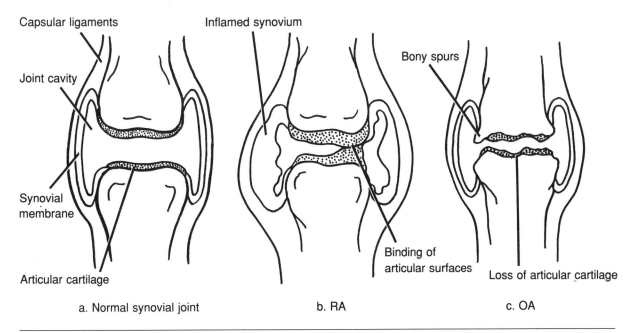

Figure 2.10 Structure of a normal joint (a), effects of rheumatoid arthritis (b), and effects of osteoarthritis (c).

Rheumatoid Arthritis. Rheumatoid arthritis, which is systemic in nature, is one of the most severe types of arthritis. In most circumstances, rheumatoid arthritis progressively worsens.

During acute stages of rheumatoid arthritis, fever, poor appetite, weight loss, and anemia may be present. Lymph glands and the spleen may become swollen and joints become inflamed and painful. During this stage, as a result of the symptoms, the individual tires easily and mobility is severely restricted.

Rheumatoid arthritis usually affects more than one joint and is usually symmetrical, affecting the same joint on each side of the body. The inflammation occurs in the synovial membranes that cover a joint capsule and spreads throughout the joint. Eventually the cartilage surrounding the bones is destroyed and scar tissue is formed. With time the bones can become fused, dramatically reducing the range of motion of that joint. Muscle spasms around the joint can also cause pain and, in some cases, joint distortions also contribute to the reduced range of motion. Joints in the arms, hands, hips, legs, and feet are predominantly those affected.

Rheumatoid arthritis also is characterized by periods of remission. During these periods many of the symptoms disappear. Over time, when joint and bone damage have resulted, the disabling effects of rheumatoid arthritis are permanent.

The treatment program for rheumatoid arthritis may include medications, rest, exercise, posture rules, splints, walking aids, heat, surgery, and rehabilitation. The medications most frequently used are aspirin, gold salts, and cortisone.

Juvenile Rheumatoid Arthritis. Juvenile rheumatoid arthritis (JRA) is the most common form of arthritis in children. In many ways its symptoms are similar to adult rheumatoid arthritis. During a period of flare-up, the child suffers severe joint pain and fever. Other secondary symptoms may also be present. In many cases medical treatment prevents permanent disability.

Osteoarthritis. Osteoarthritis is the most common type of arthritis. This condition is primarily a result of joint overuse and most commonly affects the weight-bearing joints of the knees, hips, and spine. Usually, only one joint is affected. Inflammation is rarely present.

In osteoarthritis the cartilage that covers the articulating surfaces of the bones that form the joint becomes damaged and deteriorates with time. In some cases the cartilage is completely worn away, resulting in direct contact between articulating bones. If this occurs, then bony spurs form that cause pain in the surrounding soft tissues. The major symptoms of osteoarthritis are pain, muscle fatigue, and joint stiffness.

Pain can result from several factors. As the joint breaks down, it creates pressure on the surrounding nerve endings. Bony spurs cause pain in the soft tissues. Surrounding muscles become tense due to the pain, which further increases discomfort and muscle fatigue. In addition, periodic swelling may occur, which will also increase the joint discomfort.

Over time, as joint use decreases, the muscles become deconditioned. Joint stiffness results from the reduced mechanical efficiency of the joint and from the increased muscle tenseness. This stiffness eventually reduces the range of motion in that joint.

The cause of osteoarthritis is not precisely known. Medical authorities believe the two most likely reasons are genetics or joint deficiencies that render the joint more susceptible to degeneration due to normal stresses on it. It is believed that some individuals are genetically inclined to age more quickly and that some of their joints may have a decreased capacity to withstand normal wear and tear. In other cases, osteoarthritis may develop in people who have experienced joint trauma or who were born with some degree of mechanical inefficiency at the joint.

Treatment for osteoarthritis involves rest, special exercises, heat, surgery, and in some cases, drugs to relieve pain. Because there is no cure for this disorder, an individual with osteoarthritis must maintain a treatment regimen throughout life. In a limited number of cases, physicians advise joint replacement surgery for people with constant pain and permanent disability as a result of the arthritis.

Ankylosing Spondylitis. Ankylosing spondylitis is a progressive disease of the vertebral column. The disease creates pain and stiffness in the spine. In advanced cases the spine becomes rigid, creating an increased anterior curvature of the trunk and forward stooped posture. The condition usually begins in the lumbar and sacral areas, causing low-back pain and pain in the legs. Treatment usually includes medication and exercise.

Exercise Implications

Movement impairments due to arthritis primarily occur because of pain, muscle fatigue, and joint stiffness. Although movement may increase pain, most physicians prescribe regular exercise as part of the treatment in the belief that regular exercise will increase functionality. Prolonged inactivity tends to increase stiffness.

Remember that muscles surrounding the joint become tense in reaction to joint pain, which increases the discomfort and reduces the ROM of the joint. To help counteract this symptom, people with arthritis need to perform flexibility exercises daily. Static stretching is recommended to allow the muscles to adjust slowly, thereby eliminating the trauma on joints imposed by bouncing. Teach people with arthritis appropriate stretches and stretching techniques for the affected joint. Always have them incorporate a good stretching routine (after warming the joints) before every workout, and periodically have them measure joint ROM to provide rewarding feedback for improvements gained from flexibility training.

Due to pain, many individuals with arthritis move their affected joints less frequently. As a result, the muscles become deconditioned and cardiovascular fitness declines. Consequently, activity produces fatigue more quickly. To counteract this negative cycle of deconditioning, recommend muscular endurance strengthening exercises (low resistance, high repetitions) for the muscles at affected joints. Low-impact, no-impact, or seated aerobic dance exercise is useful to improve aerobic fitness.

There are several considerations when making adjustments to help relieve pain. One is to always include a good warm-up. Second, reduce the impact of weight bearing on the affected joints. Using positions such as sitting, or mediums such as water, that reduce weight bearing on joints during exercise is a preferred way to exercise. A third factor is heat. Warm environments improve the performance of people with most types of arthritis. Exercise in a warm pool is optimal. A fourth consideration is to carefully monitor the total amount of work performed for each exercise session. Regular exercise at moderate intensity helps maintain joint function. However, each person with arthritis has an exercise tolerance beyond which pain will be increased. Any significant increase in pain during exercise indicates that the exercise should be stopped. In addition, question participants about any increases in pain between exercise sessions. If this occurs, reduce the exercise intensity during subsequent workouts.

Other Disorders Affecting Peripheral Structures

Osteogenesis imperfecta (OI), or "brittle bone disease," is caused by defective bone, ligament, and dermal tissues. With this condition, bones are easily broken and joint tissues have a reduced toler-

ance to stretch, causing joint instability. You may want to recommend a strength-building program to improve joint stability, although you must be careful to prevent excessive stress on bones and joints.

People with OI should also minimize impact with exercise training. Seated aerobics, swimming, and water exercise are ideal modes for conditioning the cardiorespiratory system.

Arthrogryposis is a nonprogressive, congenital disability characterized by muscular weakness. This disorder affects the structure and function of some or all joints. Muscle tissues that normally surround the joint are replaced by fatty and connective tissue. Common postural effects are inward rotation of shoulders, elbow extension, forearm pronation, and flexion and outward rotation of hips, knees, and ankles. Limb deformities also are common with arthrogryposis. Exercise training should focus on developing ROM and strengthening weak muscles around impaired joints. Swimming is a valuable mode of conditioning for people with this form of disability.

Visual Impairment

The vast majority of people who are blind received that diagnosis because of a severe decrement in their visual acuity. People are considered legally blind if the acuity measure in their best eye, after correction, is 20/200 or worse. This implies an ability to see at only 20 ft what the normally sighted see at 200 ft. Although people who are blind may have some degree of light perception, for the most part their eyesight is nonfunctional. The person who is blind must learn to function in a world that relies heavily on vision for gathering information. Because sight is so important for guiding movement, visual impairment can impair mobility, and you must address the effects of limited mobility with your exercise clients who are blind.

People who acquire their blindness after early childhood (adventitious type) are often better movers than those who have a congenital disorder because mature movement patterns developed before the loss of sight. After learning to function without sight, movement patterns return to near normal. People born with blindness usually experience delays in developing movement patterns, some remaining awkward throughout life. People with the adventitious type of blindness are able to construct a more accurate mental image of space, which helps them relate to the environment more easily.

Most individuals with blindness do not see total darkness. What little they can see is referred to as residual vision. In some cases residual vision may be useful. If an individual can see sharp contrasts (e.g., white on a green background) this residual vision may be used as a directional aid or as a way to identify equipment. However, for the most part, you must provide strong verbal cues for guidance. Chapter 12 offers suggestions for modified teaching strategies with clients who are visually impaired (see pp. 174-175).

A major challenge associated with visual impairment is orientation, the ability to spatially relate to the surrounding environment. Until people become oriented, they display tentative movements and a sense of being lost in space. Assisting people who are blind in a new environment by giving tours of the area and alerting them to any alterations once the environment becomes familiar helps orient them to the space. You can use auditory and tactile cues to orient the person with a visual impairment during activities that require movement or a change in position.

Mobility training teaches people with visual impairment how to use other senses, hearing and touch, to orient themselves in their environment; how to use a sighted person as a guide; and how to use a cane in walking. As a person with blindness becomes more mobile, self-stimulatory movements, known as blindisms, begin to disappear. These actions, which include rocking, finger waving, and hand shaking, are believed to be outlets for individuals with repressed movement.

Exercise Implications

The movement capabilities of people with blindness are similar to those in people without visual impairment. However, because the loss of sight creates some restrictions, it is important that you develop skills to orient the person to the activity space and that you use effective auditory and tactile cues to describe movement patterns and directions.

Individuals with blindness from birth or early childhood may display less confidence with movement; they will experience more success in an exercise program if you introduce simple movement patterns before you build complex movements. More complex movements are appropriate for people with adventitious blindness if you provide effective cuing and practice time for building patterns.

Developing and maintaining aerobic fitness is especially important for individuals with visual impairment, who typically move with less efficiency and at a greater energy cost. When selecting music to accompany an exercise session, you might consider using instrumental music, which will compete less with your verbal commands than music with strong vocals.

Resistance training and stretching require little modification as long as the client with a visual impairment has had adequate time to become familiar with the equipment and learn the exercises. Be sure to offer exercises appropriate for maintaining good postural alignment, if needed. Avoid recommending high-intensity exercise for people with glaucoma because small blood vessels of the eye are susceptible to rupture.

Summary

This chapter has presented the characteristics, classifications, and general exercise implications for some of the more common physical disabilities that you are likely to encounter in your exercise programs. We have organized disabilities according to the site of injury. This system considers whether a disorder is due to impairments to the nervous system (the brain, spinal cord, peripheral nerves) or to structures outside the nervous system, such as with bone or joint impairments. We discussed disabilities resulting from progressive disorders separately to highlight additional considerations and precautions. As an exercise leader, you must be familiar with this basic information before recommending or leading exercise programs for people with physical disabilities. Refer back to this information as you read the chapters in the remainder of the book that apply principles of exercise science, exercise conditioning, and program management.

Part II

Exercise and Training: Effects of Physical Disability

All the systems of the body that interact to regulate movement and adapt to exercise stress influence the ability to exercise and respond to exercise training. Physical disability may challenge any or all of these systems. As an exercise instructor, you should not only be familiar with the basic structure and function of the musculoskeletal, neuromuscular, metabolic, endocrine, and cardiovascular systems, but also with the influences a disabling condition imposes upon them. This will enable you to modify the exercise prescription for your clients with disabilities appropriately and ensure that their training is both safe and effective. Furthermore, such familiarity will enable you to share realistic expectations with your clients about the potential outcome of their long-term training efforts.

Part II provides a base of exercise science and conditioning principles relevant to disability upon which you can build exercise and technique modifications. Chapter 3 examines how disability might alter the basic structure, function, and anaerobic performance of skeletal muscle. We also review neuromuscular control of movement, anaerobic metabolism, and adaptations to anaerobic training in this context. Chapter 4 takes a specific look at the physiology of aerobic exercise conditioning and presents potential effects disability may have on oxygen consumption ($\dot{V}O_2$), temperature regulation, and aerobic training adaptations. We also present a comparison of physiologic responses to upper and lower body exercise.

The information presented in Part II supplements your knowledge of basic anatomy and exercise physiology. Refer to any general text on these subjects (such as those listed in the Recommended Readings list) for review. Your preliminary understanding of the principles of exercise science as applied to the nondisabled population will greatly enhance your understanding of the information presented here in these chapters.

Recommended Readings

Alter, M.M. (1988). *Science of stretching*. Champaign, IL: Human Kinetics.

Bouchard, C., Shephard, R.J., Stephens, T., Sutton, J.R., & McPherson, B.D. (1990). *Exercise, fitness, and health: A consensus of current knowledge.* Champaign, IL: Human Kinetics.

Brooks, G.A., & Fahey, T.D. (1984). *Exercise physiology: Human bioenergetics and its applications.* New York: Wiley.

Brooks, V.D. (1986). *The neural basis of motor control.* New York: Oxford University Press.

Fleck, S.J., & Kraemer, W.J. (1987). *Designing resistance training programs*. Champaign, IL: Human Kinetics.

Franklin, B.A., Seymour, G., & Timmis, G.C. (Eds.) (1989). *Exercise in modern medicine*. Baltimore: Williams & Wilkins.

Frustace, S.J. (1988). Poliomyelitis: Late and unusual sequelae. *American Journal of Physical Medicine*, **66**(6), 328-337.

Glaser, R.M., & Davis, G.M. (1988). Wheelchair-dependent individuals. In B.A. Franklin, S. Gordon, & G.C. Timmis (Eds.), *Exercise in modern medicine*. Baltimore: Williams & Wilkins.

Lasko-McCarthey, P.M., & Knopf, K.G. (1992). Adapted physical education for adults with disabilities (3rd ed.). Dubuque, IA: Eddie Bowers.

Marieb, E.N. (1991). *Essentials of human anatomy and physiology* (3rd ed.). Redwood City, CA: Benjamin/Cummings.

Mathers, L.H. (1985). *The peripheral nervous system: Structure, function and clinical correlations*. Menlo Park, CA: Addison-Wesley.

McArdle, W.D., Katch, F.I., & Katch, V.L. (1991). *Exercise physiology: Energy, nutrition and human performance* (3rd ed.). Philadelphia: Lea & Febiger.

McAtee, R.E. (1993). *Facilitated stretching*. Champaign, IL: Human Kinetics.

Sawka M.N. (1986). Physiology of upper body exercise. In K.B. Pandolf (Ed.), *Exercise and sports sciences reviews*, **14**, 175-210. New York: Macmillan.

Sharkey, B.J. (1990). *Physiology of fitness* (3rd ed.). Champaign, IL: Human Kinetics.

Shephard, R.J. (1990). *Fitness in special populations*. Champaign, IL: Human Kinetics.

Tesch, P.A. (1988). Skeletal muscle adaptations consequent to long-term heavy resistance exercise. *Medicine and Science in Sports and Exercise*, **20**(5), S132-S134.

Vogel, J.A. (1988). Introduction to the symposium: Physiological responses and adaptations to resistance exercise. *Medicine and Science in Sports and Exercise*, **20**(5), S131.

Chapter 3

Skeletal Muscle Physiology and Anaerobic Exercise

Patricia D. Miller, MA
The Fitness Factor, Morgantown, WV

Exercise implications with physical disability, as briefly introduced in the preceding chapter, are largely determined by how a disabling condition alters the basic structure and function of bodily systems that regulate movement and respond to exercise. In this chapter, we examine how disability affects the structure, function, and neuromuscular control of skeletal muscle. We also look at anaerobic capabilities of muscle and ways a disabling condition might influence responses to resistance training.

Knowledge of the basic structure and function of the musculoskeletal, neuromuscular, and metabolic systems is a prerequisite to understanding how exercise affects these systems and, furthermore, how disability may affect the capacity for anaerobic work, namely resistive exercise. As an exercise leader working with individuals with physical disabilities, it is also important that you know how physical disability may affect physiologic responses to exercise. Without this knowledge, it would be difficult to offer an effective (and safe!) program to your clients with disabilities.

Structure and Function of Skeletal Muscle and Connective Tissue

The musculoskeletal system provides support for upright posture and generates force for movement and locomotion. Muscle also provides a major source of heat for maintaining body temperature. Skeletal muscles are interlaced with connective tissue, capillaries, and nerves. Bones, muscles, and connective tissue articulate to permit specific types of movement at each joint in the body, depending on the nature of the articulation. Capillary blood flow through muscle transports oxygen and fuel to support metabolism and remove by-products following contraction. Nerves provide a means for sensing changes within muscle (such as changes in length, tension, and joint position) and initiate voluntary and involuntary muscle contractions as directed by the brain or mediated by reflex mechanisms.

Physically disabling conditions may alter the structure and therefore the function of skeletal muscle, connective tissue, and the neuromuscular system. These alterations, in turn, influence the capacity for movement, range of motion (ROM), and the magnitude of force that muscular contractions generate. For example, any impairment that causes the soft tissues of the joint to shorten at their resting length can cause a joint contracture to develop. A contracture is defined as an adaptive shortening of muscle and connective tissue that reduces the movement range at a joint. Contractures may be transient and partially or totally reversible, or they may be irreversible if normal soft tissues are replaced by large amounts of inextensible fibrotic or bony tissue. Spasticity, or resistance to passive stretch from the central nervous system, also causes a type of contracture and reduces joint range of motion. Table 3.1 lists several causes of joint contractures.

Connective Tissue and Joint Structure

Connective tissue is arranged in and around individual muscle fibers (endomysium), bundles of fibers (perimysium), and entire muscles (epimysium) and connects with bones by way of tendons across one or more joints.

Ligaments (the tissue that connects the bones that articulate at the joint) and joint capsules are also formed by connective tissue.

Smooth biomechanical function of each joint depends upon the integrity of all the tissues that form

Table 3.1 Causes of Joint Contractures

Condition	Cause
Immobilization	Casting or splinting
Decreased mobility	Inactivity or prolonged sitting
	Pain
Paralysis	Connective tissue or neuromuscular diseases
Weakness	
Spasticity	Brain injury
Muscle imbalances	Spinal cord injury (complete or incomplete)
Pain	
Edema	Tissue pathology due to trauma (replacement of soft tissue with dense fibrous tissue)
Inflammation	
Ischemia	
Hemorrhage	
Surgery	
Laceration	
Burns	

the joint structure. Physical disabilities such as arthritis, osteogenesis imperfecta, and amputation can cause pain, inflammation, or permanent structural deformities in joint tissues and thereby significantly alter movement capabilities in the affected areas. Joint structures may also be surgically altered to improve stability or modify attachment of tendons and ligaments to compensate for conditions associated with disabilities and further affect movement range. Any disability that causes joint contractures may also, over time, induce changes that cause permanent loss of movement range.

Connective tissue is normally composed of different substances that contribute to its ability to function within and around movable joint structures (Kisner & Colby, 1990):

Collagen provides stability, strength, and stiffness; elongates with light stretch; and resists deformation with increasing tension.

Elastin provides extensibility.

Reticulin provides tissue bulk.

Ground substance reduces friction and cross-linking between fibers.

Tendons, ligaments, and joint capsules have varying amounts of collagen and elastin, which affect their stiffness and extensibility, respectively. Inactivity, aging, and immobilization decrease the collagen content and increase the ratio of elastin fibers in connective tissue, which decreases the strength of the tissue.

Properties of Skeletal Muscle

Normal function of skeletal muscle is described by four characteristic properties (Tortora, 1986):

Excitability: the ability to react to stimuli, such as those provided by the nervous system

Contractility: the capability for shortening and thickening

Extensibility: the capacity for lengthening or stretching

Elasticity: the ability to return to the resting length after short-term deformation

An additional characteristic of muscle is plasticity, which refers to its ability to maintain a new resting length after a stretch force has been applied under certain conditions. Plasticity is also characteristic of noncontractile connective tissue. Plasticity is the quality that enables the soft tissues of the joint to elongate with stretching to improve flexibility.

The capabilities of muscle tissue for the properties just described depend upon not only the structure of the joint tissues but also the integrity of the neuromuscular system.

Fast- and Slow-Twitch Muscle Fibers

Muscle fibers are generally classified as being either slow-twitch (ST) or fast-twitch (FT) according to their structural and functional characteristics. Intermediate fibers, which are a subgroup of FT fibers, are capable of performing like ST or FT fibers. The ST fibers are the fatigue-resistant fibers that support long-duration aerobic exercise. The FT fibers can generate more force than ST fibers and are recruited primarily for movements that require strength and power. Table 3.2 summarizes characteristics of ST and FT fibers.

Exercise conditioning can improve the capacity of muscle fibers to perform. Appropriate conditioning can help intermediate fibers perform more like ST or FT fibers.

The distribution of fiber types is genetically determined and may be quite different from muscle to muscle or person to person. In all people, certain muscles tend to have a greater number of one fiber type than another, corresponding to the intended function of that muscle. In general, arm muscles have a greater percentage of FT than ST fibers (Johnson, Polgar, Weightman, & Appleton, 1973). Using the arms to propel a wheelchair, then, not only relies on a smaller muscle mass for locomotion but also may rely on muscle fiber types that are less well suited for continuous work in someone who is deconditioned.

Muscular dystrophy directly affects the muscle fibers, causing their eventual necrosis (tissue death) and replacing them with fibrous connective tissue. In general, muscular dystrophy, particularly the Duchenne type, results in an eventual predominance of Type I muscle fibers (Swash & Schwartz, 1988). Some types of MD are believed to affect different muscle fiber types in varying degrees, which may affect the capacity of the remaining fibers for movement and exercise training.

Motor Neurons and the Motor Unit

Muscle fibers are directly innervated by lower motor neurons of the peripheral nervous system. A motor unit is a group of muscle fibers innervated by a single efferent motor neuron. All muscle fibers of a motor unit are of the same muscle fiber type; that is, fast- and slow-twitch muscle fibers are not combined within a single motor unit. Motor units responsible for fine motor control are composed of a small number of fibers, and they tend to be composed of more ST than FT fibers. Motor units

Table 3.2   General Characteristics of Muscle Fiber Types

	Slow-twitch	Fast-twitch	Intermediate
Labels	SO (slow oxidative) Type I	FG (fast glycolytic) Type IIb	FOG (fast oxidative glycolytic) Type IIa
Aerobic capacity	High	Low	High
Anaerobic capacity	Low	High	Moderate
Speed of contraction	Slow	Fast	Fast
Rate of fatigue	Low	High	Intermediate
Strength of contraction	Low	High	High

used for gross movements requiring greater force and power, such as those contained in quadriceps muscles, are typically larger and tend to have a greater percentage of FT muscle fibers. FT motor units are capable of reaching greater tension nearly twice as fast as ST motor units.

Motor unit recruitment is the process of selectively activating motor units within a muscle group. The central nervous system (CNS) synchronizes recruitment of motor units, which enables movement force and speed to be graded. When a movement is initiated, recruitment progresses from small ST to larger FT motor units. Progressively larger FT motor units are recruited to generate more force as required by the demands of the activity. Even with forceful movement, all motor units are generally not activated, especially in deconditioned muscle. Prolonged muscular contraction against a constant submaximal load causes a progressive increase in recruitment of motor units over time as smaller motor units fatigue.

Paralysis occurs when a majority of the motor units in a muscle group become nonfunctional. Muscle weakness due to paresis (partial paralysis) occurs when one third or more of the motor units within a muscle group lose their ability to contract (Cobble & Maloney, 1985). In addition to limiting strength and function, muscle weakness may create imbalances between muscle pairs that can destabilize a joint. Paralysis or paresis may be caused by impairment to upper motor neurons of the central nervous system (such as with brain injury, spinal cord injury, or multiple sclerosis), impairment to lower motor neurons (such as with polio), or dysfunction directly within the muscle (as with muscular dystrophy).

Paresis may be accompanied by the "sprouting" of additional motor neurons in an attempt to reinnervate nonfunctioning motor units. The result is the formation of larger than normal, in some cases giant, motor units. There is some evidence that progressive weakness may be caused by chronic overwork of paretic muscles with fewer than normal functional motor units or with muscle groups that have been restructured with larger than normal motor units. This is one proposed explanation for postpolio syndrome, characterized by onset of fatigue, pain, and weakness with exertion, that occurs in about 25% of polio survivors decades after they initially contracted the polio virus.

Neuromuscular Control of Movement

The neuromuscular system regulates movement by linking sensory information derived from the periphery with commands from the central nervous system. The central nervous system (CNS) is composed of the brain and spinal cord. Motor neurons in the CNS are referred to as upper motor neurons. The peripheral nervous system (PNS) contains the cranial nerves and lower motor neurons that emanate from the spinal cord. Movement can be reflexive (an involuntary motor response to a stimulus) or voluntary. Both types of movement normally involve a hierarchy of motor control from afferent and efferent peripheral nerves to nerves of the spinal column and control centers in the brain at the highest level of the hierarchy. Excitatory responses stimulate motor neurons to contract skeletal muscle. Inhibition is a protective mechanism that dampens or overrides excitation to control movement. Disabilities that involve injury to upper motor neurons (in the brain and spinal cord) may disrupt normal excitation and inhibition, which can impair the coordination and strength of muscular actions. Figure 3.1 depicts the hierarchy of movement control as affected by movement disorders.

Afferent and Efferent Neurons

Afferent sensory neurons and efferent motor neurons innervate skeletal muscle. Afferent neurons detect stimuli to and changes within skeletal muscle and connective tissue. External stimuli, such as pain or pressure, and internal stimuli, such as changes in muscle tissue length, tension, and joint position, provide sensory information. Afferent neurons send messages to the brain in ascending tracts by way of the spinal cord or interact directly

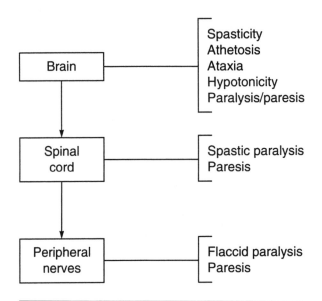

Figure 3.1 The hierarchy of motor control and levels of nervous system disorders.

with efferent motor neurons and bypass control from higher brain centers. Efferent neurons activate or inhibit a muscular response.

Reflex actions, such as the stretch reflex and inverse stretch reflex, involve interaction between afferent and efferent neurons, and they can be modulated by higher brain centers. Direct afferent-efferent interaction at the level of the spinal cord (without influences from the brain), known as the simple reflex arc, is demonstrated by the knee jerk response to a patellar tendon tap, which is used in a clinical setting to evaluate neuromuscular function. The reflex arc may become the only mechanism of control if CNS input to skeletal muscle is interrupted, as may occur with SCI. The reflex arc is responsible for muscular contractions that occur in paralyzed muscles of people with spinal cord injuries when peripheral nerves remain unimpaired. Figure 3.2 depicts relationships between afferent and efferent neurons.

Stretch Reflexes

The stretch reflex and inverse stretch reflex are mechanisms that regulate movement and protect muscle from damage due to excessive stretch or tension. These reflexes can result from direct interaction between afferent and efferent lower motor neurons, although higher brain centers may regulate their effects.

Two sensory receptors within skeletal muscle, the muscle spindle and Golgi tendon organ (GTO), are responsible for detecting and responding to changes in muscle length and tension, respectively. The muscle spindle regulates the stretch reflex, which facilitates contraction of a muscle being stretched. The muscle spindle also inhibits contraction of antagonists, for example, relaxing the triceps during a biceps contraction. This reflexive action, called reciprocal inhibition, helps regulate

movement and maintain posture and joint position.

In contrast, the GTO invokes the inverse stretch reflex, which inhibits contraction of the muscle that is shortening and initiates contraction of the antagonist muscles. The GTO responds to changes in tension due to muscle shortening or passive stretching that organs in tendons and ligaments detect. This is a protective mechanism to prevent injury that can result from excessive tension in a contracting muscle. For example, when performing a biceps curl against heavy resistance, the GTO can inhibit the biceps from achieving a maximal contraction and cause the triceps to contract for further protection. Table 3.3 summarizes the actions of the muscle spindle and GTO.

Quick, forceful, and ballistic actions (such as with a bouncing stretch) activate the stretch reflex, which may actually cause microtrauma to muscle and connective tissue. A slow stretch stimulates the GTO, which may facilitate relaxation of the muscle being stretched. The proprioceptive neuromuscular facilitation (PNF) stretching technique described in chapter 8 is based on the role the stretch reflex and the inverse stretch reflex play during a stretch.

With disabilities involving impairment to upper motor neurons (such as with injuries to the brain or spinal cord), the muscle spindle may function unchecked by the CNS. This lack of inhibition from the brain results in spasticity, a hyperactive stretch reflex, resulting in exaggerated contractile responses to stretch. Spasticity is also associated with hypertonicity or an elevated resting muscle tone. Hypertonicity and a hyperactive stretch reflex impair movement coordination and cause joint contractures, both of which have implications for exercise training.

When disabilities such as poliomyelitis damage peripheral nerves, stretch reflexes become

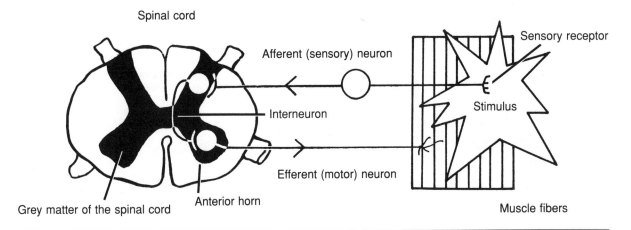

Figure 3.2 Schematic drawing of the reflex arc.

Table 3.3 Actions of the Muscle Spindle and Golgi Tendon Organ

	Muscle spindle	Golgi tendon organ
Stimulus	Rapid increase in length (within muscle)	Increase in tension (within tendon) generated by a strong stretch or muscle contraction

Reflex	Stretch reflex (myotatic reflex)
	  Contraction of stretched muscle
	Reciprocal inhibition
	  Relaxation of antagonist
		Inverse stretch reflex (inverse myotatic reflex or autogenic inhibition)
		  Inhibits contraction of agonist
		  Facilitates contraction of antagonist

Purpose	Protection from overstretching Regulate movement, joint position	Protection from excess tension

nonfunctional. The resulting flaccid paralysis is characterized by complete lack of movement and extreme muscle atrophy.

Voluntary Muscular Contraction: Regulation From the Brain

Voluntary control of skeletal muscles regulates smooth, forceful, and coordinated movement. Voluntary muscular contraction requires the integration of the musculoskeletal system and the central and peripheral nervous systems. Afferent neurons transmit information about joint position and movement to the brain, which organizes movement patterns and transmits appropriate facilitory and inhibitory messages back to skeletal muscles.

Various regions of the brain are responsible for controlling different aspects of motor function and gross movement. Table 3.4 lists the three primary regions responsible for control of voluntary movement. Impairment to any of these regions because of brain damage affects the potential for movement, balance, and movement coordination. For example, damage to the cerebellum, which is the primary area responsible for sensing body position and movement, may cause ataxia. Someone with ataxic cerebral palsy has impaired balance and kinesthetic sense, the ability to detect the position of body parts in relation to each other or other objects.

Determinants of Muscular Force

The number and type of contracting muscle fibers, as well as the rate and synchrony of motor neuron firing, determine the amount of force generated during a muscular contraction. The potential a muscle group has for developing maximal force

also is influenced by the speed of the movement and the length of the muscle.

All-or-None Principle

Unlike cardiac muscle, individual skeletal muscle fibers are incapable of grading their force during a singular contraction. Grading refers to incremental increases in tension. When adequate energy and neural input are present above a minimum threshold level, all muscle fibers in a motor unit contract simultaneously and maximally. This is referred to as the all-or-none principle. The greater the number of motor units that are stimulated to contract,

Table 3.4 Regions of the Brain That Control Movement: Effects of Brain Damage

Region	Function	Effects of brain damage
Cerebral cortex	Control conscious, specific, volitional movement	Impaired control of voluntary movement Spasticity
Basal ganglia	Control posture and gross movements	Involuntary movement Athetosis Tremors Rigidity
Cerebellum	Integrate information from other motor areas of the brain to regulate balance and coordination	Impaired kinesthetic sense Ataxia Incoordination Hypotonia

the greater the strength of the resulting contraction.

Cross-Sectional Area of Contracting Fibers

The amount of force that individual skeletal muscle fibers can generate varies from fiber to fiber. Large muscle fibers are capable of generating greater force than smaller fibers so the strength of contraction of an entire muscle is relative to the total cross-sectional area of the contracting fibers, which is determined by the number and size of motor units activated simultaneously. Force is thereby "graded" by excitatory and inhibitory input from the brain. Muscle contractions that generate maximal force require neural input to as many motor units as possible. In general, the maximal force that can be generated by a muscle is related to the cross-sectional area of the contracting fibers. However, with paresis (weakness due to partial paralysis) fewer neurons are available to activate motor units, lowering an entire muscle's potential for generating force. Also, with some types of muscular dystrophy, certain muscle groups may hypertrophy (enlarge) as they progressively become weaker. The increased cross-sectional area in these muscle groups is due to the replacement of contractile proteins in muscle fibers with connective tissue, which adds bulk but reduces the potential for generating force.

Force, Velocity, and Length Relationships

An inverse force-velocity relationship (Figure 3.3) describes the decreasing ability of a muscle group to move rapidly through a movement range as resistance increases. Maximal movement velocity is highest when an action is not resisted. Conversely, greater force can be generated with lower velocity movements. Isometric contraction, during which no movement occurs at all, can produce maximum force. Power, defined as work produced per unit of time and quantified as the product of force and velocity, is also optimized under certain conditions. Maximal power output has been found to occur with movement at approximately 30% of maximal force, which corresponds to about 40% of maximal velocity. Spasticity is a velocity-dependent condition that increases with increasing movement velocities. Fast movements increase this hypertonic condition and can dramatically reduce movement range.

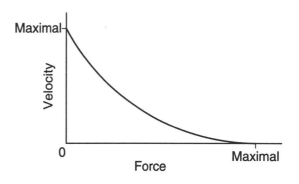

Figure 3.3 Force-velocity relationships with dynamic muscular contractions.

The length-tension curve identifies the relationship between the length of a muscle and its capacity for generating force. With dynamic exercise, when a muscle begins to contract at a length 1.2 times its resting length, it is capable of generating maximal force. This principle comes into play when you prestretch a muscle immediately prior to contraction during resistance training. Specific joint angles within the range of motion during a contraction also generate maximal force. The optimal joint angle of maximal strength varies from muscle to muscle, but it generally lies somewhere in the middle of the movement range and is influenced by the distance between the joint and the point on the bone where the muscle attaches. For example, maximal tension with an isometric contraction at the elbow during flexion may be achieved at an angle of slightly less than 100 degrees, whereas at the knee joint the angle for optimal tension during flexion is approximately 105 degrees (Komi, 1979). Muscles are weakest at the beginning and end points of the joint range of motion during a contraction. With this principle in mind, training should include exercises to work muscles at both extremes of their range to improve the overall strength of the muscle group. When contractures limit joint range of motion, the length-tension relationship of the muscle decreases, resulting in "tight weakness" and lowering the potential for strength development (Kisner & Colby, 1990).

Metabolism and Anaerobic Exercise

Metabolism in skeletal muscle converts chemical energy (stored as adenosine triphosphate, ATP) to mechanical energy for muscular contraction. The chemical compound ATP is broken down within the muscle fiber to release energy. ATP, a renewable source of energy, can be reformed in the absence or presence of oxygen (through anaerobic or aerobic metabolism, respectively) and reused as energy for subsequent muscular contractions. Figure 3.4 depicts a simple model of this complex, continuous cycle of biochemical reactions that break down and regenerate ATP.

Anaerobic simply means "without oxygen." Anaerobic metabolism does not require oxygen for the biochemical reactions that produce ATP. FT fibers are well equipped structurally to function anaerobically. Anaerobic exercise is typically of short duration (up to several minutes) and moderate to very high intensity. Examples of anaerobic exercise include resistance training, pushing a wheelchair up a steep incline, and high-strength sports such as gymnastics or power lifting. Keep in mind that most activity is supported by a combination of aerobic and anaerobic metabolism; the demands of the activity determine the relative contribution of each type.

Energy and Fuels

Anaerobic metabolism that supports high-intensity efforts or sudden and rapid muscular contractions utilizes either ATP-CP (a high energy phosphate compound) or glycogen, both stored within the muscle, to regenerate ATP for later use. Neither of these metabolic pathways requires oxygen (O_2). Metabolic processes that utilize oxygen are too slow to meet the needs of sudden and intense efforts.

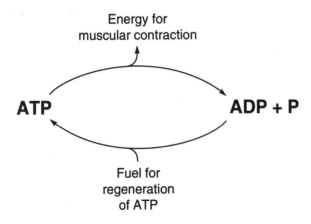

Figure 3.4 Metabolism and energy for muscle contraction.

Maximal intensity efforts rely on ATP-CP, which splits to release energy. ATP-CP is the most readily available source of energy, but it is also the most quickly depleted—maximal efforts drain stores of ATP-CP within 3 to 10 s. It takes several minutes to replenish ATP-CP supplies within the muscle so they are available again for repeated high-intensity muscular contractions. Glycolysis, the breakdown of glucose, is a second anaerobic metabolic process that supports high-intensity efforts without the presence of oxygen. It is, however, a precursor of aerobic metabolism. Lactate, which becomes lactic acid, is one of the by-products of glycolysis. Lactate may then be metabolized for a much greater yield of ATP if sufficient oxygen is present. However, when the demand for immediate energy, such as that from high-intensity exercise, exceeds the supply of oxygen, glycolysis predominates as the primary source of energy production to fuel the effort. Exercise primarily supported by glycolysis is not limited by the supply of available glucose or glycogen, but by the accumulation of lactic acid in and around the muscle and other complex mechanisms, which affect the muscle's ability to contract. With moderate- to high-intensity exercise, the relative contribution of glycolysis to the total yield of ATP limits the duration of the effort. Intense efforts supported predominantly by anaerobic metabolism may be maintained for up to several minutes. Figure 3.5 depicts the relative contribution of metabolic processes in muscular contractions of varying duration.

Acute Effects of Anaerobic Exercise

The acute and chronic effects of anaerobic and aerobic exercise training are significantly different because of differences in the physiologic systems and processes being stressed. (For a discussion of aerobic exercise physiology, refer to chapter 4.) The degree to which someone can tolerate anaerobic efforts depends on muscle fiber type distribution and conditioning level as well as the presence of disease or disability.

Temporary responses to resistive exercise (acute effects) will involve both peripheral changes within the muscle and central changes that affect cardiac and circulatory function. On a peripheral level, lactic acid accumulates within the muscle in response to high-intensity exercise. Muscular contractions may also restrict blood flow, beginning at 15% to 20% maximum voluntary contraction (MVC), preventing the transport of oxygen into the muscle and removal of waste products from the site. Complete occlusion occurs at approx-

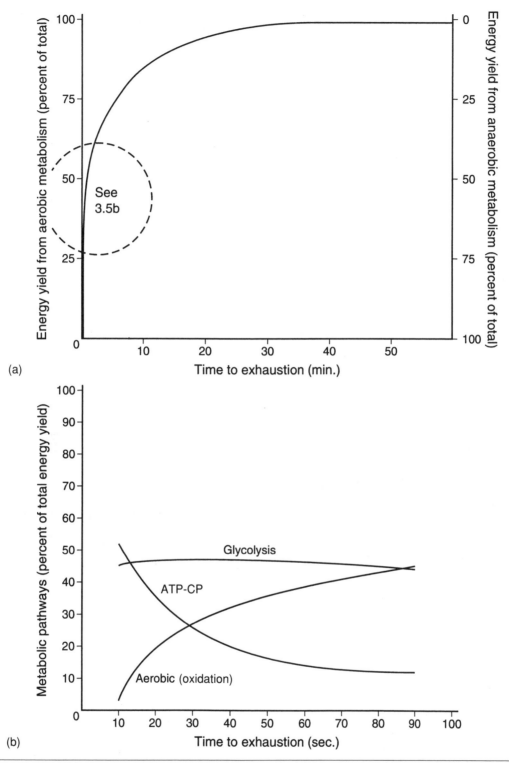

Figure 3.5 Relative contribution of aerobic and anaerobic metabolism with maximal exercise of varying durations. (a) Data adapted from McCardle, Katch, & Katch (1991); (b) adapted from Astrand & Rodahl (1977).

imately 70% MVC. This effect will be most pronounced with static or isometric work.

High-intensity efforts also have a central effect, resulting in an increase in heart rate, breathing rate, and blood pressure. Compared to aerobic exercise, anaerobic resistive exercise causes a greater increase in heart rate relative to the oxygen cost of the effort (Hurley et al., 1984). This corresponds to higher blood levels of lactic acid that signal the increase in heart rate and breathing rate. Feelings of dyspnea (breathlessness) are exaggerated when the chest cavity is affected by postural deformities or intercostal muscle paralysis, which limits expansion of the chest cavity. Increases in blood pressure also accompany resistive work, perhaps partly due to resistance to blood flow created by the contracting muscles (perfusion pressure). Blood pressure increases are most pronounced with high-intensity, large-muscle-group activity, isometric work, concentric contractions, and breath holding. Heart rate and blood pressure increase most dramatically when repetitions are performed at 70%, 80%, and 95% of MVC (Fleck & Dean, 1987; MacDougall, Tuxen, Sale, Moroz, & Sutton, 1985). People with elevated resting blood pressure or a history of stroke, heart disease, or circulatory problems may need to avoid high-intensity efforts.

Adaptations to Resistance Training

Over time a resistance training program may induce central (neural) and peripheral (muscular) adaptations (see Table 3.5). The degree, nature, and rate of the adaptations depend on the features of the training program. Chapters 5 and 6 address principles of resistance training and program design. Neural adaptations involve enhanced coordination of movement and improved recruitment of motor units. Peripheral adaptations may include increases in muscle size (hypertrophy) and strength, improved capacity for producing energy anaerobically, and increases in connective tissue strength and mineral content of bone. Central changes, involving heart and circulation, are less pronounced. With physical disability, the degree of adaptation with resistance training is related to the person's ability to utilize muscle effectively. The potential for positive gains from resistance training decreases with any condition that reduces joint range of motion (such as pain, spasticity, or structural joint deformities) or impairs innervation of motor units (such as movement incoordination, paresis, or disorders involving progressive loss of functional motor units). Figure 3.6 summarizes physiologic effects of resistance training with disability.

Neural Adaptations

Initial increases in muscular strength and endurance with a resistance training program primarily result from improved neural function because of improved coordination and motor learning (Rutherford & Jones, 1986) as well as from improved ability to recruit a greater number of motor units (Moritani & deVries, 1979). Neural changes appear to be most pronounced during the first 3 to 5 weeks

Table 3.5 Physiologic Adaptations to Anaerobic Exercise Training

Variables	Adaptations
Neural factors	Increase motor unit recruitment
	Increase synchronization of motor unit recruitment
	Decrease inhibition of agonist
Peripheral changes	Increase muscle size
	Increase capillary number (with high repetitions, moderate load)
	Decrease capillary density (with heavy resistance)
	Increase strength of connective tissue
	Increase bone density
Cardiovascular functions	Decrease resting HR (slight)
	Increase left ventricular wall thickness
	Unchanged resting BP
	Decrease exercise BP (slight)

of training. Adaptations with resistance training are specific to the pattern of motor unit recruitment of the task. In the absence of measurable hypertrophy (muscle enlargement), neural adaptations are evidenced by increases both in peak force and in the rate of force development, depending on the nature of the training program (Sale, 1988). Training may also result in an increased ability to more fully recruit the motor units in a muscle group and maintain optimal firing rates, whereas untrained people may only be capable of recruiting lower threshold motor units. Further, resistance training may be responsible for a decrease in protective inhibitory mechanisms that limit tension development, such as that of the GTO. It would be of interest to know how a resistance training program affects neural adaptation in people with impaired motor control, such as with cerebral palsy (CP) or other types of brain injury, but research in this area is quite limited.

Peripheral Adaptations

Tesch (1988) outlines current knowledge of peripheral adaptations in skeletal muscle with resistance training. Heavy resistance training increases muscular strength and muscle size. This effect is caused by hypertrophy of myofibrils, although some research indicates that high-intensity training may also cause hyperplasia (an increase in the number of fibers). The type of fiber affected by resistance training appears to be a function of the training protocol. With high-load, low-repetition work, adaptations predominate in FT fibers. High-volume,

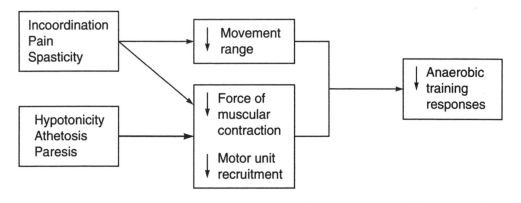

Figure 3.6 Possible effects of disabling conditions on anaerobic exercise training.

moderate-intensity exercise training (incorporating more repetitions at a lower exercise load) may also hypertrophy ST fibers (Tesch, 1988). Resistance training may affect the number of capillaries within skeletal muscle as well, with slight increases possibly resulting from moderate-intensity, longer duration anaerobic training. High-intensity, exhaustive anaerobic exercise, on the other hand, appears to actually decrease capillary density because of the increase in muscle size, although the total number of capillaries may be unaffected. Resistance training has also been found to increase the tensile strength of connective tissues surrounding muscle and joints and the bone mass in limbs subjected to exercise stress. These changes may be important for reducing the risk of injury with strenuous activity.

Central Adaptations: Cardiovascular Function

Fleck (1988) reviewed research evaluating the effects of resistance training on the cardiovascular system. Resistance work imposes a pressure overload on the heart in contrast to the volume overload imposed by endurance exercise training. This corresponds to an increase in the size of the left ventricular walls of the heart. Some research has demonstrated a slight, but nonsignificant, decrease in resting heart rate following a resistance training program. Other studies have indicated that blood pressure decreases during resistive exercise after training, but resting blood pressure does not appear to be affected.

Muscle Fatigue, Soreness, and Overwork

Muscle fatigue, a transient condition, is defined as the decreased capacity of a muscle to maintain a required or expected force or power output (MacLaren, Gibson, Parry-Billings, & Edwards,

1989). Subjectively, you can feel fatigue peripherally within the working muscle or centrally as a whole body sensation. Peripheral fatigue is sensed locally as pain or burning. Whole body fatigue is subjectively felt as an overall aching sensation or feeling of heaviness and complete exhaustion.

The causes of fatigue, as yet not clearly defined, are related in part to the duration and intensity of the exercise. Exercise of very high intensity that results in muscular fatigue in less than 30 s causes rapid accumulation of lactic acid in and around the muscle and depletion of ATP-CP stores, which are essential for efforts requiring immediate energy. Lactic acid, a by-product of anaerobic metabolism, accumulates in the muscle and increases the acidity of the local environment, rendering it unfavorable for muscular contraction. Accumulation of lactic acid with resistive work accompanies several other intracellular changes that may be more directly responsible for muscle fatigue. As lactic acid accumulates in the blood, heart rate and breathing rate increase dramatically.

Moderate- to high-intensity exercise causes fatigue anywhere from approximately 30 s to nearly an hour, depending on the relative contribution of anaerobic metabolism to the total energy yield. With low- to moderate-intensity endurance activity, which relies predominantly on aerobic metabolism, glycogen must be present. During long-duration activity, depletion of stored muscle and liver glycogen eventually prevents individual muscle fibers from contracting, despite the availability of oxygen. The phrase "hitting the wall" has been used to describe the perceived whole body fatigue that may occur about 2 hr or more into long-duration exercise, probably due to glycogen depletion and other factors such as dehydration and elevated body temperature.

The development of fatigue also depends on someone's fitness level and may be affected by the presence of disability. Fatigue occurs more rapidly in people with muscles that are weak due to deconditioning than it does in trained individuals. Physical disorders can affect "central drive" (in the CNS), transmission of nerve impulses in the peripheral nervous system and at the neuromuscular junction, or processes within the muscle (Edwards, 1986) to cause early onset of fatigue with exertion. MS, which affects the CNS, may reduce central drive to motor neurons and thereby contribute to early fatigue with exertion. MS may also cause body temperature to rise, further contributing to central fatigue with exertion. Myasthenia gravis, also characterized by excessive fatigue, involves impaired neuromuscular transmission. Muscular dystrophy provides an example of fatigue caused by dysfunction within muscle fibers.

Other mechanisms may also contribute to excessive fatigue with disability. In general, fatigue is more rapid when fewer muscle fibers are available to generate force. Muscle weakness, associated with some brain injuries, MS, incomplete spinal cord injury, polio, and muscular dystrophy, is caused by the limited number of muscle fibers available for recruitment to meet the demands of exercise. With cerebral palsy, all muscle fibers may be fully functioning, but because recruitment patterns are disturbed, more motor units than are actually required to perform a desired action may be recruited. This also leads to early onset of fatigue with activity. With spasticity, hypertonicity may further limit the duration of exercise because of restricted muscle blood flow, delaying the transport of oxygen to the muscle and the removal of lactic acid and other waste products as they accumulate.

Muscle soreness involves mechanisms that are not completely understood, the details of which are beyond the scope of this text. Symptoms of immediate postexercise muscle soreness can occur following exercise as a result of overexertion. This sensation normally subsides within an hour if adequate blood flow circulates through the muscle. Delayed muscle soreness may occur 24 to 48 hr following exercise and may last for several days to a week. Various theories have been proposed to explain this phenomenon, the most accepted attributing it to mechanisms that result from microtrauma to muscle and connective tissue. Eccentric contractions (tension during muscle lengthening) are believed to be more

Table 3.6 Effects of Specific Disabilities on Skeletal Muscle Structure and Function

Location of injury	Common disabilities	Muscle structure or function that may be affected
Central nervous system		
Brain	Cerebal palsy Head injury Stroke Multiple sclerosis	Movement coordination: processing information from motor and sensory nerves, regulating excitation/inhibition Reflexes Muscle tone Muscle length
Spinal cord	Spinal cord injury (SCI) Spina bifida	Transmission of impulses from sensory and upper motor neurons Reflexes
Peripheral nervous system		
Lower motor neurons	Poliomyelitis SCI (below cauda equina)	Transmission of impulses from lower motor neurons Muscle mass Peripheral structures
Peripheral structures		
Muscle	Muscular dystrophy	Muscle metabolism Muscle mass
Joint/connective tissue	Arthritis	Joint structure Extensibility
Bone	Amputation	Fiber arrangement Fiber length

likely to result in delayed muscle soreness than concentric exercise.

Overwork is the cumulative effect of excessive exercise stress over time, and it may cause temporary or permanent deterioration in muscle function. In athletes, overwork is referred to as overtraining, and it causes staleness or a decline in motivation and performance. With disability, overwork weakness can cause a decline in daily function. Partially innervated muscle, as with polio and incomplete spinal cord injury, is more susceptible to overwork. Remember that one theory for postpolio syndrome is that giant motor neurons (created by nerves sprouting to compensate for loss from the polio virus) have been subjected to years of overuse and eventually begin to lose their ability to function (Halstead, 1990). For these reasons, people with progressive disorders and with diseases affecting lower motor neurons should avoid overwork.

Summary

The structure and function of the musculoskeletal system determines its capacity for movement and exercise. Disability may alter normal characteristics of muscle and connective tissue, thereby reducing the system's ability to function. Muscle fiber types and neuromuscular control of involuntary (reflexive) and voluntary (conscious) movement influence the performance capacity of each muscle group. The recruitment patterns of motor units and biomechanical features of the movement pattern determine movement force. Table 3.6 reviews several disabilities affecting skeletal muscle structure and function.

Anaerobic exercise performance depends on the integrity of the musculoskeletal system and regulation of movement by the nervous system, which in turn determine the motor coordination and power output of the effort. It is important to understand the effects disability may have on the basic structure and function of skeletal muscle in order to develop safe and effective exercise programs. In this chapter, the focus was on anaerobic exercise. In chapter 4 we will look at the effects of disability on aerobic exercise and responses to training.

Chapter 4

Physiology of Aerobic Exercise

Stephen F. Figoni, PhD, RKT
Wright State University

As an exercise leader, you are well aware of the importance of aerobic exercise training for maintaining cardiovascular health, reducing risks of developing diseases associated with inactivity and sedentary living, and maintaining appropriate body composition. The benefits of aerobic conditioning extend further for people with disabilities—they play a critical role in maintaining independence, functional capacity, and mobility.

This chapter provides a foundation in disability-specific exercise science principles that, together with your understanding of physical disability, will give you the theoretical basis for decisions you will have to make when designing and leading aerobic exercise programs for people with physical disabilities. We will review physiologic responses to aerobic exercise that may be affected by physical disability. We will examine acute responses as a function of the three systems that support oxygen consumption: intake, transport, and utilization. We then will look at expected long-term training adaptations to aerobic conditioning in the presence of disabling conditions. Because physical disability often impairs the ability to use a large muscle mass during exercise, it also is important to understand how small-muscle-mass activity affects exercise responses, both acute and chronic. We will address this topic with a discussion about upper body and lower body exercise and training adaptations. Finally, we will look at temperature regulation and muscle fatigue and soreness in certain physical disabilities.

Benefits of Aerobic Conditioning

In addition to functional impairment, physical disability may reduce a person's ability to exercise and develop physical fitness. Inadequate physical fitness can then contribute to mobility impairment and predispose the person with a disability to other medical complications associated with immobility. Immediate consequences may include muscular weakness and obesity, which may interfere with walking, wheelchair propulsion, and transfers. The resulting sedentary lifestyle encourages obesity, hypertension, osteoporosis, high blood cholesterol, and diabetes, factors that put both able-bodied and disabled people at higher risk for cardiovascular disease. Some people become more susceptible to skin pressure sores, urinary tract infections, joint contractures, depression, and many other problems associated with physical deconditioning and immobility. These common medical problems discourage successful participation in active recreational activities and sports, further compromising physical fitness. Figure 4.1 depicts the cycle of deconditioning with physical disability. Therefore, the need for exercise training for individuals with physical disabilities is critical to prevent the vicious cycle of deconditioning, functional deterioration, and hypoactivity and to promote general health and an active lifestyle, both of which may prevent medical complications and promote maximal functional independence.

In addition to neurological causes of muscular paralysis, diseases such as muscular dystrophy can cause progressive weakness from childhood to adulthood. For people with these diseases, aerobic conditioning is important to prevent premature deconditioning and to delay functional deterioration and additional hypoactivity.

General benefits of aerobic exercise training for people with physical disabilities, whether performed with the arms or legs, may include these:

- Temporary reduction in muscular spasticity
- Increased functional independence
- Increased endurance for wheelchair propulsion and transfers
- Improved vocational productivity
- Improved performance in disabled sports
- More satisfying participation in community, social, recreational, and family activities
- Reduced psychological depression
- Improved self-image

Oxygen Consumption

Oxygen consumption or uptake ($\dot{V}O_2$) indicates the metabolic rate and energy cost of steady-state exercise. The ability to meet the increased demands

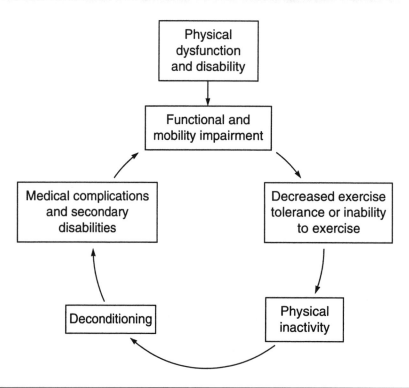

Figure 4.1 The cycle of disability, inactivity, and functional decline.

for oxygen with aerobic exercise depends upon the pulmonary, circulatory, and metabolic systems for the intake, transport, and utilization of oxygen.

Maximal oxygen consumption ($\dot{V}O_2$max) or maximal aerobic power is the highest $\dot{V}O_2$ an individual can achieve during a graded exercise test. This is the best index of overall cardiorespiratory physical fitness in able-bodied people—it depends upon the integration of the pulmonary, cardiovascular, muscular, and metabolic systems. $\dot{V}O_2$max is specific to the mode of exercise and testing protocol and is affected by the size of the exercising muscle mass.

Physiologic Systems That Support Aerobic Exercise

Figure 4.2 diagrams the flow of oxygen from the atmosphere through the heart, lungs, and peripheral tissues. The ability to use oxygen during exercise depends on the integrity of the systems that take in, transport, and utilize oxygen. Disabling conditions that limit the function of any of these

systems decrease oxygen consumption and limit aerobic capacity.

Oxygen Intake and Pulmonary Ventilation

The pulmonary system consists of the lungs, the airways that take air into the lungs, and several muscles that inflate and deflate the lungs. The pulmonary system brings oxygen-rich air from the atmosphere into the lungs. Oxygen (O_2) diffuses from the lungs through small blood vessels and attaches to red blood cells in the blood. The arterial circulation delivers the O_2 to exercising muscles. Carbon dioxide (CO_2) and metabolic waste products diffuse from the exercising muscles into the venous circulation and flow back to the lungs, where CO_2 is exhaled back into the atmosphere.

Pulmonary ventilation is a limiting factor in aerobic exercise only in cases of pulmonary disease, asthma, or extreme ventilatory muscle paralysis. With injury to the spinal cord above the fifth cervical level, part of the diaphragm muscle is paralyzed, severely limiting inspiratory capacity. Similarly, injury at the thoracic level with spinal cord injury or possibly with polio and multiple

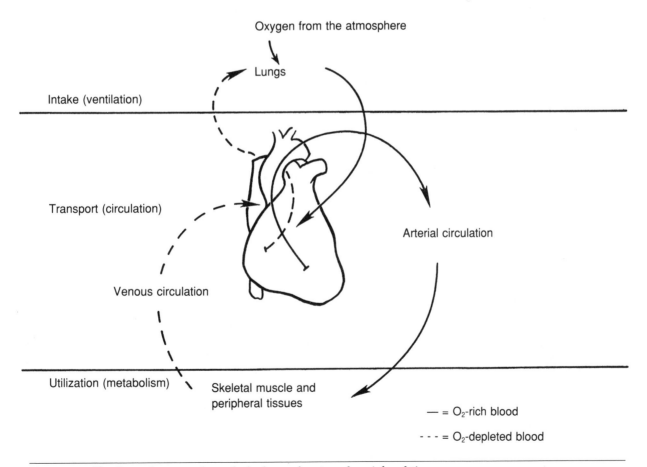

Figure 4.2 The flow of oxygen through the lungs, heart, and peripheral tissues.

sclerosis (MS) paralyzes other ventilatory muscles such as the intercostals and abdominals, limiting expansion of the rib cage, expiratory capacity, and vital capacity.

Oxygen Transport

Maintaining the supply of oxygen to exercising muscles is the key to endurance exercise. In this regard, the circulatory system plays a critical role in transporting arterial blood with O_2 and nutrients to exercising muscles and venous blood with CO_2, heat, and metabolic waste products away from exercising muscles.

Normally, blood circulates from the heart and pulmonary system (central circulation) to the muscles and body organs via arteries (arterial circulation) and back to the heart and lungs by way of the veins (venous circulation). The metabolic rate and the sympathetic division of the autonomic nervous system (ANS) control cardiac output and blood flow. Sympathetic input to the heart, which regulates heart rate and force of contraction, begins in the T1 to T5 segments of the spinal cord (Mathers, 1985). Blood flow to exercising muscle is increased during activity by widening of the small arterioles to the capillaries in muscle in response to the shortage of O_2 and accumulation of metabolic waste products. To maintain blood pressure (BP), blood flow to inactive muscles and organs during exercise is reduced by narrowing of the small arterial blood vessels. Disabilities and medical conditions that impair the function of the central, arterial, and venous circulation reduce aerobic exercise capacity.

The Heart and Central Circulation.

The heart is the muscular organ that pumps blood through the body and to and from the lungs. Normally, the ANS controls the heart rate (HR) and cardiac output (volume of blood pumped per minute). Cardiac output ($\dot{Q}$) is calculated as the product of heart rate (HR) and stroke volume (SV). SV is determined by the contractile force of the heart muscle (myocardial contractility) and volume of blood returned with each heart beat. Heart function depends on the electrical system to regulate the rate, synchrony, and myocardial contractility. When the ANS is impaired at or above the T1 to T5 level of the spinal cord, maximum HR and myocardial contractility may be reduced, which restricts the maximal exercise heart rate to approximately 120 beats per min, attenuates BP responses to exercise, and limits the circulation of blood through the body. ANS impairment may also decrease venous tone in the legs, which prevents adequate return of blood to the heart. Lowered venous return further

reduces $\dot{Q}$. ANS dysfunction is commonly associated with quadriplegic spinal cord injury (SCI) and is occasionally seen with high-level paraplegia or MS.

Arterial Circulation.

Two primary responses of the arterial circulation to exercise are an increase in the delivery of O_2-rich blood to exercising muscles and diversion of blood flow from nonexercising tissues and organs to the central circulation. Arteriole diameter controls blood flow within many organs and skeletal muscles. In turn sympathetic or parasympathetic stimulation (ANS regulation) influences the diameter of arterioles, causing vasoconstriction or vasodilation, respectively. A decrease in O_2 concentration and accumulation of waste products and lactic acid in capillaries of exercising muscle stimulate the ANS to respond by increasing the flow of blood to these tissues to provide more oxygen and remove waste products. The ANS reduces blood flow in the inactive muscles and viscera (digestive system, kidneys, skin, etc.) and diverts it to the central (heart/lung) circulation. If vasodilation of active muscles is uncompensated by vasoconstriction in inactive organs, the arterial BP falls, resulting in inadequate pressure to circulate blood effectively to vital organs. Normally, the diastolic BP (which represents the overall arterial pressure in the body between forceful heart contractions) remains constant or decreases very slightly during exercise. The systolic pressure generally rises from a resting pressure of 120 mmHg to a range of 160 to 220 mmHg, indicating an increase in pressure from the central circulation to deliver blood as needed with exercise.

Physical conditions that impair the structure of arteries or sympathetic control of arterioles can reduce the ability of the arterial circulation to deliver blood and O_2 to exercising muscles. This reduction limits aerobic capacity and induces fatigue at lower exercise levels. For example, peripheral vascular occlusive disease (a long-term complication of diabetes resulting in hardening and narrowing of the arteries in the extremities) can prevent increases in blood flow to exercising leg muscles. Inadequate O_2 causes pain in these muscles and restricts exercise tolerance. ANS dysfunction may impair sympathetic control of the arterial circulation. Exercise hypotension (low BP) is associated with ANS impairment due to an inability to maintain arterial BP during higher levels of aerobic exercise, especially in upright postures. Hypotensive symptoms may include extreme fatigue, pallor, nausea, dizziness, confusion, or perhaps fainting.

Another negative effect of sympathetic nervous system impairment, common in individuals with

SCI, is vasomotor dysfunction or improper control of blood vessel diameter in the limbs or viscera. This condition prevents the normal blood flow diversion away from nonexercising muscles and inactive visceral organs to exercising muscles with exercise. This encourages maldistribution of the O_2-rich arterial blood to organs that do not need increased circulation during exercise and restricts the circulation of blood and O_2 to exercising muscles. Inability to regulate BP and blood flow impairs the ability to perfuse vital organs, including the brain and exercising muscles, and limits exercise tolerance and endurance.

Injury to spinal cord nerves at or above the midthoracic level (T5) also can affect adrenal gland function. The adrenal glands produce hormones called catecholamines (epinephrine and norepinephrine) that circulate throughout the body and act upon the heart and arterial circulation to facilitate cardiovascular adjustments to exercise. Inadequate production of these hormones during exercise further impairs HR acceleration, blood flow distribution, and BP maintenance. Catecholamines also aid in the mobilization and delivery of fats from adipose tissue to exercising muscles during aerobic exercise. It is not yet clear if catecholamine deprivation impairs the muscle's ability to utilize fat for fuel during endurance exercise.

In summary, if the O_2 demands of exercising muscles exceed the ability of the heart and circulation to supply needed blood and O_2, then aerobic metabolism will be limited, inducing fatigue and reducing the work capacity of the muscle.

Venous Circulation. The venous circulation has two main functions—to return blood from exercising muscles back to the heart and lungs and to store the majority of the blood volume at rest. Under steady-state conditions, the increased rate of production of metabolic waste products (CO_2, lactic acid, heat, etc.) in muscles is balanced with the increased rate of removal via the venous blood. An important chemical challenge for the venous system is to regulate the acidity of the blood by preventing the accumulation of CO_2 and hydrogen ions (H^+) in the muscle. In large amounts, H^+ makes the blood more acidic and interferes with biochemical reactions required for muscle contraction. As venous blood circulates through the lungs, the blood is replenished with O_2 as CO_2 is discharged from the body.

Any condition that produces peripheral sympathetic impairment of the ANS may result in vasomotor paralysis and poor venous tone.

At rest, the venous system contains about 70% of the body's total blood volume. Thus, the veins act as a reservoir for blood, which can be mobilized and circulated to muscles in times of need, such as during exercise. The veins have flexible walls and are not as muscular as arteries. However, they do possess some tone at rest to prevent overfilling (pooling) with blood. The sympathetic nerves narrow the diameter of the veins (vasoconstriction) slightly by reflex during upright posture and exercise to help redistribute blood from the veins to where it is more needed. Normally during leg exercise, contracting leg muscles further support and squeeze the leg veins to help pump venous blood upward against gravity toward the heart. This phenomenon is called the skeletal muscle venous pump and is an important mechanism for returning blood to the heart (venous return). Some leg veins also have one-way valves to prevent backward flow of blood when leg muscles are not contracting. Contraction and relaxation of the diaphragm muscle during breathing also helps pump blood to the heart and constitutes the thoracic pump of the venous system. Despite the capacity of the venous system to hold large quantities of blood, assistance from several other organs is needed to increase venous return to maintain the appropriate $\dot{Q}$ required during exercise. Any condition that produces peripheral sympathetic impairment (such as high-level SCI and some cases of MS) may result in vasomotor paralysis and poor venous tone. Paralysis of skeletal muscles can further limit venous return via the skeletal muscle and thoracic pumps. The resulting poor venous circulation and blood pooling may

- impair the dissipation of heat from exercising muscles (encouraging excessively high muscle and body temperatures),
- inhibit the removal of metabolic by-products, resulting in accumulation of CO_2 and H^+ in the muscle, and
- induce dizziness as a result of low arterial blood volume.

All these effects limit exercise tolerance and capacity. Venous pooling can further induce higher than normal venous BP in the legs and encourage swelling (edema) of the ankles and feet. Because the heart can only pump as much blood as the venous circulation returns to it, below-normal venous return limits $\dot{Q}$, thereby limiting central circulation as well.

Extreme physical inactivity from prolonged sitting, immobilization, or bedrest could result in chronic venous pooling or venous stasis (stationary venous blood) as well as more serious medical complications such as blood clots in the leg veins or lungs.

Several measures may be considered to improve exercise tolerance in people with impaired sympathetic function or extreme deconditioning. These include exercising in a horizontal posture (as in water), using compressive abdominal binders and support stockings, full hydration (fluid intake), and minimizing use of substances that have diuretic or hypotensive side-effects such as alcohol, caffeine, and some antispastic muscle relaxants. These measures may help prevent excessive venous pooling and hypotension, especially in people with quadriplegia, and thus they may allow more normal circulatory responses during exercise.

Disabilities that cause hypertonicity, such as spastic cerebral palsy, occlude or limit the flow of blood and O_2 into exercising muscle and delay the removal of metabolic by-products following contraction, limiting the muscles' capacity to perform aerobic work. This condition also results in higher than normal BP responses with exercise due to the static nature of the muscle tension generated in both agonist and antagonist muscles during voluntary movement.

Oxygen Utilization and Aerobic Metabolism

Once O_2 has been taken in through the lungs and transported via the arterial circulation to the muscles, it is utilized for oxidation during aerobic exercise. This process, aerobic metabolism, involves the oxidation (burning) of fuels to release adenosine triphosphate (ATP)—the direct energy source for muscle contraction. An adequate supply of O_2 and fuels such as glucose, glycogen, or fatty acids must be available in muscle cells for oxidation. Concentrations of aerobic enzymes must be sufficient to facilitate the many chemical reactions needed to utilize O_2 to produce energy aerobically.

Aerobic metabolism usually satisfies the energy requirements for low- to moderate-effort muscle contractions because the rate of O_2 demand does not exceed the rate of O_2 supply. Aerobic metabolism produces far more energy per molecule of glucose than anaerobic metabolism. Thus, aerobic metabolism is the preferred source of energy for activities requiring large amounts of energy over a prolonged period of time. Oxidation delays fatigue and maintains the highest possible level of steady-state exercise. Reliance upon anaerobic metabolism leads to rapid muscle fatigue and cessation of exercise due to the discomfort of lactic acid accumulation. Examples of aerobic activities include low- to moderate-intensity walking, jogging, cycling, aerobic dance, wheelchair pushing, and swimming.

Conditions that affect the ability of skeletal muscle to utilize oxygen for aerobic metabolism limit

aerobic capacity. Muscular dystrophy (MD) is believed to affect metabolic processes and eventually cause loss of contractile fibers. As the disease progresses, fewer and fewer muscle fibers are available to utilize oxygen to provide forceful contraction for movement. With extensive muscle paralysis (due to MS, polio, and brain or spinal cord injury), less O_2 is utilized during exercise, which reduces the stress placed on the central circulation and limits the potential adaptations that may result from aerobic exercise training. Deconditioning also limits the capacity of muscle tissue to utilize oxygen and limits aerobic exercise performance.

Table 4.1 provides a summary of the components of $\dot{V}O_2$ and conditions that may limit them.

Maximal Oxygen Consumption

For the purposes of this chapter, maximal O_2 consumption ($\dot{V}O_2max$), or maximal aerobic power, will be defined as the highest volume of O_2 an individual can consume per minute. In absolute terms, $\dot{V}O_2$ values are expressed in liters of O_2 per minute (L/min); in terms relative to body weight, $\dot{V}O_2$ is expressed in milliliters of O_2 per kilogram body weight per minute (ml/kg/min). $\dot{V}O_2max$ is specific to the exercise mode (e.g., walking, running, cycling, wheelchair pushing, arm-cranking, swimming) and to the testing protocol used during graded exercise testing conducted by qualified professionals in a laboratory setting with specialized equipment. $\dot{V}O_2max$ is frequently estimated with graded submaximal exercise tests, assuming linearity (parallel changes) between $\dot{V}O_2$, exercise work load, and HR responses. In the presence of disability, such estimations may be inaccurate with formulas developed for able-bodied subjects.

In able-bodied individuals, $\dot{V}O_2max$ is the best index of overall cardiorespiratory physical fitness because it depends upon the integration of the pulmonary, cardiovascular, muscular, and metabolic systems. $\dot{V}O_2max$ among people with physical disabilities varies depending upon the size of exercising muscles, training status, and functional ability of the cardiovascular and musculoskeletal systems. In people who use only upper body musculature, as in arm-cranking or wheelchair exercise, $\dot{V}O_2max$ is more indicative of the size and training status of the arm muscles. In general, the higher the $\dot{V}O_2max$ using a particular exercise mode, the more fit the person is for endurance exercise using that mode.

Shephard (1990) has reviewed a variety of studies that examined $\dot{V}O_2max$ test results of people with disabilities. Trained people with paraplegia or lower limb amputation and able-bodied people

Table 4.1 Physiologic Systems That Support $\dot{V}O_2$: Effects of Disabling Conditions

System and function	Disabling factors	Disability
Oxygen intake		
Pulmonary function	Paralysis of respiratory muscles	Quadriplegia
• Ventilation		
Oxygen transport		
Cardiac function	ANS impairment (HR)	SCI at or above T1 to T5, MS
• Heart rate	Pharmacologic agents	
• Stroke volume	Decreased exercising muscle mass	All disabilities
• Cardiac output	Lower extremity paralysis	SCI, polio, MD, MS
	Spasticity	Brain injury, incomplete SCI
	Deconditioning	Any disability
	Cardiac dysfunction	MD
Arterial and venous circulation	ANS impairment (BP, venous tone)	SCI above T1 to T5, MS
• Blood flow distribution	Paralysis—blood pooling	SCI, MD, MS
• Arterial blood pressure	Spasticity (decreased blood flow)	Brain injury
	Deconditioning	Any disability
Oxygen utilization		
	Impaired muscle metabolism	MD
	Decreased exercising muscle mass	All disabilities
	Decreased neuromuscular control	Brain injuries
	Decreased ROM	Brain injuries, arthritis
	Deconditioning	Any disability

can achieve $\dot{V}O_2$max values of 2 to 3 L/min (29-43 ml/kg/min, for a 70-kg person) during maximal-effort arm exercise. Untrained people with more severe disabilities typically attain a $\dot{V}O_2$max of less than 1 L/min (14 ml/kg/min, for a 70-kg person). This is in contrast to able-bodied runners who may be able to attain $\dot{V}O_2$max values of 3 to 6 L/min (43-86 ml/kg/min, for a 70-kg person), depending upon their training status. Table 4.2 includes specific examples of $\dot{V}O_2$max values (estimated from modified submaximal test protocols) for individuals with different disabilities, derived from a study by DiRocco (1986).

Acute Adjustments to Aerobic Exercise

During exercise, several physiologic systems of the body must interact effectively to maintain function on a "healthy" level. This process of maintaining a balance within the internal environment and adjusting to stress is called homeostasis. The physiologic purpose of an exercise session is to temporarily challenge homeostasis and stress several body systems to levels above those to which they are accustomed. That is, an exercise session must cause acute (short-term) physiologic adjustments to increased demands for energy and physical work above the levels needed during rest or sedentary daily activities. The results of repeated exercise training sessions are chronic (long-term) physiologic adaptations that allow a person to exercise at a higher intensity and for a longer duration without serious threats to health. Thus, through systematic training, people can achieve their full potential for aerobic fitness and performance.

With an acute bout of aerobic exercise, HR, SV, $\dot{Q}$, and pulmonary ventilation ($\dot{V}_E$) increase in response to the need for more oxygen in exercising muscle. Blood flow is redistributed to working muscle, away from visceral organs to exercising muscle. With increasing body temperature, blood is directed toward skin vessels where vasodilation and sweating allow heat to be dissipated.

Effects of Disability on Acute Physiologic Responses

Physical disability may alter the magnitude of physiologic responses to aerobic exercise, especially with limited trainable muscle mass and impaired ANS function.

Table 4.2 Aerobic Capacity of People With and Without Physical Disabilities

Disability	$\dot{V}O_2max$ (ml/kg/min)	
	Males	Females
Lower limb amputation (arm)	18-27 (11)	14-21 (5)
Lower limb amputation (leg)	18-37 (26)	21-36 (14)
SCI—paraplegia (arm)	9-30 (33)	10-27 (12)
SCI—quadriplegia (arm)	9-24 (31)	10-22 (4)
Cerebral palsy (arm)	9-25 (11)	12-22 (6)
Cerebral palsy (leg)	30-35 (3)	
Polio (arm)	12-29 (9)	12-27 (12)
Polio (leg)		24-28 (6)
Multiple sclerosis (arm)	20-34 (6)	23-25 (5)
Multiple sclerosis (leg)		19-33 (8)
Able-bodied, ages 30-39 (arm)	23-35	21-32
Able-bodied, ages 30-39 (leg)	38-50	33-45

Note. Values are for arm or leg ergometry as indicated. Numbers in parentheses represent number of subjects.
Data from *Aerobic capacity of individuals with physical disabilities* by P. DiRocco, 1986, unpublished data.

Limited Trainable Muscle Mass

Many physical disabilities prevent the use of a large muscle mass during exercise either because of impaired skeletal muscle coordination or because of an inability to fully recruit the motor units of large muscle groups for activity. Brain injuries, such as cerebral palsy and head injury, may impair movement coordination. Other types of injuries to the brain or motor neurons (SCI, stroke, MS, or polio) may cause hemiplegic, paraplegic, or quadriplegic conditions of paralysis or paresis that limit access to otherwise unimpaired muscle. Pain and joint stiffness from conditions such as arthritis limit range of motion, which also reduces the mass of muscle utilized during exercise. With the muscular dystrophies, progressive loss of muscle fibers also decreases the amount of muscle available for aerobic exercise. Loss of one or more limbs with amputation, especially in the lower extremities, also decreases the volume of trainable muscle.

Impaired Cardiovascular or Autonomic Function

Several disabilities are associated with impaired cardiovascular function or autonomic control. This category includes disorders that impair circulation or spinal cord nerves at or above the T1 to T5 levels. Blood may pool in the extremities during exercise as a result of paralysis, which prevents the skeletal muscle pump in the legs from assisting with the return of blood to the heart and decreases $\dot{Q}$. The magnitude of the training adaptations induced by aerobic exercise is directly influenced by the nature and extent of impairments that affect

utilization of muscle and ANS regulation of cardiac and circulatory function. Some highly trained athletes with paralysis, however, can achieve $\dot{V}O_2max$ values that exceed those attained by sedentary, age-matched, able-bodied peers.

Anaerobic Threshold

Certain disabling conditions also influence anaerobic or lactate threshold. Normally, lactic acid is produced in excess with exercise at or above approximately 55% to 65% of $\dot{V}O_2max$ in unconditioned persons (McArdle, Katch, & Katch, 1991). Any disability that limits the volume of muscle mass available to reach a given absolute work load decreases the relative lactate threshold. In other words, more lactic acid is produced for exercise using a smaller muscle mass. This also causes a corresponding increase in HR, BP, and breathing rate for a given absolute work load. In general, disorders that reduce $\dot{V}O_2max$, such as paralysis, paresis, arthritis (with decreased range of motion), impaired neuromuscular control, or amputation, have similar effects on lactate threshold, HR, BP, and $\dot{V}_E$ relative to the magnitude of the impaired muscle mass. Exercise with spastic muscle may also induce greater increases in lactate accumulation, HR, and BP in response to ischemic conditions caused by static muscular contractions.

Effects of Pharmacologic Agents

Our discussion of aerobic exercise physiology to this point assumes that the exercising individual is not influenced by medications that modify physiologic responses to exercise. However, many people with physical disabilities, just like the able-bodied population, take common drugs and medications as part of ongoing medical treatment or to produce desired psychological or physiologic effects. Many drugs and medications alter physiologic responses to exercise. Appendix A presents a brief summary of the effects of pharmacologic agents on cardiovascular functions at rest and during exercise. For additional information, refer to more comprehensive references on this subject such as American College of Sports Medicine (1991).

Temperature Regulation

In response to environmental conditions of heat and cold, the body dissipates or conserves body heat. Some conditions associated with physical disability also may affect the body's thermoregulatory mechanisms that normally respond to environmental conditions and the build-up of heat in the body with exercise.

Impaired Thermoregulation

Strenuous exercise with large muscle groups places a metabolic heat load upon the body. If exercise is combined with environmental conditions such as high temperature and humidity, the body's core temperature could rise to dangerously high levels (hyperthermia). High-level SCI and ANS dysfunction can impair sweating and skin blood-flow mechanisms, keeping the body from losing heat through evaporation and radiation. If sweating is inadequate, less sweat can evaporate to cool the skin of the trunk and limbs. If peripheral circulation is impaired, blood will not be diverted to the skin for radiation to the surrounding environment. Inadequate fluid intake and dehydration compound heat stress problems by further impairing the general circulation and encouraging fatigue, heat exhaustion, and heat stroke. Poor venous circulation also may impair the dissipation of heat from exercising muscles, encouraging excessively high muscle and body temperatures. Some people with multiple sclerosis are very sensitive to heat because of poor fitness and autonomic impairment.

Similarly, people with general sympathetic dysfunction may not tolerate cold environments well because blood flow cannot be diverted from the skin to the core to conserve body heat. In addition, a small deconditioned muscle mass may not be sufficient to generate enough body heat to maintain normal body temperature at rest or during exercise in the cold unless proper clothing is worn for insulation to retain heat.

Effects of Environmental Heat and Cold

In addition to the impact physical dysfunctions may have on the body's ability to regulate body temperature, environmental heat and cold may also affect exercise responses and performance. Heat and cold have different effects upon spasticity. Heat tends to reduce or relax spasticity, allowing for greater range of motion with exercise. Cold, in contrast, may decrease movement ranges and prevent the individual from reaching target levels of exercise intensity. An optimal temperature for exercise for people with spastic cerebral palsy (CP) would strike a balance between being warm enough to minimize spasticity but not so hot that motor inefficiency would generate an excessive metabolic heat load.

Exercise in cold environments is also not recommended for people with rheumatoid arthritis or osteoarthritis because range of motion (ROM) normally increases with elevated body temperatures. A warm pool is the recommended medium for exercise with these conditions.

Aerobic Training Adaptations

In able-bodied people, aerobic and cardiovascular fitness are synonymous. Both types of fitness indicate the ability to perform aerobic exercise at a high level of $\dot{V}O_2$ accompanied by substantial and appropriate cardiovascular responses. An important assumption from the outset is that the active muscle mass is large enough to guarantee that the limiting factor during the determination of $\dot{V}O_2max$ is $\dot{Q}$. If that is not the case, maximal cardiovascular function and training-induced changes in it cannot be determined.

Strictly speaking, most physical disabilities that reduce the active muscle mass because of paralysis, paresis, neuromuscular impairment, or degenerative disorders preclude determination of actual maximal cardiovascular function. However, tests of cardiovascular responses to submaximal exercise may be useful in assessing cardiovascular fitness. Submaximal tests are safer and more practical, and they generally suggest changes in maximal cardiovascular function that may not be directly measurable.

Regardless of the muscle mass used during exercise, aerobic fitness can be assessed. The primary index of aerobic fitness is $\dot{V}O_2max$. Keep in mind that the $\dot{V}O_2max$ measured during exercise of small muscle groups is not necessarily the highest possible $\dot{V}O_2max$ measurable under ideal conditions (i.e., with a large muscle mass). Therefore, factors other than central circulation and cardiac output, namely, peripheral factors related to a relatively small exercising muscle mass, limit $\dot{V}O_2max$. When inadequate muscle mass limits $\dot{V}O_2max$, some cardiovascular reserve capacity remains unused even though the muscles are fatigued during maximal-effort exercise.

Changes in aerobic fitness are normally evidenced by many anatomic, physiologic, and morphologic training adaptations that are apparent during rest, submaximal exercise, and maximal exercise. Training responses for the general population without disabilities are well known. Box 4.1 summarizes the basic physiologic adaptations to chronic (long-term) aerobic training.

Effects of Physical Disability

The two main physiologic prerequisites for developing a high level of aerobic and cardiovascular fitness are a large, functional, active muscle mass and functional cardiovascular and autonomic control systems. Thus, with exercise of large muscle groups (such as that involving use of the leg muscles) and normal cardiovascular function, an increase in $\dot{V}O_2max$ is accompanied by increases in central circulation (cardiac output). That is, the pumping capacity of the heart increases.

Central Versus Peripheral Adaptations

Very little research has been done to document central training responses as compared to peripheral training responses with various disabilities. At present, most study has centered on people with SCI paraplegia (Shephard, 1990), yet information on this subject remains inconclusive. The following discussion outlines general principles you should keep in mind as you try to develop realistic expectations about aerobic trainability of people with various disabling conditions.

With disorders that prevent exercise of large muscle groups, increases in $\dot{V}O_2max$ are relatively small; the mechanisms accounting for this increase are likely to be peripheral. For example, maximal arm-crank exercise or leg exercise with small, weak legs probably stresses the heart to some unknown extent, but the heart is not likely to be the primary limiting factor. The exercising muscle itself (i.e., the muscle size and blood flow) is the main limiting factor. Thus, although small muscle exercise training may induce mild cardiovascular conditioning responses as evidenced at rest or during submaximal testing, improvements in peripheral muscular adaptations are much more likely to occur. These beneficial muscle changes probably include increased muscle blood flow and O_2 delivery inside muscle tissue and increased stores of glycogen and enzymes necessary for both aerobic and anaerobic metabolism.

Nearly everyone can improve strength, endurance, and aerobic fitness to some degree in a chosen exercise mode. However, the less the muscle mass and cardiovascular and autonomic integrity, the

---

FOR REVIEW . . .
Physiologic Adaptations to Chronic Aerobic Exercise Training

At rest:

- Decreased resting heart rate (HR)
- Increased stroke volume (SV)
- Possible decrease in systolic blood pressure

With submaximal exercise (at a given work load):

- Decreased HR, BP, ventilation ($\dot{V}_E$), and blood lactic acid
- Increased SV

With maximal exercise:

- Increased $\dot{V}_E$, SV, cardiac output ($\dot{Q}$), $\dot{V}O_2max$

General structural and functional adaptations:

- Increased blood and heart volume
- Increased muscle capillaries, mitochondria (oxygen processing units in muscle cells), aerobic enzymes, stored fuels, and ATP
- Increased ability to redistribute blood flow to exercising muscles, dissipate heat, and tolerate exercise in hot and humid environments
- Decreased time for postexercise HR recovery

lower the expected initial exercise tolerance, aerobic exercise capacity, and eventual aerobic training responses. For example, even people with quadriplegia may have the potential for increasing their maximal $\dot{Q}$ following an arm-training program. Exercise training may hypertrophy remaining innervated arm and diaphragm muscles, increasing their needs for blood flow. Any increase in venous return from the arm vasculature during maximal-effort arm exercise training may increase maximal $\dot{Q}$. Is this increased exercise $\dot{Q}$ a true central cardiovascular training effect in terms of increased intrinsic capability of the heart to pump blood, or did this adaptation merely increase the capability for venous return via increased arm muscle size and peripheral training adaptations? The point is that any person with a physical disability who trains with a small muscle mass is probably inducing beneficial peripheral training adaptations that enhance venous return although the true limits of $\dot{Q}$ are not approached.

Comparisons of Upper Body and Lower Body Exercise

A large number of mobility-impaired individuals have disabilities affecting the legs, precluding leg exercises such as walking, running, and cycling. Thus, they rely upon the arm musculature for all voluntary exercise such as arm-cranking and wheelchair propulsion. Physiologic responses during arm exercise differ from those during leg exercise in several respects, primarily because of the size of the exercising muscle mass and the degree of sympathetic activity (if sympathetic function is intact in the person who is exercising).

Voluntary Exercise

Because the normal arm muscle mass is about two thirds the leg muscle mass, the maximal power output, $\dot{V}O_2$, and $\dot{Q}$ elicited by maximal arm exercise are proportionally less than during maximal leg exercise. Despite the smaller active muscle mass, maximal HR and systolic arterial BP during arm exercise, however, are only slightly lower than the maximal values during leg exercise due to the higher level of sympathetic stimulation elicited by arm exercise. Maximal diastolic arterial BP during arm exercise usually exceeds the maximal values during leg exercise due to the greater inactive muscle mass that vasoconstricts during arm exercise.

Compared with leg exercise at low to moderate workloads, arm exercise produces a lower cardiac stroke volume and anaerobic threshold, but higher $\dot{V}O_2$, HR, BP, $\dot{V}_E$, and blood lactic acid levels. Thus, at given submaximal workloads, arm exercise requires a greater energy cost and produces greater cardiovascular and pulmonary stresses than leg exercise. Additionally, arm exercise does not increase SV and $\dot{Q}$ (it doesn't "volume-load" the heart) as effectively as leg exercise. Therefore, arm exercise is not the exercise mode of choice for central cardiovascular conditioning unless no alternative modes are feasible. Table 4.3 summarizes the differences between physiologic responses with arm and leg exercise.

Several factors may explain the differences in physiologic responses between voluntary arm-cranking and leg-cycling exercise. First, the lower mechanical efficiency of arm exercise (i.e., higher energy expenditure per unit of power output) may be due to the smaller muscle mass available for performing work. Although isometric contractions of hand, forearm, trunk, and hip muscles necessary to stabilize the body during arm exercise increase $\dot{V}O_2$, they do not contribute to the external work. Second, arm exercise in the upright sitting posture induces venous pooling in the inactive legs, and blood pooling in the lower extremities reduces SV. Rapid accumulation of lactic acid accompanies higher sympathetic tone throughout the body, inducing vasoconstriction in the nonexercising legs

Table 4.3 Physiologic Responses With Arm and Leg Exercise in Able-Bodied Subjects

Physiologic variables	Values with submaximal exercise	Values with maximal exercise
Systolic arterial blood pressure	Arm less than leg	Arm less than leg
Diastolic arterial blood pressure	Arm greater than leg	Arm greater than leg
Ventilation and heart rate	Arm greater than leg	Arm less than or equal to leg
Stroke volume	Arm less than leg	Arm less than leg
Cardiac output and oxygen consumption	Arm greater than or equal to leg	Arm less than leg
Anaerobic threshold	Arm less than leg	

and increasing HR and BP responses. Lastly, the higher ratio of fast-twitch to slow-twitch muscle fibers in the arms may contribute to their metabolic differences and the relative inefficiency of upper body work.

Separate arm and leg exercise tests do not predict the exercise capacity of the other exercise mode well. Even though results from arm testing should not be compared to those predicted for leg exercise, arm testing can provide a tool to evaluate the general function and work capacity of the upper body in whatever exercise mode selected.

An initial training work load of approximately one half that used for leg exercise is usually appropriate for arm exercise, depending upon the functional and training status of the arms and legs. Exercise training with the arms at 60% to 80% arm $\dot{V}O_2$max or at 70% to 85% HRmax is also likely to elicit measurable physiologic responses and improved arm exercise capacity. However, specificity of training is probably evident in arm and leg exercise. In more physically fit individuals, physiologic changes following an endurance training program are usually restricted to the specifically trained arms or legs, with most of the training responses due to peripheral factors such as increased muscle blood flow and cellular changes in the trained muscles rather than to central cardiovascular changes. On the other hand, less fit people have shown crossover benefits to untrained limbs, suggesting that both central and peripheral changes are possible.

It is important to note that people with autonomic dysfunction may produce much less sympathetic response during arm exercise than people with physical disabilities who have a fully functioning sympathetic nervous system. Qualified professionals should evaluate sympathetic responses in people with autonomic impairments to determine the tolerance to and safety of various exercise modes for them.

Electrical Stimulation Exercise

Recent technological advances have allowed some individuals with SCI who have significant sensorimotor loss above the 12th thoracic segment to perform leg-cycle ergometry using electrical stimulation (ES) of paralyzed quadriceps, hamstring, and gluteal muscle groups. This instrumentation was developed for therapeutic purposes to prevent or reverse multisystem deterioration following SCI, including leg muscle atrophy and spasticity, osteoporosis, and skin pressure sores. Additionally, higher levels of cardiovascular fitness were thought possible because ES cycling activated large paralyzed muscles of the legs.

After several months of training, most people with SCI using ES technology are able to cycle for 30 min at approximately 10-watts power output (0.25 kp load at 42 rpm pedaling cadence), eliciting a $\dot{V}O_2$ of about 1 L/min, $\dot{Q}$ of about 9 L/min, and HR of about 100 bpm (Figoni, 1990). This is roughly equivalent to able-bodied walking exercise at 3 to 4 mph or arm-cranking at 50 watts. Thus, ES cycling appears to be a viable alternative for mild cardiovascular training for people with paraplegia, and it may be a superior alternative for people with quadriplegia who have more limited voluntary arm exercise capacity.

Although no research to date has documented improvements in peak cardiopulmonary function resulting from voluntary arm-crank exercise training, research has shown increased peak cardiopulmonary function resulting from ES leg-cycle training (Hooker et al., 1992). Significant increases in several important peak variables were noted after ES leg-cycle training, including power output, $\dot{V}O_2$, $\dot{V}_E$, $\dot{Q}$, and HR during exercise. However, no significant changes in peak arm-crank performance were found to result from this training, supporting the concepts of specificity of lower limb training, local sites of fatigue for upper extremity muscular exercise, and peripheral circulatory training adaptations in people with SCI during short-term training.

More advanced ES exercise systems employing combined arm and leg (hybrid) exercise with more effective stimulation of a greater number of muscle groups are currently being developed and evaluated.

Muscle Fatigue and Factors Limiting Aerobic Exercise Capacity

Muscle fatigue is the failure to maintain a required or expected force or power output. Muscle fatigue is a normal phenomenon, but its causes are many and varied. Specific causes of fatigue during aerobic exercise depend upon the demands of the exercise (i.e., mode, intensity, duration, and frequency of muscle contractions) and the abilities of the individual performing the exercise (i.e., physical fitness and the presence of specific pathologic conditions that interfere with neuromuscular, cardiovascular, or pulmonary function). Central mechanisms of fatigue involve the brain and spinal cord. Fatigue may result from impaired motivation, neural motor drive, motor unit recruitment, or spinal reflexes. On the other hand, peripheral mechanisms of fatigue entail transmission of electrical impulses through peripheral nerves and muscle cells along with biomechanical and metabolic events in contracting muscle fibers. Physical conditioning normally improves cardiorespiratory endurance and resistance to fatigue.

Muscle mass (i.e., exercise mode) plays a major role in development of fatigue during maximal aerobic exercise, especially if a small muscle mass (relative to leg exercise for able-bodied people) is utilized. The overall available muscle mass for exercise is limited by neuromuscular impairments that result in paralysis, such as with SCI, MS, MD, and brain injuries (stroke and head injury) or by amputation of lower extremities. When about one half or more of the normally functioning muscle mass is exercising at peak capacity, the limiting factor for maximal aerobic power is the central circulation (i.e., cardiac output, or the ability of the heart to deliver sufficient blood and O_2 to a large exercising muscle mass) (Rowell, 1986). If only the arms are used for exercise, the relatively small muscle mass is not large enough to drive the cardiovascular system to the limits of its ability to pump blood and deliver O_2, and more O_2 can be delivered to exercising arm muscles than can actually be utilized. Therefore, the inability of a small muscle mass to utilize large quantities of O_2 and return large quantities of venous blood from the peripheral circulation to the heart limits maximal-effort aerobic arm exercise. Dysfunctional musculature, such as with paresis, paralysis of entire muscle groups, and impaired motor control, compounds these problems.

During prolonged exercise, the sites of fatigue shift toward the exercising muscles themselves, regardless of the size of the exercising muscle mass. If low- to moderate-intensity exercise is performed long enough (depending on the muscular fitness of the individual), fuel sources such as blood sugar and muscle glycogen are depleted. Muscle contractions and movements then become more and more difficult and painful to perform. Although some effort and stress is inherent in exercise training during a 20- to 40-min workout, extremely fatiguing exercise is unnecessary for general health and physical fitness.

With spasticity, such as that caused by spastic CP, metabolic processes within the muscle may be unaffected; however, because impaired motor control may limit coordinated and repetitive use of muscles, full muscle relaxation between muscle contractions may be prevented. Besides interfering with intended movements, incomplete relaxation may reduce muscle blood flow, leading to early onset of peripheral muscular fatigue and limiting exercise capacity. Energy costs ($\dot{V}O_2$) and physiologic stresses (HR and BP) of exercise movements may be very high relative to the power output. Although this response to exercise may provide beneficial stresses to the cardiopulmonary systems, higher intensity exercise may be contraindicated by abnormally high BP or increased spasticity.

Depending upon the condition, medical or therapeutic interventions may enhance abnormal neuromuscular or cardiopulmonary function, and you should explore these options with a physician. In any case, physical conditioning is usually essential to improve muscular endurance and resistance to fatigue. As an exercise leader, you must understand each client's abilities and limitations to provide appropriate exercise prescriptions and recommendations.

Summary

The basic principles of aerobic exercise physiology for people with physical disabilities are similar to those for able-bodied people. Aerobic metabolism in exercising muscles provides energy for endurance exercise and cardiovascular conditioning. Availability of O_2 is essential for aerobic metabolism—this process involves taking in O_2 through the lungs (ventilation), transporting O_2 through the arterial and venous circulation, and utilizing O_2 within the muscle fibers. The type and severity of disability, however, redefine the upper limits of maximal aerobic power ($\dot{V}O_2$max) due to decreases in muscle mass and alterations in cardiovascular responses with exercise. The functional status of the sympathetic nervous system determines the extent to which cardiovascular responses may aid O_2 transport to support high levels of aerobic metabolism. Physiologic adjustments during exercise of small muscle groups suggest that peripheral training adaptations within the muscle fibers may be the primary source of increases in $\dot{V}O_2$max. A smaller muscle mass may be insufficient to effectively stress the cardiovascular system to yield central adaptations with training. Central compared to peripheral aerobic training effects are largely unknown for most people with physical disabilities, especially the most functionally impaired. Nevertheless, enhancing peripheral muscle capabilities, strength, and endurance contributes to health, physical fitness, and functional performance of people with physical disabilities.

Part III

Designing Accessible Fitness Programs

Developing fitness programs for your clients with physical disabilities involves integrating your knowledge of disability and the principles of exercise science (from Parts I and II) with the skills necessary for modifying and individualizing exercise routines and techniques. Part III applies exercise principles to the actual exercise setting. It offers guidelines for designing safe and effective exercise programs for both general types of disabling conditions and specific physical disabilities. This information will help you develop appropriate and individualized training programs for each of your clients.

Chapter 5 introduces general guidelines for adapting standard principles of fitness conditioning for resistance training, stretching, and aerobic exercise. Chapter 6 reviews the variables of resistance training programs while chapter 7 offers suggestions for modifying programs that use stretch bands to meet the needs of your disabled clients. Chapters 8 and 9 examine principles of flexibility training and methods for modifying stretching techniques. Chapter 10 presents a series of exercises for developing muscular fitness that emphasize safety and how to modify techniques for specific conditions associated with disability. Chapter 11 introduces a system for modifying aerobic dance exercise routines also based on condition-specific needs.

Recommended Readings

Alter, M.M. (1988). *Science of stretching*. Champaign, IL: Human Kinetics.

American College of Sports Medicine. (1991). *Guidelines for exercise testing and prescription*. Philadelphia: Lea & Febiger.

American Council on Exercise. (1991). *Personal trainer manual*. San Diego: Author.

Basmajian, J.V., & Wolf, S.L., (Eds.) (1990). *Therapeutic exercise*. Baltimore: Williams & Wilkins.

Corbin, C.B., & Lindsey, R. (1985). *Concepts of physical fitness*. Dubuque, IA: Brown.

Fleck, S.J., & Kraemer, W.J. (1987). *Designing resistance training programs*. Champaign, IL: Human Kinetics.

Franks, B.D., & Howley, E.T. (1989). *Fitness leader's handbook*. Champaign, IL: Human Kinetics.

Gordon, N.F. (1993a). *Arthritis: Your complete exercise guide*. Champaign, IL: Human Kinetics.

Gordon, N.F. (1993b). *Stroke: Your complete exercise guide*. Champaign, IL: Human Kinetics.

Grimby, G., & Einarsson, G. (1991). Post-polio management. *Physical and Rehabilitation Medicine*, **2**(4), 189-200.

Heyward, V.H. (1984). *Designs for fitness—A guide to physical fitness appraisal and exercise prescription*. New York: Macmillan.

Kisner, C., & Colby, L.A. (1990). *Therapeutic exercise: Foundations and techniques*. Philadelphia: F.A. Davis.

Lasko-McCarthey, P.M., & Knopf, K.G. (1992).

Adapted physical education for adults with disabilities (3rd ed.) Dubuque, IA: Eddie Bowers.

McAtee, R.E. (1993). *Facilitated stretching*. Champaign, IL: Human Kinetics.

Sapega, H.A., Quedenfield, T.C., Moyer, R.A., & Butler, R.A. (1981). Biophysical factors in range-of-motion exercise. *The Physician and Sportsmedicine*, **9**, 57-65.

Sinaki, M. (1987). *Basic clinical rehabilitation medicine*. Philadelphia: B.C. Decker.

Van Gelder, N., & Marks, S. (Eds.) (1987). *Aerobic dance-exercise instructor manual*. San Diego: IDEA Foundation.

Chapter 5

Exercise Prescription: Adapting Principles of Conditioning

Stephen F. Figoni, PhD, RKT
Wright State University
Kevin F. Lockette, PT, CSCS
Rehabilitation Hospital of the Pacific, Honolulu
Paul R. Surburg, PhD, RPT
Indiana University

Principles of exercise conditioning apply theoretical concepts of exercise science to the actual exercise experience. The so-called exercise prescription is really a recommendation for an appropriate quantity and mode of exercise that can safely allow an individual to reach fitness goals. The American College of Sports Medicine (ACSM) offers guidelines for developing an exercise prescription defined by the mode, intensity, duration, frequency, and progression of exercise training (ACSM, 1991). These guidelines are based on research that shows that a certain minimal level of exercise is required before significant training benefits can be realized. Always individualize exercise recommendations for your clients by combining general principles with specific information about the client, including the initial level of fitness, health and medical history, physical abilities, personality traits, and personal goals. With clients who have physical disabilities, it is also critical that your exercise prescription take into account their movement abilities and the safety precautions associated with the disability.

Recommending exercise programs for people with disabilities should be an ongoing process. You must continually modify the prescription according to how each person responds to the training program. This is especially important with people who have progressive disorders or who may experience a decline in function following exercise. You must maintain continual contact with each participant to determine if, in fact, your recommendations need to be modified. It is also best that you periodically reassess each client to evaluate progress or readjust the exercise prescription.

In this chapter, we present guidelines for modifying basic principles of conditioning for the development of health-related physical fitness, as established by ACSM. We will review principles of overload, specificity, progression, and consistency and detail the overload principle as applied to resistance training, stretching, and aerobic conditioning. We will also identify several conditions common to a variety of physical disabilities that must be considered when you recommend exercise programs for people with disabilities.

Basic Principles of Conditioning

Principles of conditioning define a range of recommendations to guide the exerciser toward achieving specific goals. In this chapter, we offer principles for achieving health-related physical fitness, specifically related to disease prevention and improved ability to function in daily activities (Pate, 1988). Some clients may be interested in improving performance in a certain sport or activity, others may wish to improve their abilities to perform daily skills, and others may want to improve their mobility and independence. You can manipulate the variables of the exercise prescription to direct each person toward achieving specific goals. You also must adjust the principles of conditioning—overload, specificity, progression, and consistency—to meet the individual needs of all clients based on their abilities or disabilities.

Overload

The principle of overload in exercise training implies that structural and functional adaptation of some unit or system of the body will occur if it is repeatedly stressed to a level beyond which it is normally accustomed. Overload is more completely defined by these four variables:

Frequency: how often the exercise is performed

Intensity: to what degree the system is stressed

Duration: the period of time the system is stressed

Mode: the general type of activity that is undertaken

The mode of training determines the nature and magnitude of the conditioning response. For example, aerobic conditioning that utilizes large muscle groups rhythmically and continuously induces changes in cardiovascular function. By contrast, small-muscle-mass activity against heavy resistance is unlikely to result in a similar type of change.

Modifying With Resistance Training

Several variables can be manipulated to alter the outcome of a resistance training program. In addition to the basic variables of frequency, intensity, and duration, resistance training overload also is influenced by rest between training sessions and recovery between exercise sets. Progressive resistive exercise (PRE) refers to programs that employ progressive increases in overload or resistance with exercise training. Be careful when determining overload for people with progressive

or neuromuscular disorders and remember that a PRE program may be inappropriate in some cases. Overworking the muscles in multiple sclerosis (MS), for example, can cause excessive fatigue that temporarily decreases the person's ability to perform daily functional activities such as dressing, walking, and wheelchair use (Olgiati, Burgunder, & Mumenthaler, 1988). In neuromuscular diseases and postpolio syndrome, overwork can possibly cause permanent loss of muscle fiber function (Peach, 1990). Program goals for people with these disorders may be restricted to strength maintenance, which can be achieved without PRE, especially as the diseases progress. Consult the individual's physician and therapist for guidance before designing the strength program. Table 5.1 summarizes guidelines for recommending the variables of overload with resistance training.

The frequency of resistance training depends in part on the duration and intensity of the exercise sessions. It should vary from several daily sessions to three to seven periods per week, depending on the participant's needs, interests, and functional abilities. In general, positive gains in muscle strength or endurance require a minimum of 2 to 3 days of resistance training per week (ACSM, 1991). A maintenance program can be effective with as little as one training session per week. One day of recovery is recommended between days of training for each muscle group to prevent overwork from limiting progress. More frequent training should alternate muscle groups, such as upper body and lower body exercises, or alternate high- and low-intensity training. More frequent but shorter training sessions may be appropriate for people with extreme weakness or fatigue who can only tolerate light loads. Training with these conditions generally requires medical supervision, especially when pain is present.

The frequency principle of the resistance training prescription is generally unaffected by conditions associated with disability. Conditions that involve periods of flare-up may interrupt training frequency, however. If special transportation needs prevent some people from accessing your facility, train them in a mode of exercise, such as with stretch bands, that they can use at home to maintain the desired frequency of training.

You can determine the intensity and duration of resistance training by manipulating the interdependent variables of load, reps, sets, and recovery. (See the review box for a summary of basic definitions.)

Subjectively, a participant can determine the appropriate exercise load with resistance training by the amount of resistance that causes a burning

Table 5.1 Variables of Overload With Isotonic Resistance Training

Variable	Recommendations	Modifications
Frequency	2 to 3 days/week (1 day/week for maintenance)	Arthritis (affected joints): daily
Intensity and duration		
Reps	3 to 7: STR 8 to 12: STR/END 12 to 20: END	Arthritis (unaffected joints), neuromuscular disorders and progressive conditions, *weakness: low load/moderate to high repetitions
Sets	3 to 5	Arthritis (affected joints): 2 to 3 reps, low load daily
Load	Heavy: STR Moderate: STR/END Light: END	Stroke: moderate to low load/moderate to high reps
Recovery	2 to 4 min Less than 2 min	

STR = strength, END = muscular endurance
*With paresis, resistance training (in the fitness program) is indicated only when the intended movement can be isolated.

FOR REVIEW . . .

Variables of Resistance Training: Definitions

One-repetition-maximum (1RM)—the maximum force that can be generated or weight that can be lifted in a single effort

Load—the amount of resistance used for each repetition, quantified as a unit of weight or resistance

Repetition (rep)—the singular effort that is required to resist a force or move a weight through a range and return to the starting position

Set—a series of consecutive repetitions separated by recovery periods

Recovery—a period of rest between sets

---

sensation associated with the onset of local muscular fatigue or with isotonic work by the inability to move a weight through the range of motion (ROM) at the end of one set of repetitions. The exercise load can also be calculated as a percentage of the one-repetition-maximum (1RM)—the most a participant can lift with a single effort. However, for most people in a general fitness program, attempting to perform a maximal lift imposes risks for injury that contraindicate its use for determining an appropriate exercise load. The important point about exercise load is that someone with normal function should perform each set of repetitions at a load that will result in muscle fatigue in an intended number of repetitions.

Each client's fitness level, functional abilities, and personal goals determine the appropriate training load. Low training loads, recommended for beginners to prevent injury, strengthen tendons and ligaments in preparation for heavier loads during later stages of the training (Fleck & Falkel, 1986). People who have joint instability, weakness,

or a risk of high blood pressure (such as may be the case following a stroke) should also use low workloads. Heavy training also may be inappropriate with spastic muscles because it can increase spasticity and thereby decrease range of motion (ROM) and functioning after exercise. As always, individualize your recommendations and maintain a strong focus on safety. Observe how your clients move when a training load is initially prescribed to ensure that the load is not so great that it encourages the use of substitute motions, especially toward the end of the set. Substitution is generally a clear indication that the training load is too high.

Duration of isotonic resistance training (in which resistance is provided through the range of motion at a constant tension) for each muscle group can mean the number of sets and repetitions performed or the length of time for one set of exercises. Duration is useful for calculating work-rest intervals to achieve a specific training effect. With isometric work (applying resistance without movement), duration also can imply the amount of time (s) for each contraction. Gains in strength with isometric work are achieved with a minimum contraction time of 6 s. However, following a stroke people should avoid isometric contractions for longer than 6 s because of potential increases in blood pressure beyond safe limits (Gordon, 1993b).

Depending on the goal of the program, three to five sets of exercises consisting of 3 to 20 repetitions for each set are recommended. Optimal strength gains are generally realized with a maximum of 5 to 7 reps, although this type of training imposes greater risks for injury. Protocols that use 12 to 20 repetitions (with a lighter load) typically target development of muscular endurance.

Regardless of the specific purpose of the program, to achieve training overload the load selected should cause muscle fatigue with the intended number of repetitions. However, remember that people with progressive conditions, joint instability, pain with movement, or a likelihood of developing disabling fatigue with intense training should avoid exercising to fatigue regardless of the number of repetitions performed for each exercise. These people should perform resistance training at a submaximal level.

The duration of the recovery period between sets also affects the outcome of the training program and is related to the specific fuel system targeted. According to Stone, O'Bryant, Grahammer, McMillan, and Rozenek (1982), recovery periods of between 2 and 4 min should be used for general strengthening routines. To stress the glycolytic system, they recommend shorter rest periods of a minute or less. These shorter rest periods are utilized more frequently with sport-specific and muscular endurance training.

Another method of evaluating recovery periods is to determine the work to recovery ratio appropriate for the goals of the program (Graves, Welsch, & Pollock, 1991). This system compares the time required to perform a set of repetitions to the rest period. Longer rest periods are optimal for pure strength training with ratios as high as 1:12 (15 s of effort to 3 min of recovery). Muscular endurance routines involve ratios as low as 1:1 (60 s of effort to 60 s of recovery). A 1:4 ratio combines strength and endurance training. People prone to functional decline with fatigue, as with progressive disorders such as MS or postpolio syndrome, should extend rest periods as needed.

In summary, the variables of set, reps, load, and recovery of the resistance training overload are interdependent. Participants achieve overload by combining higher work loads with fewer repetitions or combining a greater number of repetitions with lower workloads. However, there is a direct relationship between the strength of the training stimulus (higher workloads) and risk for injury. With this in mind, use caution when designing programs for people with impaired joint or muscle function. The objective of the resistance training program should be the highest rate of muscular development possible with the lowest risk of inducing functional decline. Chapter 6 provides more information about developing muscular strength, endurance, and power through resistance training.

Modifying With Stretching

Muscles and connective tissue must be overstretched to produce adaptive lengthening. The frequency, intensity, and duration of flexibility training are the variables of overstretching that influence the outcome of the stretching program. As with training for other components of physical fitness, the variables of overstretching are interdependent and specific to the stretching mode or technique.

Unlike aerobic conditioning or resistance training there currently does not appear to be one set of widely accepted principles of conditioning for flexibility development. Table 5.2 summarizes recommendations for stretching and suggested modifications with disabling conditions.

The beginner starting a new stretching program should work out three times per week, gradually increasing frequency to daily, but not at the expense of comfort. You may have to monitor this gradual increase in flexibility training closely for people with disabilities, especially if they have low fitness levels or contractures, such as hip flexor contractures with lower extremity amputation.

Table 5.2 Variables of Overload With Static Stretching

Variable	Recommendations	Modifications
Frequency	3 times/week (minimum), may gradually increase	Increase frequency with contractures, spasticity, arthritis
Intensity	Subjective sensation of tension 3 to 5 repetitions	Low load with spasticity
Duration	6 s to 12 s for warm-up 10 s to 30 s (or more) for flexibility	Longer duration with spasticity

Some people with disabilities such as spastic cerebral palsy or rheumatoid arthritis may already be stretching daily and should incorporate several stretching sessions throughout the day to maintain an optimal level of functioning. The intensity of a stretch is determined by the degree of stretch, the length of time a stretched position is held, and the number of repetitions performed. Degree of stretch is subjectively determined by a feeling of tension in the stretched muscle. Recommend that your clients avoid stretching to the point of pain. Any of the following aftereffects indicate that the intensity of the stretch was excessive:

- Muscle vibration
- Persisting pain
- Muscle quivering
- Loss of ROM

The duration or length of time to hold a muscle in a stretched or elongated position varies depending on the purpose of the activity and technique employed. A 6-s static stretch is sufficient during a warm-up to prepare the muscles and joints for activity. This duration is relatively effective to temporarily elongate muscle and connective tissues. Longer duration, low-force static stretches are recommended for achieving more permanent elongation. People with spasticity or coordination problems should employ gentle, less intense stretching and maintain a stretched position for 30 s or more to prepare for more vigorous activity. This duration allows the person ample time to get into the desired stretching position and to concentrate on relaxing to achieve effective results.

There is no agreement about a recommended number of repetitions for each stretching exercise—in part, repetitions depend on the stretching technique employed. The American College of Sports Medicine (ACSM, 1991) recommends 3 to 5 repetitions of static stretching exercise for the general population. Some protocols may suggest up to 15 repetitions of shorter duration stretches, especially with the proprioceptive neuromuscular facilitation (PNF) technique. People who are just beginning an exercise program should begin with fewer repetitions and increase the number as tolerance allows.

Modifying With Aerobic Conditioning

The pulmonary, cardiovascular, and aerobic metabolic systems of the exercising skeletal muscles contribute to the ability to use oxygen (which is in greater demand with aerobic exercise). To improve aerobic fitness, conditioning must progressively overload these systems. Table 5.3 includes general recommendations provided by the American College of Sports Medicine (1991) and modifications that may be appropriate for different disabling conditions.

The recommended frequency of aerobic training is 3 to 5 days per week. This principle is generally applicable to all persons, with or without a disability. Exercising fewer than 3 days per week for the extremely deconditioned individual may yield slight benefits or may be sufficient to motivate an individual to adopt an exercise program as part of a lifestyle change, so this level of aerobic exercise should not be discounted as an important first-stage conditioning program. Conversely, exercising for more than 5 days per week may impose the risk for overtraining injury, fatigue, and "staleness," which can limit future success with the conditioning program.

Table 5.3 Variables of Overload With Aerobic Conditioning

Variable	*Recommendations	Modifications
Frequency	3 to 5 days per week	Allow rest with progressive, high-fatigue disorders
Intensity		
HR method	55% to 90% HRmax (dependent on baseline fitness) 70% to 85% average range	Low intensity with progressive, high-fatigue disorders, deconditioned participants, stroke; modified formula for upper body work
RPE method	12 to 16 (20-point scale) 4 to 6 (10-point scale)	Use with ANS impairment, incoordination
Duration	15 to 60 min	Intermittent with limited muscle or exaggerated HR responses (spasticity, athetosis)

*Recommended ranges from *Guidelines for exercise testing and prescription* by American College of Sports Medicine, 1991, Philadelphia: Lea & Febiger.

A day of rest between exercise sessions may be advisable for people who are beginning exercise programs or for people with progressive conditions such as MS or postpolio syndrome. Extremely deconditioned people may benefit from several low-intensity exercise sessions of 5 min duration daily during the first several weeks of conditioning (ACSM, 1991).

In the exercise class setting, heart rate (HR) and subjective rating of perceived exertion (RPE) methods are easily used to assess aerobic exercise intensity. The simplest method for determining an appropriate exercise intensity is to calculate a percentage of the estimated maximal heart rate (HRmax). For many able-bodied individuals, the calculation 220 − age may suffice to estimate HRmax during leg or whole body exercise. During upper body exercise, the calculation 200 − age approximates the age-related HRmax because arm exercise is generally associated with maximal heart rates of approximately 90% to 93% of the HRmax with leg exercise (Shephard, 1990). A broad range of exercise intensity, between 55% and 90% of HRmax, is recommended for improvements in cardiorespiratory fitness, depending on the health and fitness status of the individual. In general, the healthy individual benefits from exercise at a target heart rate range of between 70% and 85% of HRmax. Deconditioned people may need to restrict exercise intensity to the lower ranges of the scale, whereas highly fit people may need to exercise at a heart rate nearer the recommended upper limits to achieve overload. Figure 5.1 provides examples of heart rate calculations. Exercise involving spastic arm muscles or excessive use of overhead arm movements may exaggerate the HR response, rendering it a less reliable indicator of the appropriate training level.

Some people may be unable to evaluate exercise intensity by HR because of an attenuated HR response due to impairment of the autonomic nervous system (ANS). This impairment may occur with high-level spinal cord injury (quadriplegia), MS, or as a result of certain medications (see Appendix A for examples of pharmacologic agents). People with impaired coordination also may have difficulty taking a pulse to determine HR during exercise. The RPE scale is a useful alternative measure for determining exercise intensity (Borg, 1982). Table 5.4 shows two RPE scales (ACSM, 1982). The recommended target zone with use of the 20-point scale is between 12 and 16; with the 10-point scale, the target zone is between 4 and 6. Regardless of the method used to determine exercise intensity, the ability to converse comfortably during the activity is generally an indication that the effort is not excessive. This subjective evaluation is referred to as the "talk" test.

People whose symptoms of fatigue increase with exertion (such as individuals with MS or postpolio syndrome) should keep exercise intensity in the lower ranges of the target zone with both HR and RPE determinations. This recommendation is also appropriate for persons with circulatory problems or a history of stroke and heart disease. People identified as at risk in prescreening assessment should obtain medical clearance and guidance or participate in programs specifically developed to monitor their conditions. HR response during exercise may be limited because a lowered mass

---

Leg or whole-body exercise   (220 minus age) × % HRmax = target heart rate

Upper-body exercise   (200 minus age) × % HRmax = target heart rate

Example: The target heart rate range (70% to 85% HRmax) for a healthy 30-year-old person performing whole-body or upper-body exercise:

	Calculations			
	Whole body exercise		Upper body exercise	
	Lower limit (bpm)	Upper limit (bpm)	Lower limit (bpm)	Upper limit (bpm)
Age	220 − 30	220 − 30	200 − 30	200 − 30
Predicted HRmax	190	190	170	170
Exercise intensity (%HRmax)	× .70	× .85	× .70	× .85
Target heart rate range (bpm)	133	161	119	144

Figure 5.1 Calculating exercise heart rates with upper body and whole body exercise.

Table 5.4 Scales for Subjective Ratings of Perceived Exertion

6 to 20 Rating Scale		0 to 10 Rating Scale	
Scale	Description	Scale	Description
6		0	Nothing at all
7	Very, very light	0.5	Very, very weak
8		1	Very weak
9	Very light	2	Weak
10		3	Moderate
11	Fairly light	4	Somewhat strong
12		5	Strong
13	Somewhat hard	6	
14		7	Very strong
15	Hard	8	
16		9	
17	Very hard	10	Very, very strong
18		*	Maximal
19	Very, very hard		
20			

Note. Individuals are asked to rate how much effort, exertion, or stress they feel subjectively in each of the following categories:

- Central (breathing, temperature, sweating, dizziness, anxiety)
- Peripheral (muscle fatigue; painful, aching, or burning muscles and joints)
- Integrated (combined central and peripheral ratings, overall rating of perceived exertion)

Note. From ''Psychophysical Bases of Perceived Exertion,'' by G.A. Borg, 1982, *Medicine and Science in Sports and Exercise*, **14**, pp. 377-387. Copyright 1982 by the American College of Sports Medicine. Reprinted by permission.

of muscle is utilized during the activity. Paralysis, paresis, and limited range of motion also will lessen the degree to which exercise can be performed vigorously. Everyone must work within personal limits of comfort and tolerance to exercise; your exercise prescription must reflect any limitations.

The recommended duration of aerobic exercise training is 15 to 60 min, either continuously or in intervals, as long as intensity does not drop excessively during the recovery phases of the interval. Deconditioned persons may be unable to maintain exercise in the target zone for the recommended time and need to gradually increase the intensity and duration of the effort as conditioning progresses. A 10% increase in session duration per week (representing about 1 to 4 min) is recommended for increasing the exercise duration from 10 to 40 min.

People with limited muscle function may find more success with interval training than with continuous training. Interval training lessens the constant stress imposed on the few muscle groups that are functional for exercise. For example, a person with quadriplegia who can only utilize shoulder and arm muscles to overload the cardiorespiratory system may fatigue quickly with continuous aerobic exercise because the intensity of the effort may require more anaerobic than aerobic metabolism. Incorporating brief rest periods or periods of recovery, during which lower intensity exercise is maintained, allows work to be performed for an extended period.

Specificity

Adaptation to exercise training is specific to the nature of the exercise activity and the physiologic systems that are stressed. Training specificity extends to metabolic systems (aerobic or anaerobic), muscle-group and fiber-recruitment patterns, joint angles, types of muscular contractions, and movement velocities. Central training effects are specific to the ways in which the pulmonary, cardiovascular, endocrine, and nervous systems are utilized. For example, resistance training imposes a pressure overload whereas aerobic training imposes a volume overload on the heart. Accordingly, cardiac changes with resistance training and aerobic conditioning are quite different; aerobic conditioning induces changes that have greater implications for cardiovascular health.

Consider specific training goals in your exercise prescription and select variables accordingly. If a training goal is to improve the maximal distance traveled by wheelchair in 30 min, for example, training should emphasize long-distance aerobic wheelchair exercise, not anaerobic sprints with an arm-crank ergometer.

One contrast to the principle of specificity is evidence that supports the concept of cross-training. With resistance training, for example, adaptations may occur in a contralateral limb, though to a lesser extent, when only one limb is exercised (Houston, Froese, Valeriote, Green, & Ranney, 1983; Yasuda & Miyamura, 1983). Whether someone can achieve crossover benefits of any significance with health-fitness training to accommodate disabling conditions has not been well investigated.

Part II reviewed adaptations to resistance training and aerobic conditioning that suggested the specificity principle is relevant to disability. In general, the degree of dysfunction produced by conditions associated with disability affects the magnitude of the specific exercise response. For example, the strength-training response is inversely related to the extent of the motor-unit impairment within a muscle group with weakness (such as in polio, muscular dystrophy, or incomplete SCI). With aerobic conditioning, increases in aerobic capacity are related to the volume of muscle utilized in stressing the cardiac system. Exercising small muscle masses, such as with arm training, causes less volume overload on the heart than large-muscle activity. Accordingly, the conditioning responses with arm training tend to be more peripheral in nature.

Progression

The principle of progression, sometimes referred to as progressive overload, is the requirement that exercise training progressively increase the overload stimulus to elicit continual improvements in fitness. Because everyone has genetic limits to exercise performance, although these limits are difficult to define, the prescribed rate and magnitude of progressive increases in the training stimulus must be individualized. In other words, at some point, the exercise overload may be increased to a degree that causes soreness, injury, or symptoms of overtraining. Normally, genetic limits are only tested with elite athletes in intensive training. Limits due to disability may be more strongly influenced by the nature or stage of the disabling condition.

It is critical that you recommend progressive increases in exercise overload carefully to ensure the safety of every client, especially those with disabilities. With some progressive disorders or conditions that involve pain and abnormal fatigue with even light or moderate exercise (such as arthritis or postpolio syndrome, respectively), progressive increases in overload must be monitored carefully. Some people may not tolerate progressive overload or may need to progressively decrease training intensity with time. Be sure to obtain adequate information about each client so the exercise prescription you devise considers conditions that limit tolerance to progressive exercise overload. Remember that for some people, the primary goal of an exercise program may simply be to maintain a certain level of function or to slow decreases in function as symptoms progressively increase. Seek guidance from an appropriate medical professional whenever you have questions about the safety of an exercise prescription.

Conditions involving exacerbations or flare-ups may require an interruption in the training program. Initial reductions in the level of overload may be necessary when the program is resumed before those levels can be progressively increased. Once again, consult the physician or therapist of a client with a cyclic condition to obtain medical clearance before resuming a program interrupted by a period of exacerbation.

Consistency

Because the effects of exercise training are transient and reversible with "detraining," the principle of consistency states that training must occur on a continual and regular basis to produce or maintain training adaptations. Detraining, or loss of training benefits, occurs when exercise is discontinued. With aerobic conditioning, for example, detraining begins with more than 3 days of rest between exercise sessions. Therefore, training for physical fitness should continue indefinitely and become a permanent part of an active lifestyle if a high level of fitness and health are to be maintained.

Periodic detraining, inherent with cyclic conditions (which have periods of exacerbation and remission) or progressive conditions may prevent people from obtaining significant benefits from exercise. It is not hard to understand how clients who are motivated to exercise can become discouraged if they cannot maintain conditioning consistently. The importance of your role in helping clients develop realistic goals, cope with frustrations caused by interruptions, define alternative benefits of participation in exercise programs, and exercise consistently cannot be overstated.

Developing the Comprehensive Individualized Exercise Plan

Exercise prescriptions should be developed with individual needs, abilities, and goals in mind. Generic exercise prescriptions are not recommended, especially with clients who have physical disabilities. Developing preliminary exercise prescriptions for each client enables you to individualize training even within the context of the group setting.

When developing the comprehensive program, you should address all the exercise components of physical fitness, including resistance training, stretching, and aerobic conditioning. You must also evaluate your clients' general medical, health, and activity histories to determine if they need medical clearance or a preliminary preparatory program before initiating the fitness program. To truly individualize the exercise plan, you must also obtain information about each person's baseline fitness level, movement abilities, and personal goals. Once program goals have been set, it is important that you continually document progress and periodically reevaluate the program to make adjustments as needed.

Assessment and Screening

Before you can develop the individualized exercise plan, you must gather pertinent information about each client to allow you to choose activities and program variables to safely guide the individual toward intended fitness goals. Qualified exercise specialists or health care professionals should conduct and evaluate assessments and screenings. If, as an exercise instructor, you are not qualified to perform this function, work with someone who is qualified to obtain the information you need for your exercise classes.

Medical Clearance

Reviewing medical and health histories is the first step in the assessment process. This information can help you identify individuals at risk with exercise and determine who should be referred to appropriate medical professionals for clearance and further guidance before beginning an exercise program. The medical professional can be an invaluable resource as you develop individualized exercise prescriptions, providing advice for selecting appropriate and remedial exercises, identifying contraindicated exercises and potentially harmful symptoms during training, setting the exercise overload, and predicting the outcome of the fitness program. Medical clearance is generally essential for progressive or neuromuscular conditions, postpolio syndrome, poststroke disabilities, painful conditions (such as arthritis), amputations due to circulatory disorders, or *any condition that causes concerns about a client's safety with exercise*. In determining who must receive medical approval, it is better to err on the side of caution than to risk injuring or jeopardizing the safety of any exercise client. However, unless you require that all clients receive medical clearance, requiring only the people with physical disabilities in your integrated programs to do so may appear to be discrimination. The extent of your knowledge about disability determines whether you are qualified to decide what conditions require input from medical professionals. Remember, seek assistance if needed!

Fitness and Movement Assessments

A qualified exercise professional should conduct a fitness assessment to establish baseline levels in all parameters of fitness before setting program goals. When testing for muscular fitness with conditions that have asymmetrical effects, be sure to conduct tests on both sides of the body. Conduct periodic reassessments to evaluate program progress and redefine the program variables as needed.

Before you develop an individualized exercise prescription, note general characteristics of your client's condition and assess movement abilities and limitations. This assessment will not only highlight needs for equipment modifications, but also direct your choice of exercise and conditioning variables. Evaluate these general areas:

✓ Motor control or coordination—identify the extent and nature of any impairment (e.g., ataxia, spasticity, athetosis, etc.).

✓ Balance and trunk stability—identify any instability with resisted movement, unilateral exercises, side-to-side, or overhead movement and assess general stability with exercise from a standing or sitting position.

✓ Spasticity—determine if single joint movements can be isolated (avoid resistance training if they cannot), identify initial levels of spasticity, and note if functioning decreases or spasticity increases with specific exercises.

✓ Range of motion—identify muscle imbalances, joint instability, effects of exercise on postexercise ROM, or needs for additional stretching during the warm-up or cool-down.

✓ Pain—determine if any types of exercises or movements cause or increase pain.

✓ Muscle function—identify functional muscles that can be trained; identify needs for adapting equipment for stability and hand gripping; identify muscle groups with weakness and distinguish between weakness due to deconditioning, progressive or neuromuscular disorders, and overstretch or muscle imbalances.

✓ Sensation—identify and note muscle groups where sensation is lacking.

✓ Fatigue—identify individuals prone to excessive fatigue due to extreme deconditioning, limited muscle function, or other conditions associated with the specific disability (such as MS).

✓ Nature of the condition—identify whether a condition is progressive, static, recurrent (exacerbating-remitting), or fluctuating.

Goal Setting and Documentation

The progression of an exercise program depends on an individual's functional ability or level, health status, age, needs, and goals. Progression is extremely individualized, especially with people who have physical disabilities. By identifying conditions associated with a disability that may limit or reverse progress, you can help your client set realistic program goals.

Goal setting should be a joint effort between you and your client. Your client should clearly understand what goals are realistic and how they relate to personal abilities. By maintaining the emphasis on abilities and avoiding exclusive focus on limitations, the goal-setting process can remain positive and motivating. Develop both short- and long-term goals—realistic short-term goals that can be readily achieved help motivate an individual to stay with the exercise program.

The severity and rate of progressive disorders determine the magnitude of the training adaptations required. During the earlier and inactive stages of disease, fitness may gradually improve; however, when the disease is in an active state, the client must stop or adjust his exercise program according to his health and tolerance. An appropriate exercise program goal for someone with a progressive disorder might be to maintain fitness for as long as possible, even if improvements are not expected.

Documentation not only provides continuity and cohesiveness to an exercise program but also can serve as a motivational device. Records should designate the variables of the training protocol and indicate improvements or changes in fitness level.

Barriers to Health-Fitness Conditioning

The foundation of any fitness program is good general health. Good health allows a person to train regularly and tolerate the increasing demands of progressive training. Chronic, recurring medical complications interfere with training progression and prevent attainment of training goals. In general, people with physical disabilities must pay particular attention to personal hygiene, proper hydration, and diet, and they should avoid unnecessary medications and drugs.

Several conditions associated with physical disability may prevent a person from benefiting from exercise conditioning. You may need to address the following prerequisites to an exercise training program before developing the program itself:

- Flexibility: Adequate joint flexibility is essential because joint contractures restrict range of motion and make dynamic exercise impossible. People with spasticity may benefit from extended stretching before aerobic activity to warm the muscles and improve flexibility for the workout. People with severely restricted ROM may need to use flexibility training before starting a fitness program until their movement range can adequately allow benefits from exercise conditioning to occur.

- Muscular strength and endurance: Minimum levels of muscular strength and endurance are necessary to overcome gravity, perform progressive resistance exercises, and train for cardiorespiratory endurance. Some people with progressive conditions may be unable to train for fitness because of extreme weakness or loss of muscle function.

- Skill: Adequate skill is necessary to perform exercise movement patterns safely and effectively. You may need to consult a therapist about therapeutic procedures to remediate motor dysfunctions that prevent successful participation in an exercise program. Some people with impaired coordination may need to begin a conditioning program by practicing movement patterns that can eventually be incorporated into an exercise routine of sufficient intensity to provide a conditioning effect.

Summary

Principles of conditioning are general recommendations to help guide the development of individualized "prescriptions" for health-fitness exercise programs. Principles of conditioning are based on research that has demonstrated that positive benefits require a minimum quantity and quality of exercise. Four principles apply to any mode of exercise conditioning: overload, progression, specificity, and consistency. The variables of the overload principle (frequency, intensity, and duration) are mode-specific and can be manipulated to direct the outcome of the training program based on individual abilities and goals. The overload stimulus must be progressively increased to maintain continual improvements in fitness.

The basic principles of conditioning are similar for people with and without disabilities. Some people with disabilities, however, must decrease the overload to keep exercise within safe limits and to prevent overwork from causing a decline in functioning. In particular, consult the physicians of clients with progressive and neuromuscular disorders for guidance before developing the exercise prescription.

Evaluate each person individually to identify risks or barriers that may hinder progress before you develop the exercise prescription. Fitness and movement assessments will help shape the base program and set realistic goals. Periodic reassessment is essential to evaluate progress and fine-tune the exercise plan. Some people may be unable to benefit from fitness training initially because of poor health, extreme weakness, limited flexibility, or lack of appropriate motor skill. With guidance from the health care professional, in many cases these barriers can be reduced through preliminary "therapeutic" training that will eventually enable the person to participate in the fitness program. The remainder of Part III presents recommendations for specific modes of exercise training relevant to disability to help guide you with developing and instructing health-fitness exercise programs.

Chapter 6

Resistance Training: Program Design

Kevin F. Lockette, PT, CSCS
Rehabilitation Hospital of the Pacific, Honolulu

Resistance training, traditionally referred to as strength training or weight lifting, is a general description of all modes of exercise that improve anaerobic muscular function and performance. The variables of a resistance training program can be manipulated for a variety of goals, including improvements in muscular endurance, strength and power; muscle hypertrophy; muscle balancing; and flexibility. These goals can be achieved through training with a variety of modes of resistance and training systems.

As a fitness instructor for people with disabilities, you must know not only the basic principles of resistance training and program design, but also appropriate precautions and considerations for developing programs that are effective for people with physical disabilities. This chapter reviews muscle contractions and capabilities, adapted principles of conditioning, resistance training program variables, and guidelines for program development.

Resistance training stresses the anaerobic energy systems and results in peripheral adaptations, affecting muscle and connective tissues (Stone, 1988; Tesch, 1988). In contrast, aerobic or endurance training stresses aerobic metabolism within the muscle and the cardiovascular system, resulting in central changes that include adaptations in the heart and circulatory system (Sherker, 1991). However, all body systems (neural, endocrine, skeletal, muscular, cardiovascular, etc.) interact and can be affected by both anaerobic and aerobic exercise in differing degrees (Vogel, 1988).

Benefits of Resistance Training

Resistance training is commonly undertaken to develop physical fitness and sport-specific skills. In medical rehabilitation programs, this training is used for occupational and physical therapy. Resistance exercise also helps prevent orthopedic (skeletal muscle and connective tissue) injuries. Research indicates that resistance training not only increases muscular strength and endurance, but also promotes growth or increases in strength of ligaments, tendons, joint cartilage, and connective tissue sheaths within the muscle. Increases in bone mineral content also have been found; these increases further help prevent skeletal injuries (Fleck and Falkel, 1986).

Many misconceptions surround the use of resistance training and the training potential of people with physical disabilities. However, resistance training can enhance fitness development and increase function and independence. Research has shown, for example, that resistance training can help some people who have had a stroke or with cerebral palsy increase strength and functional skills such as walking, sports performance, and activities of daily living (Holland & Steadward, 1990; Inaba, Edberg, Montgomery, & Gillis, 1973; McCubbin & Shasby, 1985). With some progressive disorders, resistance training can help maintain strength and prolong a higher level of function as the disease progresses (Milner-Brown & Miller, 1988).

Performance Capabilities of Muscle

A review of terms commonly used to define types of muscular contractions, performance outcomes, and the roles of muscle in movement follows.

Muscular Contractions

Concentric contraction refers to muscle shortening during a contraction or the development of tension, as in the up-phase of the biceps curl. An eccentric contraction occurs when the muscle contracts while it is lengthening, as in the down-phase or negative phase of the exercise.

Isometric exercise refers to muscle contractions performed without joint movement, such as pushing against a wall or other fixed object. An isometric contraction occurs without mechanical work being performed. Isometric exercises are appropriate for individuals when joint movement is painful; however, this type of work only strengthens the muscle within a narrow range of the joint angle being trained. An isotonic contraction refers to dynamic exercise (joint movement) with constant tension. In reality, the tension within the muscle varies because of variations in the strength curve during isotonic exercise. To clarify confusion that has resulted from the pure definition of this term (*iso-*, same; *-tonic*, tension) the terms dynamic constant resistance and dynamic variable resistance have been introduced. The word *dynamic* indicates that movement results from muscular contraction (as opposed to isometric work). Constant resistance is distinguished by an unchanging external load, such as with free weights, throughout the range of motion (ROM). Variable resistance refers to exercise in which the external load varies throughout the ROM, such as with the cam-shaped systems or manual resistance. With variable resistance there is an attempt to correct for changes in the muscle's ability to generate force at different joint angles by varying the external load, thereby equalizing the internal muscular tension throughout the ROM.

Isokinetic exercise involves movement at a constant angular limb velocity. The external resistance (i.e., the equipment) controls the velocity of the movement and the participant controls the tension. A few specialized machines deliver this type of training; however, isokinetic machines are quite expensive and are primarily used as an assessment tool or in the sports medicine and rehabilitation setting.

Strength, Muscular Endurance, and Power

Skeletal muscle is capable of generating force for movements that require strength, muscular endurance, or power. Muscular strength refers to the maximum force a muscle can generate during a single effort or contraction. With dynamic work, muscular strength can be measured by the amount of weight that can be moved through a distance during one maximal repetition, referred to as a one-repetition-maximum (1RM) or maximal voluntary contraction (MVC). Muscular strength is necessary for activities such as performing a transfer independently.

Muscular endurance refers to a muscle's ability to repeatedly perform submaximal muscular contractions over a short period of time (Graves, Welsch, & Pollock, 1991), typically less than 3 to 4 min. To perform repeated contractions, a lighter work load is necessary. Muscular endurance is generally measured as the number of repetitions that can be completed with 50% to 60% of the 1RM (Pate & Lonnett, 1988). In contrast, cardiorespiratory endurance relies on aerobic metabolism for exercise that can be continued indefinitely, such as long-duration walking, jogging, or long-duration wheelchair exercise. Exercise is generally supported by both anaerobic and aerobic metabolism simultaneously. The predominance of one type of metabolism over the other depends on the duration and intensity of the activity. Muscular endurance falls somewhere in the middle of a continuum with muscular strength and aerobic endurance at each end. Many daily activities utilize muscular endurance, including wheelchair propulsion up short, steep inclines; outdoor wheelchair propulsion on uneven surfaces; and short-distance, high-intensity ambulation with or without an assistive walking aid such as a cane or crutches. Any continuous, short-duration effort of moderate to high intensity that relies predominantly on anaerobic metabolism requires muscular endurance.

Muscular power refers to the speed or rate of a muscular contraction (work performed per unit of time). Muscular power is required when force must be generated quickly. Contractions requiring muscular power are typically seen in short bursts of explosive activities such as popping a wheelchair over a curb and pushing up to a standing position with crutches from sitting, and in field events such as throwing a shot put, discus, or javelin.

Muscle hypertrophy refers to an increase in muscle size or, more specifically, an increase in the diameter of the muscle fiber. Until recently, increases in muscular strength have been attributed solely to hypertrophy. However, recent evidence suggests that increases in overall muscle size and strength can be due to hyperplasia, or an increase in the number of muscle fibers (Tesch, 1988).

Muscular Involvement During Movement

A muscle group can assume different roles during movement to facilitate an intended action. When muscle acts as a prime mover or agonist, it supplies the primary force for an intended action. For example, with elbow flexion, the biceps and brachialis muscles are the prime movers. Assistors are muscles that contribute to the action, particularly when the prime mover must move against heavy resistance. Assistors do not normally supply the primary force for the movement. The brachioradialis, for example, assists with elbow flexion when the forearm lifts a heavy load.

Antagonist muscles directly oppose the action of the prime mover. Antagonists are normally inhibited from contracting initially to ensure smooth movement during activation of the prime mover. Contraction of antagonists, however, may be facilitated at the end of the movement to protect the joint from injury during fast, vigorous movements; during a movement to reduce the velocity of contraction with directional changes; and throughout a movement to provide control and precision. For elbow flexion, the triceps muscles are the antagonists. With spastic cerebral palsy, lack of inhibition in antagonist muscles can cause significant movement incoordination and jerky actions. This is due to a hyperactive stretch reflex that responds to the slightest changes in the length of the triceps muscle causing reflexive forceful contraction.

Stabilizers are muscles that contract to support or stabilize bones in adjacent joints. This contraction anchors the bone so the bone acts as a fixed segment, allowing movement to occur in the intended bones. Muscles of the shoulder and shoulder girdle, for example, contract when the elbow flexes against a heavy resistance to protect the shoulder joint and fix the scapula in an appropriate position. Muscles more distal to the action, such as those of the trunk and hips, also contract isometrically to stabilize the body when the action is performed from a sitting position.

Synergists are muscles or muscle groups that contract simultaneously to perform a desired movement and rule out undesired actions. Synergy occurs, for example, when a desired action involves a two-joint muscle, such as with a standing kick. During the preparatory phase, the hamstrings contract to cause hip extension and knee flexion, shortening the muscles at both joints they cross. This action lengthens the rectus femoris, increasing its potential for generating greater force during contraction. When knee extension alone is desired from a sitting position (caused by contraction of the rectus femoris), the hamstrings contract as a synergist to prevent hip flexion. Without the action of the hamstrings, the rectus femoris muscle normally causes both knee extension and hip flexion because it crosses both the hip and knee joints.

"Helping" synergy is another type of synergy that occurs when two or more muscles with the same intended action (but that also activate opposing unintended actions) contract simultaneously to eliminate either of the two unintended actions. For example, when all three muscles of the hamstrings group contract simultaneously to extend the hip, inward or outward rotation of the thigh is neutralized. Rotation would occur if only one of the group contracted alone.

With paralysis and paresis the normal teamwork that initiates intended actions and provides support and protection for surrounding joints may be disrupted. Prime movers, assistors, antagonists, stabilizers, and synergists may be affected in differing degrees by a disabling condition. Paralysis of trunk and shoulder muscles, such as muscles that normally fix or move the scapula, can create challenges for other upper body movements. It is important that you assess the integrity of all major muscle groups for each client to ensure that the exercises you prescribe can be performed as intended and do not compromise joint stability.

With loss of muscle function, actions normally supported by specific muscle groups can often be performed with use of assistors and substitute muscles. For example, someone without triceps function can perform shoulder abduction with extended elbows by externally rotating the shoulder and passively locking the elbows into extension, thus allowing the intended movement to be performed. Some substitute actions may place excessive stress on muscles not intended to support such actions. For example, wheelchair propulsion and crutch walking place great demands on musculature not normally intended for locomotion. This can have implications for the strength training program, requiring strengthening substitute muscle groups, maintaining muscle balance, and avoiding potential overuse injuries. You may wish to consult with a client's therapist or physician for guidance in developing a resistive exercise program if loss of muscle function alters normal movement patterns.

Variables of Program Design

When designing a resistance training program, you can manipulate several training variables to yield specific desired training outcomes. These variables are training volume, exercise selection, modes of resistance, and training systems.

Training Volume

The total amount of work performed during an exercise session is referred to as the training volume. Training volume can be quantified by multiplying repetitions times sets times load. Each of these elements was defined as variables of the overload principle with resistance training in chapter 5. People with progressive disorders and neuro-

muscular diseases should generally use a lower training volume to prevent excessive fatigue or overwork weakness from interfering with daily functioning. Training volume for people with any disability is related to the amount of muscle mass available for training. Conditions such as paralysis, hemiplegia, impaired motor control, and limited joint function may decrease the trainable muscle mass to varying degrees.

Circuit resistance training programs consist of a series of low- to moderate-intensity exercises with minimal rest between each exercise. These programs are designed to increase strength, muscular endurance, and power (Gettman & Pollock, 1981). Circuit resistance training is popular because it maximizes equipment usage, is time efficient, and can be an enjoyable, sociable activity. Although it is not the most effective method for maximally increasing strength or endurance, its advantage is that it combines both.

The variables of training volume are interdependent variables that you can manipulate to achieve different training outcomes; that is, training can target development of muscular strength, muscular endurance, or power. To develop muscular strength, an exercise load should be used that fatigues the muscle with between four and eight repetitions (Poliquin, 1989). An appropriate exercise load is between 80% and 90% of the 1RM. The American College of Sports Medicine (1991) provides similar guidelines, suggesting that maximal gains in strength result from programs that utilize three sets of no more than 5 to 7 repetitions for each movement. Muscular strength routines are exceptionally good for individuals using wheelchairs (such as those with spinal cord injury) who must overcome their own body weight for pressure relief, transferring, or general activities of daily living. When prescribing exercise programs to develop muscular strength, be aware that lifting heavy loads can cause the participant to move into inappropriate or even unsafe postural alignment, especially with the last repetition of the set. Training with heavy loads should be done with a partner or assistant.

Muscular endurance routines are appropriate for most beginners. Poliquin (1989) suggests that the beginning program consist of three to five sets of 8 to 20 repetitions. This amount allows for safety and provides the beginner an opportunity to learn proper technique and control. Poliquin further recommends a minimum of 8 repetitions per set for the first year of training prior to moving on to higher loads. Muscular endurance routines can generally be performed with loads of 65% of the

1RM. For resistance training to improve muscular strength and endurance, 75% of the 1RM can be used for 8 to 12 repetitions. People with limited muscle mass, such as with quadriplegia or some progressive diseases, may have to further modify such routines by lowering the number of repetitions according to their physical fitness levels and tolerance to exercise stress. They may also have to limit each set to a submaximal level (i.e., not exercising to the point of muscular fatigue) by lowering the load to avoid the risk of overstressing unimpaired motor neurons and muscle fibers.

Muscular strength and power routines require fewer exercises, heavier loads, fewer repetitions, and longer recovery intervals. Power routines use loads that fatigue the muscle with between one and three repetitions. Training for muscular power is generally not necessary for developing health fitness. However, such routines can be used for specific goals such as pushing up to standing with long leg braces, and they are used with sport-specific training (shot put, discus, javelin).

Exercise Selection

Select specific resistive exercises to reflect the goals and intended outcome of the overall program. Also consider the client's needs and movement capabilities. Several basic considerations are applicable to choosing exercises for the general population, and additional considerations apply to choosing exercises for people with various conditions associated with disabilities.

Muscle Balancing

The exercises you select for the training program and for each training session should consider muscle balance. Maintaining balanced strength between muscle pairs is essential for preventing injuries and for maintaining optimal range of motion and good body alignment.

Certain conditions associated with physical disabilities may challenge someone's ability to maintain muscle balance in certain muscle pairs. Many individuals who use wheelchairs overdevelop anterior shoulder muscles (pectoralis major and minor, and anterior deltoid muscles). Overstretch weakness in back musculature is also a common phenomenon with chronic sitting. Overuse of the anterior muscles from performing most daily activities in front of the body further increases imbalances in strength. When choosing resistive exercises for people who use a wheelchair, focus attention on strengthening muscles of the posterior shoulder and shoulder girdle. Combine those exercises with additional stretching for the muscles of the anterior shoulder.

Spasticity (abnormal increase in muscle tone), which is common with some types of cerebral palsy, head injury, stroke, and incomplete spinal cord injury, can also provoke muscle imbalances. Spasticity in a muscle group may habitually place the limb in a position that shortens the muscle on one side of the joint and lengthens it on the opposing side. For example, with spastic CP, elbow, wrist, and knee flexors often display increased tone. Over a period of time, muscle imbalances increase to further reduce joint ROM and cause joint contractures (shortening of connective tissues at the joint). When graded carefully, resistance training for muscles opposing spastic muscle groups preserve or increase ROM at the joint. Although spastic muscles are not necessarily strong, be cautious using resistance training for spastic limbs to prevent temporary increases in abnormal muscle tone that could reduce functioning. Chapter 7 offers additional considerations for modifying resistance training with spasticity.

A comprehensive training program that aims to preserve or restore muscle balance also includes stretching, especially with spasticity. Chapter 9 includes further considerations for stretching with spasticity.

With such disabilities as muscular dystrophy, differing rates of muscle atrophy in muscle pairs create muscular imbalance, particularly in postural muscles. A resistance training program of mild intensity that focuses on preserving strength in unimpaired muscles helps delay the effects of these imbalances. Because the appropriateness of resistance training is questionable with muscular dystrophy (MD), seek the advice of a physician before prescribing any type of resistive work with this disorder.

To assure muscle balance, muscle groups with opposing actions should be worked in the same exercise session. One method for achieving balance is to use a "push-pull" routine. For example, a push exercise, such as the bench press, should be followed by a pull exercise, such as rowing, that will counter the push motion (see Figure 6.1). The bench press requires use of the pectoralis major and anterior deltoid muscles through the action of shoulder flexion and transverse adduction. Bent-over rows exercise posterior deltoids with transverse shoulder abduction and extension.

Single-Joint and Multijoint Exercises

Single-joint exercises isolate muscle groups by requiring movement from only one joint, whereas

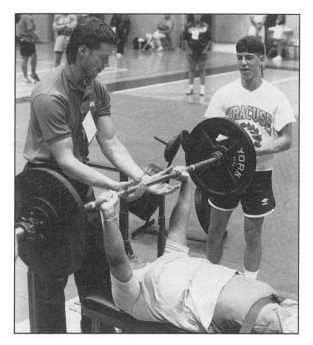

a

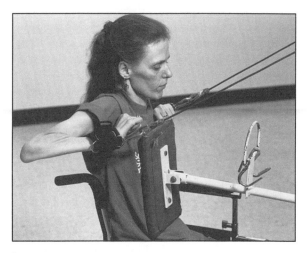

b

Figure 6.1 Muscle balancing with push-pull exercises using the bench press (a) and seated rows (b). Photos by Oscar Izquierdo.

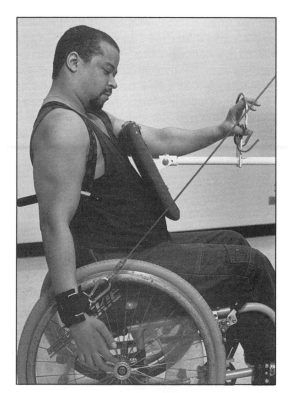

a

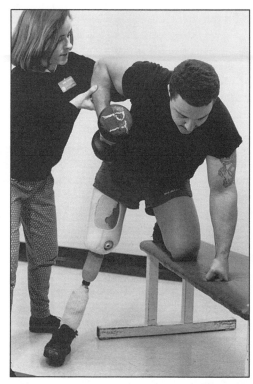

b

Figure 6.2 Examples of single-joint and multijoint exercises with resisted shoulder extension (a) and bent-over rows (b). Photos by Oscar Izquierdo.

multijoint exercises require movement at two or more joints. Resisted shoulder extension is an example of a single-joint exercise (see Figure 6.2a). The bent-over row is a multijoint exercise that requires movement at the shoulder and elbow joints (see Figure 6.2b). Multijoint exercises are often preferred over single-joint exercises because they are more time efficient and more typical of daily, general activities or sport skills. Multijoint exercise trains several muscle groups simultaneously, which minimizes the chances of developing muscle imbalances. Single-joint exercises may be preferred when weaker areas require special attention or when beginners are learning proper technique. People with impaired coordination (which is common with cerebral palsy, closed head injury, stroke, and multiple sclerosis) may find more success with simple, single-joint exercises because these exercises enable them to maintain balance and concentrate on proper technique throughout the exercise ROM.

Unilateral and Bilateral Exercises

Bilateral exercise (performing exercises with limbs on both sides of the body simultaneously) targets more proximal (shoulder and pelvic girdles) and torso strength than unilateral exercise (performing exercises with the extremity or limb on only one side of the body). Bilateral exercise may be useful for people with minimal torso control (ataxia) or with balance impairments such as those sometimes seen with multiple sclerosis and closed head injury. Increases in proximal strength may allow improved coordination and movement with the distal extremities or limbs (arms and legs). People with hemiplegia and moderate to severe coordination and balance impairments may require unilateral

exercises to maintain trunk stability and balance during exercise. Unilateral exercise is also useful when motor control is not equal on both sides. Figure 6.3 shows examples of unilateral and bilateral exercises.

Exercise Order

You can select an order for exercises to emphasize certain goals, to prevent fatigue from decreasing the value of the workout, or to simplify management of the group program. Traditionally, multijoint, "core" exercises that work several large muscle groups simultaneously are performed prior to working individual muscles (single-joint exercises). Performing single-joint, small-muscle-group exercise prior to large-muscle-group exercise may pre-exhaust the smaller working muscles and thus limit the intensity with which the large muscle groups can be exercised. Pre-exhaust routines have recently become popular, but their benefits have not been proven through scientific research. Another pre-exhaust system exercises synergists and assistors before exercising the prime mover, theoretically placing greater demands on the prime mover. In any case, the weakest link in the combination of muscle groups used to perform the exercise limits the potential strength stimulus.

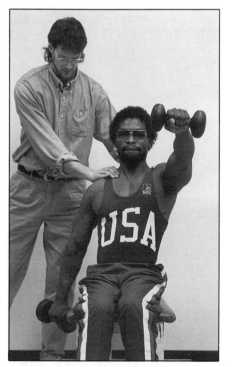

a

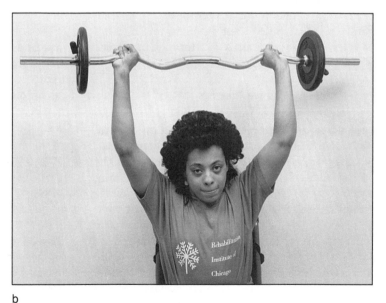

b

Figure 6.3 Unilateral (a) and bilateral (b) exercises. Photos by Oscar Izquierdo.

You can manipulate exercise order when designing the program to allow adequate recovery between sets of exercises. This is easily achieved by working one muscle group while another is allowed to fully recover. Alternating sets between agonists and antagonists, such as with the bench press and bent-over rows or upper body and lower body exercises, is recommended to allow recovery between sets. In a group program that uses resistive bands for training, a head-to-toe format may be the easiest to manage. However, you must be prepared to offer alternatives in a mixed group, such as additional upper body exercises for people with paraplegia while other class members perform leg exercises. Exercises with a similar setup, such as floor or partner exercise, also may be grouped together to help prevent delays between exercises and decrease the overall time of the complete workout.

Modes of Resistance

Mode of resistance refers to the type of external resistance applied during training. Because each mode requires different levels of independent balance and movement coordination by the user, they have been grouped into three general categories:

- Free weights
- Pulleys, bands, and manual resistance
- Machines

Each form of resistance has implications for safety, stability, and movement restriction. The needs and neuromuscular control of the participant, the availability of equipment, and general objectives of the program will determine the choice of resistance mode.

Free Weights

Resistance classified as free weights includes any device that does not restrict the user's movement, such as barbells, dumbbells, sandbags, cuff weights, or limb weight. Gravity determines the optimal line-of-pull and therefore the positioning of the body for effective use of the intended muscle group(s). Free-weight exercises can be structured to resemble daily functional actions and many sports movements, unlike exercises restricted by bands or machines. They also require synergistic action of stabilizing muscles to stabilize the torso and surrounding joints. The skills learned from free-weight resistive exercise training may also better train the neural system than exercise machines because "real life" movements are rarely limited

to actions of isolated muscles. With free-weight exercise training, the exerciser must independently balance and control the resistance throughout the complete ROM.

In cases of muscle weakness, limb weight may provide sufficient stress to fatigue a muscle with resistance training. As strength progresses, cuff weights can be added to increase resistance. In both cases, gravity still provides the force for resistance. With extreme muscle weakness, the force of gravity may actually be too great. In this situation, gravity-eliminated exercise may provide sufficient stress to exercise the muscle. Gravity-eliminated exercise involves moving the limb in an arc perpendicular to the force of gravity, for example by sliding it across a flat surface on or parallel to the floor. Figure 6.4 illustrates the position for a gravity-eliminated biceps curl.

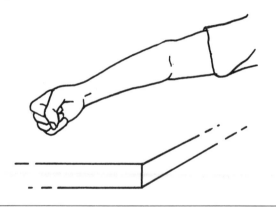

Figure 6.4 Gravity eliminated biceps curl.

Because skill, coordination, and good balance are prerequisites for safe and effective use of free weights, this mode of resistance may be inappropriate for beginners who are newly learning proper technique and control. Heavier lifts, such as with the bench press and squats, require assistance from a spotter and may not be safely feasible in a group exercise program. Free-weight resistance training may be contraindicated for individuals with impaired balance or coordination such as with disabilities resulting from injury to the brain.

Pulleys, Bands, and Manual Resistance

A second general category of resistance mode includes devices such as pulleys, stretch bands or tubing, and manual resistance. These modes of resistance restrict movement to a greater extent than with free weights, but they offer more freedom than with machines. With resistance fixed at one point, the line-of-pull is not restricted by gravity but rather by the attachment point of the device and orientation of the limb to that point. As with free weights, these devices require considerable skill and torso or joint stabilization for effective training. Unlike free weights, however, attached resistance is a safer mode of training for people with impaired balance and coordination. Manual resistance provided by a partner is another resistance mode with features similar to bands and pulleys.

Bands and pulleys are generally inexpensive, portable, and quite versatile. They are useful for group programs or for maintaining a program schedule at home when it may not be possible to work out at an exercise facility. Bands and pulleys can be used in a variety of ways. By using partners or attaching the equipment to chairs, doors, or hooks placed at different angles, virtually any line-of-pull can be achieved from any body position (see Figure 6.5). Because some nonambulatory individuals may prefer not to transfer from a wheelchair to exercise, stretch bands may offer exercising options not available with free weights that depend on gravity to determine the line-of-pull or with machines that are not wheelchair accessible.

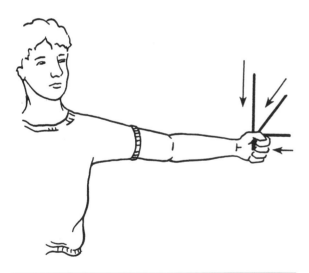

Figure 6.5 Stretch bands enable the user to modify the line-of-pull by changing the point of attachment.

A possible disadvantage of band, pulley, and manual resistance is that because it requires skill and knowledge to correctly set up the exercise to achieve an effective line-of-pull, some individuals may require the continual assistance of a skilled partner. In a group setting, it may be difficult to monitor every participant to ensure that they are performing exercises correctly and with enough tension to effectively work the muscles.

Another disadvantage of band and pulley resistance is that resistance gradually increases through the ROM, providing less resistance at the beginning of the exercise and much more stress at the end of the range. With movements requiring a large arc of motion, several sets of exercises at varying joint angles must be performed to effectively exercise the muscle through the full range. Manual resistance with a skilled partner, by contrast, can be adjusted to provide relatively equal tension throughout the range of movement.

Stretch bands or tubing, although available in different tensions, are not useful for quantitative assessment of effort or progress. Unlike with free weights or some machines, with bands and pulleys pounds of resistance cannot be used as a gauge to measure progress throughout the program. Hence, it is important that you teach each participant the feel of overload to compensate for lack of a measure of resistance in the program design. The inability to measure resistance with resistive bands may actually be an advantage for people with extreme muscle weakness or progressive disorders because the quantifiable progress that other modes of training measure cannot become a source of discouragement. Because bands and pulleys do not allow quantitative assessment, their use prevents comparison between participants—something you should discourage in any general fitness class, regardless of the mode of training used.

Exercise Machines

Resistive exercise machines provide the greatest stabilization, postural support, and restriction of movement of the three general types of resistance modes (see Figure 6.6). Because the equipment balances the weight and the seating partially stabilizes the body, resistive machines require less involvement of the small and accessory stabilizing muscles. For example, the Universal shoulder press minimizes use of the small stabilizing muscles of the shoulder girdle, which is an advantage for people with spinal cord injury who do not have independent sitting balance or have weakened rhomboids and trapezius muscles. However, it may be a disadvantage for people with fully functional trunk musculature to minimize use of these muscles because the result can be a weak area or muscle imbalance.

Resistance training with machines is also recommended for people with impaired motor control, such as with multiple sclerosis, closed head injury, and cerebral palsy, because the machines limit movement to an intended arc. Some machines, however, require bilateral movements, which may

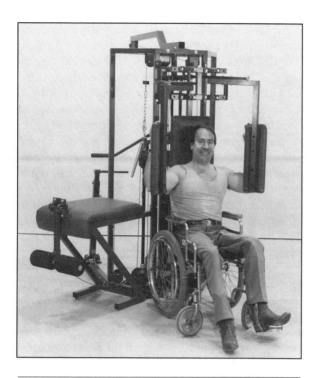

Figure 6.6 Resistance training exercise machine (The Equalizer) designed for wheelchair use. Photo courtesy of Helm Distributing, Inc.

not be appropriate for individuals with hemiplegic conditions or asymmetrical strength and control.

In general, resistive machines provide a higher degree of safety, are easier to use, and give people with impaired balance and coordination training opportunities that less restrictive modes of exercise may not provide.

Table 6.1 summarizes considerations for selecting an appropriate mode of resistance.

Training Systems

A training system is a preplanned progression of exercise sets for each muscle group. The variety of systems currently in practice is too extensive to include in this discussion, so you should consult texts, such as those suggested in the Recommended Readings, that explain scientifically based training systems. Of the myriad of systems in use, many have been designed only for serious weight trainers and may not be appropriate for a general fitness program. When selecting an appropriate system, consider the overall volume of the training session and overload applied to each muscle group. People with significant weakness, degenerative joint disease or instability, or progressive disorders should avoid high-volume, high-intensity training systems.

A brief description of several training systems follows. For each type, except the single-set system,

sets of exercises are preceded by a few warm-up sets of low-intensity repetitions.

> Single set to exhaustion: one set of exercises for each muscle group with a load selected to fatigue the muscle in a predetermined number of repetitions
>
> Multiple-set system: several sets of repetitions
>
> Heavy-to-light system: several sets of repetitions beginning with the heaviest load during the first set and progressing to the lightest load
>
> Light-to-heavy system: a reversal of the heavy-to-light system
>
> Pyramid system: combining light-to-heavy and heavy-to-light systems for each exercise.

Time limitations and the needs, capabilities, and goals of the participants will dictate your selection of an appropriate training system.

Program Development

It is generally appropriate to follow basic guidelines for resistance training development when designing programs for clients with physical disabilities. We reviewed these general guidelines in chapter 5. Precede the selection of exercise variables and the initiation of the program with assessment of baseline strength and movement abilities. Also consider characteristics and stages of the disability to ensure each client's safety. Be sure to educate your participants about the safe use of equipment, proper technique, and training protocol, and closely monitor the progression of training to make adjustments when needed. Remember that for some people with progressive and neuromuscular conditions, resistance training may be limited to a maintenance program; observe carefully to ensure that the program does not decrease function for these participants.

Initial Assessment

Before you develop an individualized program for a client, use your initial assessment to evaluate these conditions:

- Motor control and coordination
- Balance and trunk stability
- Spasticity
- Range of motion and muscle imbalances
- Baseline strength and causes of weakness
- Muscle function

Table 6.2 summarizes considerations for program design.

Table 6.1 Selecting Modes of Resistance

Mode	Characteristics	Considerations for use
Free weights	LOP determined by gravity Requires use of stabilizing muscles Requires balance, skill, and control Permits movement freedom, simulates functional movements	Inappropriate for • Excessive weakness of proximal stabilizers • Impaired balance • Impaired coordination
Pulleys, bands, manual resistance	LOP determined by fixed point Requires use of stabilizing muscles Requires *some* balance, skill, and control	Appropriate for • Impaired balance and coordination (mild) • Mobility restrictions • Group programs • Home use
Machines	LOP determined by machine Provides support, stabilization Restricts movement freedom May not permit unilateral movements	Appropriate for • Most conditions (if accessible), especially impaired balance and coordination Maximum safety

LOP = line-of-pull

Table 6.2 Resistance Training Program Design: Critical Considerations With Specific Mobility Impairments

Impairment	Disabling conditions	Critical program considerations

Motor control and coordination	Spasticity
	Ataxia
	Athetosis
	Tremors
		Warm-up: practicing motor patterns
		Movement isolation
		Positioning: reflexes
		Exercise selection:
		    single-joint and multijoint exercises
		    unilateral and bilateral exercises
		    muscle balancing
		Safety: movement restriction
		Intensity: postexercise effects

Balance and trunk stability	Paralysis Hemiplegia Ataxia	Positioning: support and balance Exercise selection: unilateral and bilateral exercises Safety: stability

ROM and muscle imbalances	Spasticity
	Contractures
	Pain
	Joint deformities
		Warm-up: stretching for ROM
		Exercise selection:
		    muscle balancing
		    unilateral and bilateral exercises
		Intensity: pain
		Movement isolation

Weakness and muscle function	Paresis
	Deconditioning
	Progressive conditions
		Exercise selection:
		    muscle balancing
		    single-joint and multijoint exercises
		Safety and intensity:
		    joint stability
		    postexercise effects
		    overwork

Muscle Soreness

Muscle soreness 2 to 24 hr following exercise is a normal response to resistance training. However, delayed soreness beginning up to 48 hr after exercise is generally an indication of excessive overload during training. Eccentric contractions produce a greater degree of delayed muscle soreness than concentric or isometric exercise (Talag, 1973).

Participants should not be alarmed about slight postexercise soreness; however, they should recognize persistent soreness as a sign of overtraining or too rapid a progression of the exercise program. Resistance training can be resumed once muscle soreness declines. If muscle soreness interferes with function, the participant should not resume the exercise program until the soreness has completely subsided. The exercise program should be reevaluated prior to restarting training.

Use extreme caution designing exercise programs for people who have progressive and some neuromuscular disorders, such as muscular dystrophy, multiple sclerosis, and postpolio syndrome. Muscle soreness with these conditions, which may involve a gradual loss in muscular strength and mass over time, is a strong indication that the exercise overload was excessive, and exercise training with excessive work loads may be associated with permanent loss of muscle function with these conditions (Bennett & Knowlton, 1958; Feldman, 1985; Johnson & Braddom, 1971; Peach, 1990).

Summary

People with physical disabilities can enjoy many of the same health-related benefits from resistance training programs as people without disabilities. Resistance training may also enhance functioning and improve mobility. After prescreening for contraindications to training and to evaluate each participant's health and fitness levels, select appropriate program variables to meet individual needs and goals. Your knowledge of characteristics of physical disabilities, safety precautions associated with disabling conditions, and principles of conditioning enable you to develop safe and effective resistance training programs for your clients with physical disabilities. The next chapter offers suggestions for modifying exercises for general disabilities and specific conditions.

Chapter 7

Resistance Training With Stretch Bands: Modifying for Disability

Kate F. Baxter, MS, PT
Woodrow Wilson Rehabilitation Center, Fishersville, VA

Kevin F. Lockette, PT, CSCS
Rehabilitation Hospital of the Pacific, Honolulu

In chapter 6 we introduced guidelines for developing resistance training programs and provided general considerations for resistance training for people with disabilities. In this chapter, we focus on appropriate modifications for using stretch bands or tubing as the mode of exercise with specific conditions and disabilities. We include both technique modifications and program variables. Although the suggestions in this chapter apply to use of resistance bands, many of the principles are also useful with other modes of resistance.

This chapter provides suggestions for the proper use of resistive bands; addresses condition-specific modifications (weakness, impaired sensation, reduced tolerance to exercise, impaired balance, and impaired coordination) and modifications for specific types of disabilities (injury to the spinal cord, postpolio syndrome, progressive conditions, arthritis, amputation, and visual impairment). For more complete information regarding characteristics of physical disabilities, refer back to chapter 2.

Using Stretch Bands for Resistance Training

Resistance training with stretch bands (or tubing) can be an effective means of improving muscular strength and endurance. As described in the previous chapter (see p. 86), stretch bands are inexpensive, portable, versatile, and useful for group programs. Your preliminary assessment of each client helps you determine whether using stretch bands is appropriate and provides you with the information you need to formulate modifications for their use. With guidance, your clients will learn techniques that will give them a safe and effective resistive exercise workout.

Resistive bands or exercise tubing can be purchased individually or in bulk in a variety of colors, lengths, and tensions. Be sure to purchase bands in lengths of 6 or 7 ft (or more)—the normal 3-ft lengths are too short for many adapted exercise set-ups. Appendix C lists suppliers of this and other types of adapted equipment.

Teach your clients how to use resistive bands properly and safely. They should be sure the bands are attached to other objects securely. When a band releases unexpectedly, it can cause injury, especially if it snaps into the face. Also, it is important to inspect equipment regularly to check for small tears and rips. Discard any bands that show such signs of wear to prevent tearing from causing an injury during the workout.

Modifying for a Safe and Effective Workout

It is essential that you work individually with each client before offering stretch bands as an exercise mode so you can formulate modifications or determine if using the bands may be contraindicated. You also must identify any joint instabilities or weaknesses in muscles used for stabilizing or gripping.

Independent use of stretch bands for resistance training may not be possible for some people. People with impaired motor coordination, for example, may be unable to properly isolate movement with the relative freedom afforded by this mode of exercise. People with limited hand and muscle function may have difficulty securely attaching the bands to achieve an appropriate line-of-pull. Often, however, simply having a skilled partner or assistant available can make this mode of resistance accessible for most people.

You may need to modify the usual anatomical attachment points when weakness compromises joint stability. In this situation, you can identify points proximal to the unstable or weak joint (such as above the wrist, knee, or ankle) for modified arrangements. For example, attach the band above the knee for a seated hip abduction exercise, instead of below. In this set-up, with the knee in a flexed position, the powerful quadriceps are active in protecting the knee during the lateral movement; placing the band just above the knee eliminates any stress on the knee joint. Alternatively, you can protect the wrist by wrapping the band comfortably to add stability (See Figure 7.1). To avoid stress on joints, it is also essential that people with an amputation avoid attaching resistive bands to a prosthesis. By experimenting and using a little creativity, you can develop ways for most people to use resistive bands comfortably and easily.

It is generally helpful if you can prepare loops or handles in the bands before beginning a class to avoid delays once the workout begins. Figure 7.2 illustrates some examples of makeshift handles. Experiment with each person to determine which modifications work best.

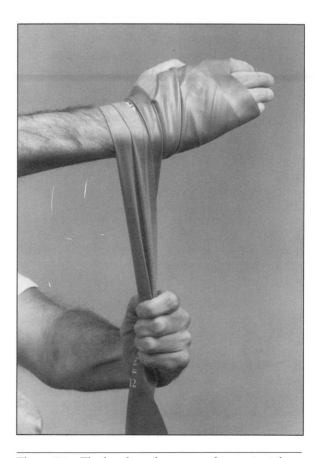

Figure 7.1 The band can be wrapped to protect the wrist and help maintain the desired neutral position.

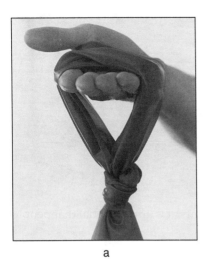
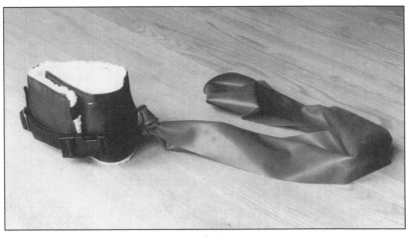

a
b

Figure 7.2 Handles and loops can be prepared in advance to accommodate gripping needs and weaknesses. Temporary loop for gripping (a) and home-made cuff for attaching stretch bands (b).

Technique Guidelines

During resistive work with stretch bands, good form and technique yield the best results and ensure the safety of all participants. In a group setting, it is essential that you are aware of each student. In some situations, it may be prudent to ask another instructor or qualified volunteer to help you monitor the class. Also, by thoroughly educating all your students about proper use of resistive bands, you share the responsibility for proper technique and effective training with participants and their assistants.

Consider offering your students the following reminders during the resistance training workout (many of these guidelines also apply to other modes of resistance training).

❏ Maintain good posture: Keep the neck and back in alignment in both sitting and standing postures.

❏ Isolate the intended movements: Avoid substitute movements to compensate for fatigue or muscle weakness if the band tension is excessive (especially at the end-point of the movement range).

❏ Maintain slow and controlled movements: Especially with the eccentric contraction, where there is a tendency to move too quickly and lose control of the movement, the end of the movement range should be distinct; discourage "flinging" actions. Counting aloud for each repetition is helpful in keeping movement speed in check. You may want to use two slow counts during the concentric contraction and four counts during the eccentric phase.

❏ Perform each repetition through the full available range of motion (ROM): However, discourage absolute full extension (locking-out the joint) at the end of the range.

❏ Maintain a neutral wrist position: Avoid permitting the band to pull the wrist into flexion or extension. Use alternative anatomical attachments for weakness as needed.

❏ Avoid breath holding: Encourage a normal pattern of breathing to prevent excessive elevations in systolic blood pressure. (Some sources recommend exhaling during the concentric contraction and inhaling through the eccentric range.)

❏ Apply tension throughout the movement range: Often, your beginners will have too little resistance at the beginning of the exercise and too much at the end to permit movement through the full range. Perform exercises for movements that involve a large available range in several arcs to ensure adequate tension at all angles of the movement. For example, with normal shoulder abduction, 180 degrees of motion is possible. Lateral raises can be performed in two or more arcs by using resistance from 0 to 90 degrees and then from 90 to 180 degrees (see Figure 7.3). The desired number of sets can be performed for each of the smaller ranges after adjusting the tension to yield the appropriate level of resistance for each arc. Although this can add time to the overall exercise session, use of smaller arcs for each movement gives people with limited functional muscle mass more opportunity for full participation in the group resistance training class.

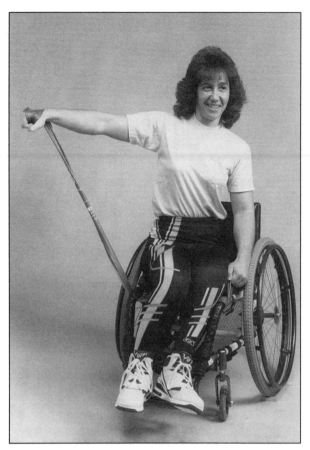

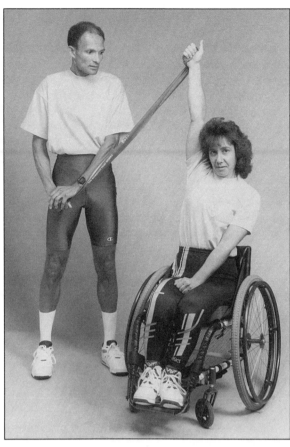

a   b

Figure 7.3 Two arcs of movement can be used for exercises with a large range of motion. Resistance can be applied through the first 90 degrees of shoulder abduction (a) and then readjusted to provide resistance for 90 to 180 degrees of movement (b).

❏ Use the correct line-of-pull: Secure the band at an appropriate angle to provide resistance throughout the movement range and to isolate the target muscle or muscle groups. A general rule for evaluating line-of-pull is to examine whether the band forms a right angle with the moving segment (arm, leg, etc.) at about the midpoint of the movement range.

Modifications for Specific Conditions

Several different disabilities may have common conditions or impairments for which general modifications with resistance training are appropriate. In this section, we look at exercise implications with weakness, impaired sensation, deconditioning, impaired balance and trunk stability, and impaired coordination.

Weakness

Chapter 3 reviewed causes of weakness (see Figure 3.1 on p. 40). It is important to know the cause of weakness before prescribing the exercise load or anticipating progress from training. If any tubing or band resistance is too great for weak muscles, the participant may use positions in which gravity alone provides resistance or may use gravity-reduced positions. For example, a person with an incomplete spinal cord injury might have quadriceps muscles that are too weak to extend the knee against resistance from a seated position (from 90 degrees of knee flexion to full knee extension). The weight of the limb against gravity alone may provide enough resistance for this exercise. The same arc of motion could also be performed lying on the side to reduce the effects of gravity if limb weight provides too much resistance. As strength improves, the participant can add band resistance to further overload the muscle.

Impaired Sensation

Impairment to sensory nerves may be associated with injuries to the brain and spinal cord. The inability to sense external stimuli may prevent an individual from detecting skin irritations or wounds. People who wear any type of brace while exercising must pay careful attention to prevent skin irritation from developing as a result of pressure or rubbing on the appliance. Other sources of skin irritation that require caution are the wheelchair or the resistive material itself.

Deconditioning

Many people with a disability who begin an exercise program are deconditioned, often secondary to inactivity caused by mobility problems associated with the disability. People who have been sedentary for extended periods have a very low tolerance to exercise. Because an exercise or fitness program should be designed to improve the quality of life and enhance functionality, prescribe and monitor exercise overload carefully to prevent undue fatigue or a decline in function. These problems are of particular concern with people who have progressive degenerative disorders.

Impaired Balance and Trunk Stability

Balance may be affected by either structural or neuromuscular impairments. Ambulatory people with lower limb amputations may experience balance problems with standing exercise. Double high AK amputations or hip disarticulation challenge sitting balance. Brain injuries that impair motor control (such as with head injury or cerebral palsy) and spinal cord injuries that cause paralysis also impair balance and trunk stability.

People who exercise from a seated position and who have limited trunk control or balance may want to exercise one side of the body at a time. To maintain balance with upper body exercise, someone in a wheelchair may either hold onto the chair or hook the nonexercising arm around the push handle of the wheelchair to increase stability (see Figure 7.4). You can wrap straps, belts, or elastic binders around the participant and the wheelchair to aid in trunk stability while performing exercises with the extremities (see Figure 7.5).

Impaired Coordination

Because movement is regulated and coordinated by the central nervous system, injury to the brain

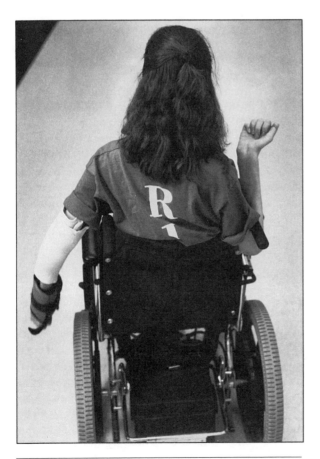

Figure 7.4 The nonexercising arm can be hooked around the push handle of the wheelchair for added trunk stability. Photo by Oscar Izquierdo.

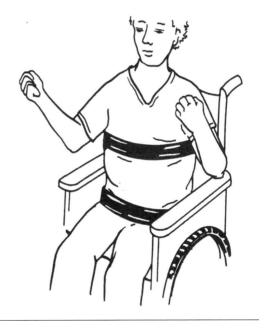

Figure 7.5 Abdominal binders can be used to aid upright posture with impaired trunk musculature.

is often associated with impaired coordination. Someone with severe involvement may require the assistance of a partner for spotting and to help with exercise set-ups.

In general, people with impaired coordination benefit from relaxation or stretching exercises before beginning resistive exercise training. Some people may need to spend additional time practicing motor patterns without resistance before attempting to strengthen muscles.

Spasticity

Considerable controversy still remains regarding the appropriateness of resistance training with spasticity. Although not substantiated with research, it has traditionally been believed that resistance training further decreases ROM or possibly increases spasticity. However, because spasticity has a neural base that involves involuntary, uncontrolled movements with the initiation of an action (causing activation rather than inhibition of antagonists) and because resistance training tends to result in increased inhibition of antagonist muscles, the validity of this traditional viewpoint can be questioned. A proper conditioning program for people with spasticity offers exercises for opposing muscle groups and ends with stretching and relaxation drills. Any temporary increase in tension in spastic muscles that may occur with increased muscular effort should not result in a decline in function or permanent increase in spasticity if the exercise program is properly prescribed and monitored. Routinely check with your clients who have spasticity during succeeding exercise sessions to determine if any decrease in function occurred following training. If a decrease does occur, adjust the exercise load to prevent further incidents.

Involved limbs may experience a temporary increase in spasticity when exercises are performed by a contralateral nonspastic limb. This increase is generally transient and should subside soon after the session. Spasms with exercise are also generally transient and should not have any significant effect on the person's ability to function after exercise. Instruct your clients with spasticity to avoid quick movements because they may cause a spasm. After a spasm occurs, allow the muscles to relax before continuing exercise.

Avoid massaging or applying pressure to the spastic muscle belly to prevent a reflexive increase in muscle tone. To provide assistance with movement during resistive work, only grasp bony structures at or distal to the joint. For example, during a biceps curl, grasp the medial and lateral bony prominence at the elbow and wrist if necessary to guide movement through the exercise.

Clients should only train spastic muscles in a general fitness class if they can isolate movement in the target muscle or muscle groups. For example, the participant should be able to perform elbow flexion without shoulder flexion occurring simultaneously. If synergistic movement patterns such as this occur, exercise training for involved muscle groups should be left to the therapist. In general, use a conservative approach with resistance training for any spastic muscle groups, and avoid high-intensity training.

During resistance training, you should always encourage proper form; however, remember that *ideal* is a relative and individualistic term. Spasticity generally decreases movement control and ROM. Be sure you are aware of each person's movement potential so you can give appropriate feedback.

When muscle weakness due to paresis accompanies spasticity, such as with hemiparetic conditions, aggressive resistance training may not be appropriate. Consult with the person's therapist or physician before recommending an exercise load with this condition.

To improve or maintain muscle balance and joint ROM, direct your focus to strengthening muscle groups that oppose tight, spastic muscles. Spastic muscle groups should be stretched with general ROM exercises (after warming the muscle) or relaxed prior to applying resistance. Chapters 8 and 9 offer further suggestions on stretching.

If you question the value of resistance training with spastic muscle groups, remember that a spastic limb is not necessarily strong, yet it still must be used for activities of daily living. Improving function, muscle balance, and voluntary control of a muscle are desired goals of a resistance training program. Although a strengthening program will not eliminate spasticity, it should not worsen it.

Athetosis and Ataxia

Athetoid movements are involuntary and unpredictable. Muscle tone can vary from hypertonic to hypotonic. People with athetosis should avoid using free weights or resistive equipment that does not provide guidance with movement patterns. The best initial exercise program for people with prominent athetoid movements might focus simply on learning movement patterns before applying any resistance.

With ataxia, muscles are hypotonic, causing difficulty with movement accuracy. Use caution to prevent excessive resistance from compromising joint function with this condition. Exercise machines can provide needed guidance with movement patterns to assist with exercise training. As with any disability, experiment with different modes and exercises with little or no resistance to determine the best choices for each individual.

Modifications for Specific Disabilities

You must remain aware of precautions and modifications for participants with specific disabilities to provide a safe and effective resistance training program. This section offers guidelines for several common disabilities. For concerns about disabilities not discussed in this book, it is imperative that you consult with the individual's therapist or physician to develop appropriate modifications.

Injury to the Spinal Cord

Disabilities that cause injury to the spinal cord (such as SCI or spina bifida) can result in spastic paralysis or paresis. Conditions associated with this disorder may include weakness, impaired sensation, deconditioning, and impaired balance. Training implications discussed in the previous section for these conditions apply. In addition, consider the following safety points and modifications with injury to the spinal cord:

❏ Caution people with quadriplegia against extremes of neck range of motion, particularly neck hyperextension.

❏ Limit trunk rotation in people whose spines have been surgically fused or stabilized with Harrington rods or other such internal rod devices.

❏ People with paralysis often use substitute actions and muscle groups to replace actions normally controlled by the muscles that become paralyzed. Because these muscles were not intended to perform the alternate action, they may need to be strengthened and balanced with other muscle groups. For example, an individual with impaired triceps function, such as with C5 and C6 quadriplegia, can often perform exercises that normally require the use of triceps (C7 level of innervation) if he externally rotates the shoulder to allow gravity to passively "lock" the elbow into extension (See Figure 7.6a). Remember,

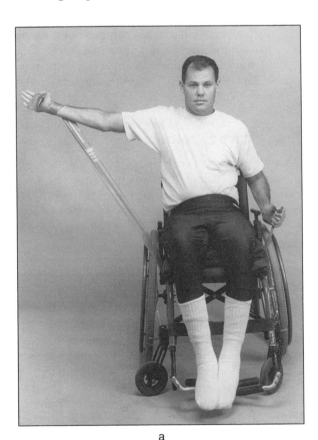

a

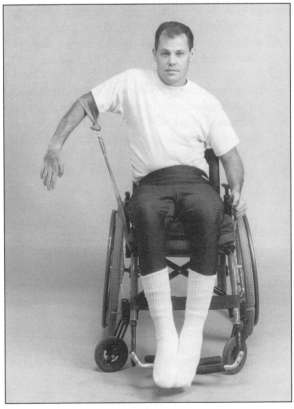

b

Figure 7.6 Alternative positions can be used for shoulder exercises with nonfunctioning triceps muscles: external rotation of the shoulder passively locks the triceps into extension (a) and alternative band placement allows middle deltoid work (b).

however, that a change in position also changes the muscle group being exercised. During upright shoulder abduction with the palms facing the floor the shoulder is in a neutral position (not requiring internal or external rotation), and the prime mover is the middle deltoid muscle. However, if the shoulder is externally rotated before performing the same exercise, the anterior deltoid and biceps muscles become the prime movers.

If triceps are nonfunctional or too weak to support elbow extension, the middle deltoid muscle can still be exercised with use of elbow splints or air casts. Another alternative is to place resistance above the elbow with cuff weights or by attaching bands or tubing just above the elbow joint, thus eliminating the need for maintaining elbow extension (see Figure 7.6b).

❏ People with impaired hand function often rely on tenodesis, a passive finger flexion response to active wrist extension, for gripping. In this case, the person should avoid applying resistance distal to the wrist joint, such as by attaching a cuff weight to the hand, because it can lead to excessive forced extension or flexion of the wrist and fingers, decreasing the effectiveness of a tenodesis grasp or resulting in musculoskeletal injuries that reduce hand function.

❏ People with lower body paralysis may have full upper body function and can benefit from a full resistance training program without restrictions. They can perform back exercises from a bent-over position in the wheelchair or regular chair.

Postpolio Syndrome

Some people experience a decline in function many years after initially contracting polio. This condition, termed postpolio syndrome, is characterized by progressive muscle weakness, fatigue, and pain with exertion (Halstead, 1990). Until further research is available on the effects of resistance training with postpolio syndrome, use caution prescribing exercises for people with this condition.

When working with individuals who have had polio, keep the following safety considerations in mind:

❏ Resistance training for symptomatic muscles in people with postpolio syndrome is contraindicated.

❏ Resistive work with nonsymptomatic muscles (as determined by clinical testing) should target development of muscular endurance through low-resistance, high-repetition sets. Before beginning the program, however, obtain clearance from the individual's physician. Increases in training volume (with increases in either load or number of reps) should be gradual, based on the person's tolerance and comfort.

❏ Proceed generally with resistance training for asymptomatic muscles affected by polio that have become weak with disuse. A safe program for people with this condition would be to engage in resistance training for 3 months to increase muscular endurance to levels that will enhance functioning. A program to increase cardiovascular endurance or functional activities of daily living should follow (Grimby & Einarsson, 1991). Long-term, continuous resistive programs are not recommended due to current uncertainties associated with this disorder.

❏ Persistent postexercise pain and fatigue are indications that the exercise intensity or volume was too great. Reduce the load to a level that does not elicit such a response, or exercise to a submaximal level rather than to the point of muscular fatigue. With persistent symptoms, discontinue training and consult the person's physician.

Progressive Disorders

Although diseases such as multiple sclerosis and muscular dystrophy remain incurable and irreversible, a resistance training program can help an individual to maintain or delay declines in function as their disease progresses. A common characteristic with progressive disorders is that with time, fewer and fewer muscle fibers are available to perform work. With MS, fatigue may become a significant symptom and can limit daily function. Stress the importance of remaining as active as possible within the limits of safety and comfort to prevent disuse weakness.

Resistance training may not be appropriate for everyone with progressive diseases; the extent of muscle degeneration and progression of the disorder determine the appropriateness of training. Consult the individual's physician before initiating any exercise program. In addition, consider the following precautions:

❏ Use caution to avoid overworking and possibly damaging apparently unaffected muscles. Limit the overall training volume for each session to prevent excessive fatigue after exercise. The resistance load with each set of repetitions (10 to 15 reps are generally recommended) should not carry the muscle to fatigue; instead approximately 70% of the load needed to fatigue the muscle for a specified number of repetitions is advisable. Encourage adequate rest as needed during training sessions.

❑ People with MS should generally avoid exercising in hot or humid environments because this may increase postexercise fatigue. If they do exercise under hot and humid conditions, exercise intensity should be further reduced.

❑ Resistance training should be significantly modified or temporarily stopped during periods of exacerbation. Obtain medical clearance before resuming the program.

❑ Carefully monitor people with progressive conditions; increase training volume or load very gradually.

Arthritis

Arthritis is characterized by joint pain with movement, especially ballistic, high-impact, and heavily resisted movements. The goal of a resistive exercise program for people with arthritis should be to improve function and range of motion without increasing pain or discomfort. Consider the following precautions when working with clients who have arthritis:

❑ To avoid unwanted stress, wear and tear, inflammation, and trauma on joints affected by arthritis, recommend a program consisting of moderate to high repetitions and very low resistance.

❑ When flare-ups occur, particularly with rheumatoid arthritis, the individual should skip several resistance training sessions before resuming the program.

❑ Isometric exercises can be used, if tolerated, in place of dynamic exercises when pain limits movement. To derive benefits through the full range of motion, static exercise at several joint angles, including each extreme of the range, should be performed. Isometric exercise is beneficial at the specific joint angle where the exercise is performed, and a carryover of plus or minus 20 degrees is possible (Knapik, Mawdsley, & Ramos, 1983). Meyers (1967) determined that static contractions of

26 s result in greater carryover to adjacent joint angles. Hence, isometric exercise may be an effective way to improve dynamic strength in people with arthritis who experience pain with repetitive movement.

Amputation

An amputated limb should be exercised to prevent contractures, maintain postural alignment, and enhance function. Because balance may be impaired with lower limb amputations, keep in mind points discussed previously regarding standing and sitting balance (see p. 95). Consider the following additional points when leading resistive exercise programs for people with amputation:

❑ Exercise the muscles of a residual limb. If the stump is too short for conventional weight machines or to accommodate resistive bands, use cuff weights. For very short above-elbow or above-knee amputations (just below the shoulder or hip joints), manual resistance may be the most efficient mode of exercise. If you include bilateral exercises in the program, additional resistance or weight may have to be applied to the amputated limb to equalize the resistance on both sides. Remember that force applied at a shorter lever-arm length provides less resistance.

❑ People with a lower extremity prosthesis often develop postural defects and muscle imbalances because they develop an abnormal gait. In the lower trunk, these problems typically involve shortened low-back and hip flexor muscles as well as overstretched abdominals. Upper body imbalances may also result, producing tightened rhomboids and middle trapezius muscles and overstretched pectorals. Strengthening overstretched and weaker muscles combined with stretching shortened muscles helps restore optimal muscle balance, possibly providing a remedy for the low-back pain that may accompany the condition.

❑ Caution people with amputation, particularly those with bilateral AK amputations, to be careful not to lose their balance during a forward lean, such as with seated back extensor or seated abdominal exercises, when the center of gravity radically shifts.

❑ When a client performs resistive exercises wearing a prosthesis, he should only apply force through the long axis of the limb. Applying resistance at an angle to the line of the prosthesis creates the danger of rubbing or shearing on the residual limb (see Figure 7.7). With this principle in mind, also avoid attaching equipment to the prosthesis with resistive exercise because the equipment may place such a perpendicular or shearing force on the limb.

❏ Encourage the individual with an amputation to check the residual limb or limbs regularly during a training program for any new skin irritations, especially in diabetics who may have decreased sensation.

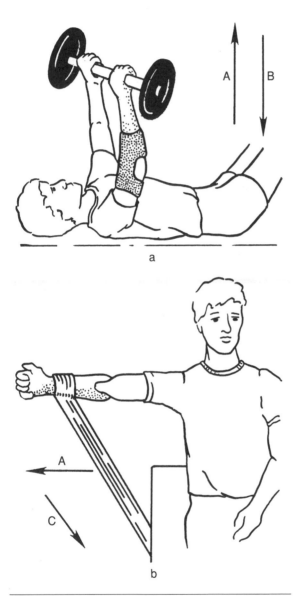

Figure 7.7 Resistive exercises with a below-elbow prosthesis: bench press with a direct line of force (a) and lateral raise with application of an improper shearing force (b). A = axis of limb, B = direct line of force, C = shearing force

Visual Impairment

Although visual impairment is not generally considered a physical disability, this condition can affect a person's movement and may require that you adapt your teaching methods. Chapter 12 includes general considerations for leading exercise programs for people with visual impairments and Hegey and Aceves (1991) offer these guidelines:

❏ Provide a thorough verbal and tactile introduction before beginning a resistance training program. Identify each muscle group to be exercised and ask the participant to locate the muscle by feeling for the attachment points and muscle belly. If the person is unsure of the muscle location, ask if he wants you to show him physically.
❏ Provide minimal physical assistance only when needed. Start with verbal cues; offer physical contact only as a supplement.
❏ Allow new participants adequate time to feel and test the equipment before beginning an exercise program.
❏ Introduce correct movement terminology from the beginning to enhance communication between you and the participant and between other participants in the program.
❏ In group programs or programs in a weight room, have a partner or assistant help the participant locate the exercise equipment and set up for each exercise.

Summary

In this chapter, we have applied the principles of conditioning and program design for resistance training (from chapters 5 and 6) to specific conditions and disabilities. We offered guidelines for exercise with stretch bands or tubing to provide a safe and effective resistance training workout. Stretch bands offer versatility for group programs and enable you to modify exercise set-ups to compensate for weaknesses or neurological and muscle dysfunction. Your ability to lead safe and effective exercise programs for your clients with disabilities depends upon your knowledge of these considerations and your ability to apply them to meet individual needs.

Chapter 8

Flexibility Training: Program Design

Paul R. Surburg, PhD, RPT
Indiana University

A holistic approach to physical fitness involves exercise training for development of strength, muscular and cardiorespiratory endurance, appropriate body composition, and flexibility. Too often, however, flexibility is the neglected component of the otherwise comprehensive fitness program. Flexibility is an especially critical component of the exercise prescription for people with physical disabilities because of its value in maintaining muscle balance and functional abilities. This chapter provides information about flexibility, range of motion, factors that influence flexibility development, and stretching techniques as they pertain to people with physical disabilities.

Benefits of Flexibility

Flexibility is a vital component of total physical fitness, providing functional, recreational, and therapeutic benefits. These benefits for people with physical disabilities may include

- enhancing performance of the activities of daily living,
- improving mobility and independence,
- maintaining or improving posture and muscle balance,
- improving performance in recreational and sport activities,
- preventing injury,
- reducing postexercise muscle soreness, and
- optimizing the ability to perform dynamic exercise for other fitness modalities.

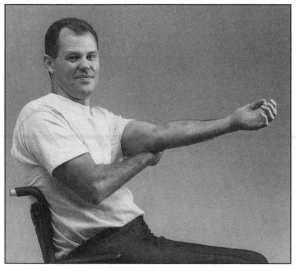

a

Flexibility and Range of Motion

Corbin and Lindsey (1985) described *flexibility* as "a measure of the range of motion available at a joint or group of joints." Alter (1988) describes two types of flexibility: static flexibility, or the degree of movement possible through a range without emphasis on speed or time of movement, and dynamic flexibility, the dynamic quality of movement through a range, considering speed, such as during physical activity. Range of motion (ROM), measurable in linear or angular units, refers to the degree of motion at a joint, and stretching is the process of elongating muscle and connective tissue to increase ROM and improve flexibility. The terms flexibility, range of motion, and stretching are not synonymous and should not be used interchangeably.

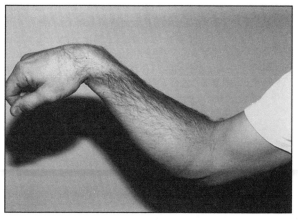

b

Figure 8.1 Functional range of motion. Optimal end-point for elbow extension (a) and functional end-point in person with spastic cerebral palsy (b).

Optimal and Functional Range of Motion

Establishing or maintaining optimal ROM should be an integral part of all physical fitness programs. However, for some people the concept of "functional range of motion" may be more appropriate at certain joints because limitations associated with the disability make full ROM impossible. The limits of the disabling condition and the ROM needed to permit adequate functioning, mobility, and independence define the functional range of motion. For example, someone with spasticity in a limb may have extremely variable joint ROM, but the upper limits will never exceed a certain percentage of the normal range (see Figure 8.1b). As an exercise leader, modify what you consider optimal and

focus instead on functional ROM as defined by individual needs and differences.

The optimal range of motion varies among individuals and is specific not only to the joint but also to the direction of movement within the joint. For example, most people have 90 degrees of wrist flexion but only 70 degrees of wrist extension. ROM may also vary in the same joints on opposite sides of the body, especially with hemiplegic conditions and spastic cerebral palsy.

Maintaining a functional ROM is very important for people with physical disabilities. With some activities, a person with a disability may have to substitute or adapt certain movements of the body that require a greater ROM at the involved joints in order to effectively perform a skill.

Joint Stability

Certain types of disabilities require judgments about an appropriate ROM for each joint. Both too much and too little flexibility may have a detrimental effect upon functioning or may result in muscle or other tissue damage. Postural or joint problems are not always the result of restricted ROM; excessive flexibility may also affect the stability of the joint. For example, with the condition genu recurvatum (hyperextended knees), excessive extensibility of the hamstrings compromises the stability of the knee joint. In this case, excessive flexibility is not an optimal condition. Destabilized joints are less protected from trauma and forceful stresses, and increments in joint laxity may lead to joint-related problems such as subluxation and dislocation.

Factors That Influence Flexibility

Factors that influence ROM and flexibility at each joint may be classified as neuromuscular or biomechanical in nature. Limitations may be accordingly classified by the source of the limitation: whether the nervous system is involved or whether limitations are due to the structure of the joint and the viscoelastic properties of joint tissues. Table 8.1 summarizes neuromuscular and biomechanical influences on flexibility development.

Neuromuscular Influences

The nervous system normally regulates stretch and tension development in the muscle. The muscle spindle and Golgi tendon organ (GTO) are the primary receptors that sense changes in the length and tension of the muscle. The neuromuscular actions of the stretch reflex, inverse stretch reflex, and reciprocal inhibition regulate muscle elonga-

Table 8.1 Neuromuscular and Biomechanical Influences on Flexibility Development

	Neuromuscular influences	Biomechanical influences
Structures and functions	Stretch reflexes • The nervous system • Muscle spindles • Golgi tendon organs	Viscoelastic properties of connective tissues Joint structure Joint position (with bi-articular muscles)
Stretching protocols	Static stretching (low load) PNF stretching Relaxation	Static stretching Tissue temperature
Limiting conditions	Spasticity	Scar tissue Adhesions Contractures Joint deformities

tion. The review box summarizes definitions for these mechanisms.

Proprioceptive neuromuscular facilitation (PNF) stretching techniques were originally developed as a neuromuscular model of flexibility development. Several of these techniques are discussed beginning on page 108.

A hypersensitive stretch reflex, as with spasticity, limits ROM and flexibility. People with spasticity may find flexibility exercises that minimize the role of the stretch reflex such as relaxation, prolonged static stretching, and PNF techniques, to be most effective.

Biomechanical Limitations

The structure of the joint and the characteristics and arrangement of the connective and contractile tissues that cross the joint limit joint ROM.

FOR REVIEW . . .

Influences of the Stretch Reflex, Reciprocal Inhibition, and the Inverse Stretch Reflex

Stretch reflex—reflexive response to stretch (detected by the muscle spindle) that causes the stretched muscle to contract; increased by a sudden, ballistic stretch.

Reciprocal inhibition—reflex action of muscle pairs that causes the antagonist of a contracting muscle to relax.

Inverse stretch reflex—response to tension in the tendon generated by a strong stretch or muscle contrac-

tion (detected by the Golgi tendon organ) that causes the tensed muscle to relax (also referred to as autogenic inhibition).

Together, these reflexes act in the normally functioning nervous system to protect the muscle from overstretching or developing excessive tension.

Joint Structure

The underlying structural composition of a joint determines its movement capabilities. These capabilities are designated by degrees of freedom, the number of different types of movement possible at a specific joint. For example, the shoulder (glenohumeral) joint has three degrees of freedom (flexion/extension, medial/lateral rotation, adduction/abduction). The shape of the articulating surfaces also affects movement range. Although the hip and shoulder are both ball and socket joints possessing three degrees of freedom, the ROM in the hip is more limited because of the greater depth of the hip socket.

Muscles that cross more than one joint also influence joint ROM. Contraction of a uniarticular muscle causes only one joint to move. A biarticular muscle affects two joints. For example, the biarticular nature of the hamstrings muscles reduces ROM at the hip when the knee is extended (see Figure 8.2). For this reason, when stretching biarticular muscles (such as the quadriceps, hamstrings, and gastrocnemius) consider the position of both joints that are crossed.

Viscoelastic Properties of Soft Tissues

Connective tissues that surround the joint have characteristic structural properties that define their ability to elongate or resist stretch, depending on the nature of the stretching force that is applied. These tissues are composed of fibrous (inelastic) and elastic elements. Viscosity (plasticity) is defined as resistance to flow and represents the non-elastic quality of fibrous tissues that provides joint stability. (Note that viscosity is reduced with elevations in temperature). The fibrous tissues are primarily collagenous and are found in ligaments, tendons, fascia, and aponeuroses (flat tendons). Collagen is also found in scar tissue, adhesions, and permanent contractures caused by corrective surgeries or chronic limitations in joint ROM. Collagenous tissue is characterized by its strength and resistance to stretch. It protects elastic tissues from overstretching. Tissues with a greater proportion of collagen than elastin have restricted ROM but provide rigidity and stability to the structures they surround. Immobilization, inactivity, and aging decrease the collagenous content in tissue and weaken it. Overstretching collagenous tissue can result in tissue sprain.

Elastic connective tissue surrounds the muscle and its various subcomponents. Elasticity allows a tissue that has been stretched to return to its resting length. Elastic tissues are more resistant to injury. However, overstretching elastic tissue can result in muscle strain.

Specific qualities of a stretch influence either the viscous or elastic nature of connective tissues. Viscosity is affected most by low-load, long-duration stretching, which favors more permanent elongation of connective tissues. Elastic properties are addressed more with high-load, short-duration stretching, favoring temporary elongation.

During flexibility training the viscoelastic properties of joint tissues must be protected. In other words, stretching must increase ROM and flexibil-

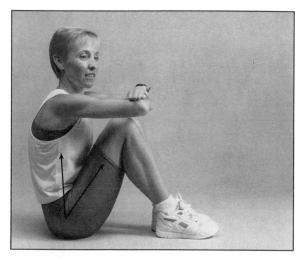
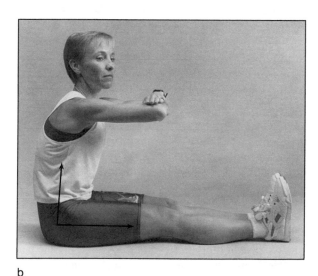

a   b

Figure 8.2 The hamstrings are a two-joint muscle group. Deeper hip flexion is permitted with knee flexion (a) than with knee extension (b).

ity without decreasing joint stability. Coping with this delicate balance in flexibility protocols is an important consideration. The hurdler's stretching exercise (Figure 8.3), for example, has been criticized because of the stress it places on ligaments of the knee, despite its effectiveness in improving joint range of motion. When the inelastic ligaments surrounding the knee are lengthened, the stability of the knee joint may be compromised.

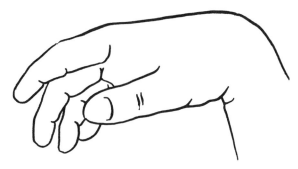

a

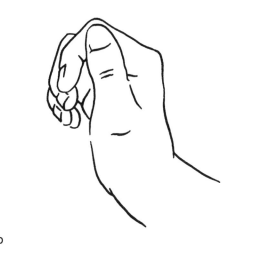

b

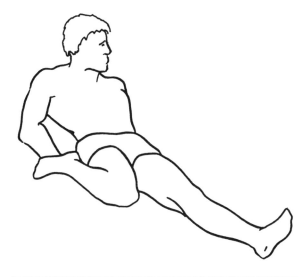

Figure 8.3 The hurdler's stretch might compromise stability of the knee joint.

Maintaining a restricted range of motion in certain muscle groups may actually be of value when a restricted ROM enhances function. For example, with paralysis of finger flexors, tenodesis permits grasping when wrist flexors maintain a certain degree of inflexibility. Tenodesis causes fingers to passively flex when the wrist is actively hyperextended (see Figure 8.4). Overstretching finger flexors while simultaneously stretching wrist flexors can greatly reduce hand function in people who rely on the tenodesis action for grasping. A certain degree of inflexibility in back extensors may also be beneficial for providing additional postural support with conditions involving paralysis of the trunk. Carried to an extreme, however, excessive tightness in the back and hip flexors may impose limitations on functioning by making activities that require reaching toward the lower extremities, such as dressing, more difficult.

In some cases, permanent elongation or deformation of specific collagenous tissues may be the primary objective of a flexibility program when adhesions, scar tissue, or adaptive shortening (contractures) occur in muscles and connective tissues.

Figure 8.4 Inflexible wrist flexors permit grasping through the tenodesis action. Passive wrist flexion (a) and passive finger flexion with active wrist hyperextension (b).

A health care professional should prescribe and carefully monitor a stretching program to elongate collagenous tissues for people with these conditions.

Additional Influences

Other factors that may influence flexibility include these:

Age: flexibility generally increases through adolescence and then begins to decline with advancing age (especially with inactivity).

Gender: females tend to be more flexible than males.

Temperature: temporary increases in intramuscular temperatures are associated with increased joint ROM.

Muscle balance and resistance training: training should be balanced between opposing muscle groups and performed through the full ROM.

Immobilization: transient increases in ROM occur when a muscle is immobilized in a lengthened position; with immobilization in a shortened position, effects are transient if the immobilization is followed by a period of stretching.

Pain with movement: people voluntarily restrict movement range with pain.

Research has not substantiated claims that body type influences flexibility. However, extreme obesity may limit ROM at certain joints.

Uses of Stretching

Stretching is used in three different contexts: for warm-up or cool-down, for progressive improvements in flexibility as part of a physical fitness or sports program, and for rehabilitation. All roles of flexibility training are applicable to people with disabilities. Table 8.2 summarizes the purposes and effects of stretching.

Table 8.2 Purposes of Stretching

Objective	Specific effects
Warm-up	Increases tissue temperature
	Slowly increases circulation
	Gradually produces normal ROM
	Improves performance
	Reduces risk of injury
Cool-down	Gradually reduces exercise intensity (decreasing stress on the circulatory system)
	Reduces tissue temperature
	Reduces development of muscle soreness
	Maintains flexibility
Physical fitness	Optimizes functioning
	Enhances performance
Rehabilitation	Restores or improves movement for independent functioning

Warm-Up and Cool-Down

As part of a warm-up routine before activity, stretching is generally more useful for preparing the body for activity than for developing long-term improvements in flexibility. With spasticity, a prolonged period of stretching during the warm-up helps increase ROM before dynamic exercises. Immediately following exercise, cool-down stretching helps the muscles recover from activity, and it may help reduce muscle soreness. With spasticity, stretching during the cool-down is essential for restoring ROM, which may have decreased during physical activity.

Physical Fitness

A second use of stretching exercises is to improve overall physical fitness or sport performance through flexibility training. The prescribed exercise program for flexibility development will vary with the goals of the individual. Stretching to improve flexibility should be performed after an adequate warm-up or after the cool-down from vigorous activity when intramuscular temperatures are still elevated.

Rehabilitation

Stretching also plays an important role in the rehabilitative process for both acute injury and chronic conditions. At one time rehabilitation programs consisted of the following sequence of exercises: passive, active-assisted, active, and resistive exercises. Although the traditional rehabilitative adage of establishing full ROM before proceeding to active or resistive exercises is no longer found in all rehabilitation protocols, developing ROM is still a major concern of most physical rehabilitation programs.

Some people with restricted ROM due to conditions associated with a disability may need to precede other forms of dynamic exercise with therapeutic stretching because of limitations that prevent them from realizing benefits with other modalities of fitness training. A health care professional must guide this type of stretching.

Stretching Techniques

A variety of techniques have been developed to improve joint ROM and flexibility in people with and without physical disabilities. Everyone involved in a physical fitness program can use these techniques except for passive stretching where sensation is absent. Only therapists or other trained medical personnel should perform this type of stretching on a person who lacks sensation.

Chapter 5 reviewed protocols for several stretching techniques. For information about the recommended frequency, intensity, and duration of stretching, see pages 70-71.

Passive Stretching

An external force—provided either manually or by a machine—accomplishes passive stretching; the individual being stretched does not participate actively. Nor do the muscles surrounding the joint being stretched with passive stretching actively contract. Passive stretching is used in a rehabilitation setting when a person is too weak to perform the exercise, lacks sensation, or is inhibited from performing the exercise by obstructive factors such as adhesions.

When someone lacks sensation, passive stretching exercises should only be administered by medically trained personnel and should not be used in the general or group fitness program. A person who lacks sensation in part of the body is incapable of providing feedback to a partner performing a passive stretch. Professionals qualified to perform passive stretching are trained to "feel" safe limits in joint range of motion to prevent causing injury during the procedure.

Active-Assisted Stretching

Active-assisted stretching involves the combined efforts of an assistant or an external force (such as gravity) and the participant. The role of each varies with the circumstances. With muscle weakness, the person being stretched may be capable of isometrically holding an elongated or stretched position after a partner has moved the extremity into the desired position. Another type of active-assisted stretching involves the participant independently assuming a stretching position and a partner applying additional stretch. In this situation the partner must understand the participant's functional ROM. Communication between partners is imperative with active-assisted stretching to prevent injury.

Allowing a body part to provide passive force for a stretch as it is pulled by gravity is a third form of active-assisted stretching. For example, the gastrocnemius can be stretched by the weight of the body by leaning forward and resting against a wall (see Figure 8.5). The active contraction of the quadriceps maintains knee extension required for effectively stretching the two-joint gastrocnemius muscle.

Active-assisted stretching allows a person to achieve a stretch not possible independently and

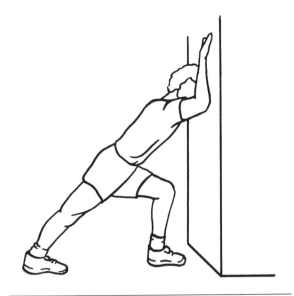

Figure 8.5 Gravity-assisted stretching of the gastrocnemius.

provides the opportunity to relax muscles not needed for the stretch. This technique can strengthen an overstretched or weak agonist muscle by stretching the opposing tight antagonists. A disadvantage with partner stretching, however, is that inappropriate use of force may cause injury.

Active Stretching

The participant's efforts alone accomplish this type of stretching. Active stretching requires the participant to contract the agonist, which places the target muscles (the antagonists) in an elongated position. This type of stretching generally does not develop as much ROM as passive or active-assisted types. A second type of active stretching involves functional activity exercises, such as walking in a pool to increase ROM of the ankle, knee, or hip. Another example is to pedal a bicycle ergometer with minimal resistance and with the seat height appropriately set to control the degree of knee extension. This type of exercise stretches the muscles that cross the knee joint without stressing anterior cruciate ligaments. Rhythmic limbering during warm-up in an aerobic dance class is another type of active stretching with functional activity. Functional activity exercises are a form of controlled ballistic stretching.

Ballistic Stretching

Ballistic stretching involves the use of momentum, such as with bouncing, twisting, or swinging movements that elongate muscles. This technique is generally *contraindicated* because sudden, forceful elongation activates the stretch reflex, which causes the target muscle to contract rather than relax. When a muscle contracts while it is being stretched, tissue damage may result. The possibility of injury is heightened in people with upper motor neuron conditions, such as spasticity.

An argument for the use of ballistic stretching is that many athletic events are ballistic in nature. Although the ballistic nature of sport cannot be denied, this facet of skill movement can be developed as a person practices the athletic skill itself. You should avoid recommending ballistic stretching in your general fitness programs.

Static Stretching

Static stretching involves slowly elongating a muscle group and maintaining a stretched position for a predetermined period of time. Static stretching may be done actively, passively, or with assistance. An objective of active static stretching is to elicit reciprocal inhibition, which dampens the stretch reflex and allows the muscle being stretched to relax.

The advantages of static stretching are that it requires less energy and is safer than ballistic stretching. Static stretching also reduces the chance of developing muscle soreness. Static stretching is appropriate for all people and is particularly recommended for people with shortened muscles due to inactivity, inappropriate positioning, weakness, or muscle imbalance.

Proprioceptive Neuromuscular Facilitation

Proprioceptive neuromuscular facilitation (PNF) is a group of stretching techniques developed by a physician, Herman Kabat (1965), and popularized in therapeutic settings by two physical therapists, Margaret Knott and Dorothy Voss (1968). PNF techniques are based on the theory that inhibitory and facilitory mechanisms of the muscle spindle and GTO can enhance ROM and flexibility. Three popular PNF techniques that are useful for physical fitness training are hold-relax, contract-relax, and rhythmic stabilization, which are depicted in Figure 8.6. In the discussion that follows, the *agonist* refers to the muscle opposing the tight muscle, and the *antagonist* is the muscle being stretched.

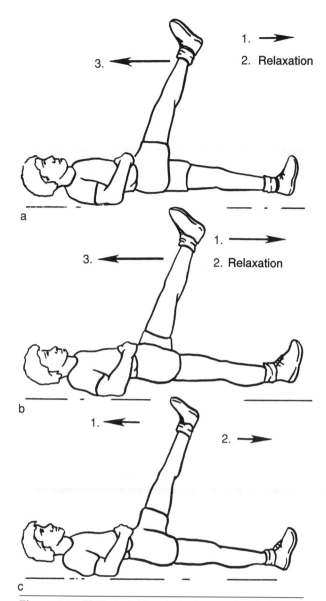

Figure 8.6 PNF stretching techniques using hold-relax (a), contract-relax (b), and rhythmic stabilization (c) techniques. Arrows for contractions are solid (long arrows for isotonic, short for isometric) and arrows for stretches are dashed. Resistance for the muscular contractions is provided by a partner.

Hold-Relax

With the hold-relax (HR) technique the participant isometrically contracts an elongated muscle for a period of 6 to 10 s. This contraction is followed by a brief period of relaxation during which an assistant slowly moves the limb into a deeper stretch. Recall from a discussion in chapter 5, however, that people poststroke generally should not hold isometric contractions for longer than 6 s (Gordon, 1993b). The hold-relax technique is based on assumptions that contraction of the antagonist will cause reflexive relaxation of the muscle because of the inverse stretch reflex stimulated by the GTO. People who have pain with resisted movement, such as individuals with rheumatoid arthritis, may prefer PNF hold-relax stretching.

Contract-Relax

PNF contract-relax (CR) stretching involves a maximal isotonic contraction of the target muscle from a stretched position against resistance provided by an assistant. During the brief period of relaxation that follows, the assistant passively moves the joint into a position of greater stretch, and the procedure is repeated. Like the HR technique, this method is also based on the mechanism of the inverse stretch reflex.

Rhythmic Stabilization

With this technique, the participant performs alternating isometric contractions of the agonist and antagonist muscles against resistance provided by an assistant, gradually increasing the strength of the contractions throughout the sequence. Repetition of alternate isometric contractions is theorized to alternate reciprocal inhibition between the muscle groups.

Effective use of PNF stretching requires training beyond that provided in this book. If you are interested in using PNF stretching techniques in your programs, seek further information and training. (See the Recommended Readings for Part III).

The three PNF techniques we described may be performed in different planes. According to Kabat (1965) and Knott and Voss (1968), PNF exercises should be done in specially sequenced diagonal and spiral patterns. The proponents of PNF believe these diagonal patterns elicit an irradiation effect that helps recruit appropriate muscle action. To successfully execute these spiral patterns, both participant and assistant must understand these techniques. Knott, Ionta, and Myers (1985) and McAtee (1993) further explain these techniques. An alternate approach for PNF techniques is to perform the exercises in the cardinal (frontal, transverse, sagittal) rather than diagonal planes (see Figure 8.7). For example, the hamstrings may be stretched in the sagittal plane using the hold-relax technique already described.

Proponents of PNF stretching believe that these techniques offer the greatest gains in flexibility development, provide greater strength and stability around the joint, and cause superior muscle relax-

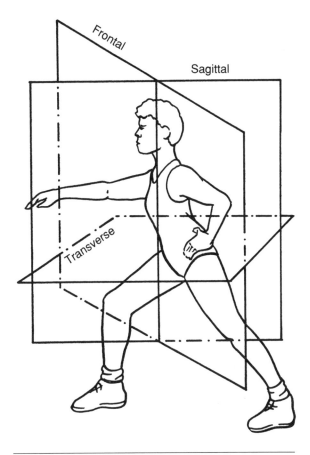

Figure 8.7 The cardinal planes—frontal, sagittal, and transverse—identify three planes of movement.

ation. Arguments against use of the techniques include their greater potential for causing injury if not properly performed, possible increases in blood pressure with the breath holding that may occur during the isometric contractions, and possible flaws in the theoretical basis of the techniques (Alter, 1988).

Relaxation

Regardless of the techniques used with flexibility training, relaxation (reduction of muscular tension) enhances the outcome of the effort. A participant can use physical and psychological techniques to relax overall or to relax specific muscle groups. Some exercise leaders use techniques to encourage relaxation before actually performing stretching exercises and controlled breathing during stretching to encourage relaxation. Alter (1988) reviewed several relaxation techniques, and a summary follows.

Physical Techniques

Several techniques physically reduce tension in a muscle, thereby enhancing relaxation. Slow static stretching induces relaxation by overriding the action of the muscle spindle that causes reflexive contraction of a muscle subjected to sudden stretch. Sufficient tension from a maintained stretch may activate the GTO, which relaxes the muscle being stretched. PNF techniques have been developed theoretically to override or take advantage of neural mechanisms that inhibit muscular tension. Other methods used to affect muscle tension include applying heat and cold, massage, and pharmacologic agents. Drugs are often prescribed with disabilities involving spasticity when the effects are severe enough to affect functioning.

Psychological Relaxation

"Mind-over-body" techniques to control muscle tension, combined with efforts to create an environment more conducive to whole-body relaxation, also have been utilized to improve flexibility. One such technique is biofeedback, a process by which a person attempts to control—through mental concentration—physiological events that are sensed electronically and converted to visual or auditory signals. The concept is based on the idea that feedback enhances the ability to voluntarily regulate functions typically controlled involuntarily. Another technique, progressive relaxation (Jacobson, 1978), involves the sequential temporary tensing and relaxing of muscle groups from one end of the body to the other. This practice was designed to increase a person's awareness of tension in all muscle groups of the body and the ability to relax them at will. Other techniques require employing a mental device such as imagery or repetition of words about relaxation in a quiet environment to reduce tension (Benson, 1980).

Breathing

Controlled breathing may facilitate relaxation and stretching, especially if it is combined with imagery (Jencks, 1977). Imagery should involve the desired outcome—in the case of stretching, lengthening of connective tissue. Controlled breathing can also help prevent breath holding, which may cause immediate problems for people with circulatory disorders. Encourage exhalation during a stretch of short duration or instruct your students to breathe "normally" during a longer stretch. To prevent hyperventilation, the period of exhalation should be longer than the period of inhalation.

Program Development

To ensure that you are offering your clients an appropriate stretching program, consider the safety, movement abilities, needs, and goals of each participant. In addition to the basic considerations for developing the exercise prescription (see chapter 5) it is very important that you educate each participant about the importance of stretching, proper techniques, and specifics of the program. It is helpful, with some individuals, if you can work one-on-one in the development and early phases of the program before integrating the person into the mainstream group setting or fitness class.

Assessment

To evaluate muscle groups in need of specific attention and to monitor the progress of the program, initial and ongoing assessments are essential. You can assess ROM with a goniometer (see Figure 8.8), which measures the degrees of movement at a joint. You can also qualitatively assess ROM by noting the position of one body part in relation to another. For example, you may note that as a person horizontally adducts the right shoulder, the hand touches the middle of the clavicle on the left side. Adequate documentation is essential for ensuring the gradual and effective progression of the flexibility program.

During preliminary and follow-up assessments, note conditions that contraindicate the use of stretching exercises. These include

- infection,
- edema,
- crepitus identified by a crackling sound or the sensation of rough surfaces working against each other,
- pain, and
- apparent joint instability.

If muscle quivering, twitching, or a decrease in ROM occur as a result of a stretching program, it may be necessary to adjust or temporarily discontinue the program. Also use caution with people who have osteoporosis, a recent fracture or immobilization, and a history of joint dislocations or subluxation (partial dislocation). For example, people with a history of shoulder dislocation should avoid placing the shoulder in an abducted, externally rotated position because ligaments that normally stabilize the joint in this position may be weakened. Ask participants' therapists or physi-

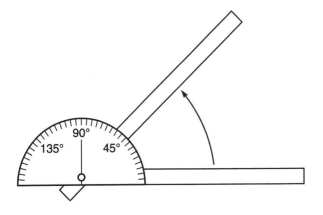

Figure 8.8 A goniometer is a protractor-like device that can be used for measuring joint range of motion.

cians for information you need to design fitness programs for your clients with joint dysfunction and instability.

Contraindicated Exercises

Recent research has found that a variety of stretching exercises are contraindicated for the general population because of their potential for jeopardizing joint stability. In addition, other exercises commonly used by the general population may reduce functioning in people with specific conditions. For example, stretching the lower back, which is an integral part of the stretching program for protecting low-back function, can reduce trunk stability in someone with paralysis of back extensors. You must be fully aware of each individual's needs, abilities, and disability characteristics to screen inappropriate stretches. The advice of a

physician or therapist can be invaluable in giving you pertinent information to ensure that you deliver a safe program for all your clients.

Summary

Flexibility development is an important component of the physical fitness program, and it may be essential for maintaining mobility and independent functioning in some people with physical disabilities. Neuromuscular mechanisms and biomechanical properties influence joint ROM and flexibility. Neuromuscular mechanisms are influenced by the muscle spindle and Golgi tendon organ (GTO) through the stretch reflex, inverse stretch reflex, and reciprocal inhibition. Addressing these mechanisms in stretching protocols may be particularly beneficial with disabilities caused by impaired neuromuscular control, such as with spasticity.

The structure of a joint and viscoelastic properties contribute to biomechanical factors that influence flexibility development, both of which can be altered with disabling conditions and tissue trauma. Table 8.3 presents a two-tiered model of stretching to address both neuromuscular and biomechanical factors influencing flexibility development.

Several common techniques are used in stretching programs that are suitable for use in the health-fitness program. Static and proprioceptive neuromuscular facilitation (PNF) techniques use active, active-assisted, and passive modes of stretching. As an exercise instructor, you must be skilled in the use of these techniques and be knowledgeable about the impact conditions associated with dis-

Table 8.3 Two-Tiered Model of Flexibility Development With Disabling Conditions

Objective	Technique	Condition
Neuromuscular tier		
Relax target muscle	Contract-relax Rhythmic stabilization Successive induction	Spasticity
Strengthen opposing muscle	Hold-relax Rhythmic stabilization	Overstretch weakness Muscle imbalances
Biomechanical tier		
Lengthen tissue	Low-load, prolonged stretching Warm-up before stretching Ice after stretching	Adhesions Scar tissue Contractures

ability may have on the outcome of the training program. Individualized flexibility programs should be developed for each person based on the advice of the health care professional, whether the participant exercises in a group setting or on an individual basis. In the next chapter, we look at specific conditions and disabilities and examine the possible influence they may have on choices you make as you develop individualized stretching programs.

Chapter 9

Static Stretching: Modifying for Disability

Paul R. Surburg, PhD, RPT
Indiana University

In the previous chapter we provided a foundation of principles for developing flexibility to guide you with decisions about modifying stretching programs for people with physical disabilities. In this chapter, we reverse the focus and look at condition-specific and disability-specific considerations for modifying stretching programs. We also offer suggestions for adapting stretching techniques and exercises.

Many conditions are common to a variety of disabilities and require similar, generalized stretching modifications. Some disabilities warrant additional specific considerations. As always, individualize stretching modifications to address the needs and goals of each person, whether your programs involve group stretching classes or one-on-one training.

Safety should remain at the forefront of all recommendations you offer your clients with disabilities. If at any time you or the participant has questions about the safety of a particular exercise or modification, consult a physical therapist or physician for advice. This is especially important if you believe that a client with braces can better perform a stretch without them.

Modifications for Specific Conditions

The following general adaptations are applicable to conditions that are common to more than one type of disability. The next section contains additional disability-specific modifications that address safety or movement concerns created by specific disabilities.

Spasticity, Muscle Imbalance, and Contractures

Certain conditions associated with physical disabilities may result in contractures (adaptive shortening of soft tissues about a joint). Contractures, in turn, may cause "tight weakness" of shortened muscles on one side of the joint and "overstretch weakness" of the opposing muscle group, both of which further contribute to a loss of joint range of motion. These imbalances may occur with disabilities that cause spasticity, such as those involving upper motor neuron dysfunction (cerebral palsy, spinal cord injury, multiple sclerosis, head injury, and cerebrovascular accident). Other disabilities that limit joint ROM due to muscle imbalance (such as incomplete spinal cord injury, muscular dystrophy, polio) or pain (such as arthritis) also may cause contractures or adaptive shortening of muscle and connective tissues over time. To restore muscle balance, an appropriate fitness program includes stretching exercises for the shortened muscles and strengthening exercises for opposing muscle groups. For example, direct the client with spastic CP who has tight elbow flexors, hip adductors, and plantar flexors to concentrate on stretching these muscle groups. As part of the stretching program it is also beneficial to include strengthening exercises for the opposing triceps, gluteus medius and minimus, and tibialis anterior muscles. Remember that resistive exercises with fitness conditioning should only be recommended when the intended joint actions can be isolated and do not involve other, unintended synergistic actions. Otherwise, you'll need guidance from the participant's medical professional. Resistive exercise must be carefully monitored because people with certain disabilities may substitute other body or joint motions for the desired actions.

Impaired Balance

People with impaired balance may need to consider alternate positions or have additional support available during certain stretches to ensure the safety and effectiveness of the exercise. These considerations often apply to people with impaired postural support due to paralysis of the trunk and lower extremity muscles or with ataxia caused by injury to the brain such as some types of cerebral palsy, head injury, or multiple sclerosis.

Balance may be improved by stretches from a seated position with the use of seat belts (ace wraps, stretch bands, or other ties). For additional support with seated exercises from the floor, direct your clients with impaired balance to sit near a wall or stationary object. As an alternative, they can substitute a prone position or hooked position lying on the side for upright postures when upright balance is precarious, as long as ROM is not hindered. During standing exercises, provide a sturdy chair for additional support or have an assistant available for spotting.

Impaired Coordination

Impaired coordination is a common characteristic of people with injury to the brain, such as CP, CVA, head injury, or multiple sclerosis. If simultaneous bilateral movements are too challenging, select exercises that they can perform unilaterally. With hemiplegic conditions, suggest using the unimpaired arm to assist the impaired side of the body in assuming the correct position for the exercise. Using partners also helps participants with impaired coordination assume stretching positions more quickly. Avoid rushing through the set-up of each stretching exercise, however, to allow people who want to participate independently plenty of time to assume the correct position.

Impaired Sensation

Some disabilities, such as hemiplegia with head injury or stroke and spinal cord injury, impair the individual's ability to receive sensory information from the extremities. Avoid passive stretching exercises for people with this condition unless you or an assistant have received appropriate training and are qualified to perform it. In many cases, the person has been taught to independently stretch areas lacking sensation. In addition to exercises you recommend for your client, encourage him to maintain the program prescribed during rehabilitation training for passively stretching target muscles.

Modifications for Specific Disabilities

The following modifications for stretching exercises are generally applicable to the specific disabilities cited, although symptoms of these disorders and the modifications they require will vary. The disabilities presented are generally listed in order of site of impairment from the brain to the periphery. We discuss progressive disabilities (MS and MD) separately because of additional considerations.

Cerebral Palsy

Recommendations for stretching modifications with impaired balance, impaired coordination, and muscle imbalances are generally appropriate for people with spastic cerebral palsy. Daily stretching is especially important—continually encourage it for people with spastic CP because flexibility enhances the ability to perform activities of daily living. The following specific stretching modifications are advised for people with spastic CP:

❏ Emphasize prolonged static stretching during the warm-up and cool-down. Stretching before aerobic or resistance training may optimize ROM and improve performance during the ensuing activity. Also, because spasticity may increase after vigorous exercise, spending additional time on stretching following the cool-down may help restore ROM.

❏ Spend additional time stretching or engaging in functional exercises with spastic muscle groups (often the flexors, adductors, and internal rotators) during flexibility training.

❏ Incorporate relaxation exercises (reviewed in chapter 8) prior to stretching to improve the outcome of the session. Consider leading flexibility exercises in a heated swimming pool (85 °F) because warm temperatures may facilitate stretching and flexibility development.

❏ Avoid eliciting hyperactive stretch reflexes in spastic muscles. With static stretching, use slow, deliberate movements. Also avoid applying pressure to the muscle belly of a spastic muscle when offering manual assistance with stretching. Pressure on the muscle belly may cause reflexive contraction of the muscle you are trying to stretch.

❏ Limit exercises to one joint at a time or progress from single-joint to multijoint exercises. For example, begin with a stretch for the wrist, add the elbow to the same exercise, and eventually include the shoulder.

❏ Avoid eliciting primitive reflexes during stretching. Because CP is a disorder involving upper motor neurons, primitive reflexes may persist. Recommend exercise positions and a seated posture to prevent initiation of these reflexes. For example, attempting to stretch elbow flexors during activation of the asymmetric tonic neck reflex will not be effective. (Recall that with this reflex, turning the head to the right causes the left elbow to flex.) Be sure to position yourself appropriately when offering assistance or giving instructions. For a review of primitive reflexes see Table 2.2 on p. 15.

Head Injury

Participation in any type of exercise program following a head injury, be it flexibility development or other components of physical fitness, should be approved by a physician because of conditions that may persist. For example, a person with a fractured nose, particularly if there is septum damage, may have difficulty with respiration, and you should monitor exercise intensity closely to prevent breathing problems.

Because head injury may significantly impair balance and coordination, the modifications described for those conditions would apply. With hemiplegia, general stretching considerations for muscle imbalances and impaired sensation also may apply. Communication or behavior problems may require that you modify your instructional approach. Additional considerations for stretching exercises with head injury are as follows:

❏ Active-assisted exercises may be useful to help people with hemiparesis assume certain stretching positions. Be sure sensation is present when a partner assists with stretching.

❏ If visual disturbances impede the execution of directed movements, provide manual guidance from a partner or assistant. Visual disturbance may also impair balance.

❏ Consider tactfully restricting someone with behavioral or judgment disturbances from providing manual assistance to another person during partner stretching.

Cerebrovascular Accident (Stroke)

Depending on the site of injury, a variety of communication disorders that can affect your instructional approach (as described in chapter 2) may be associated with a CVA. Modifications for impaired coordination and balance may also apply. Muscle imbalances and impaired sensation associated with hemiparesis also require the recommended modifications. Be aware of pain, tenderness, or numbness in people who have had strokes. Additional considerations for stretching follow:

❏ Consider alternate exercise positions for a participant with pain and tenderness in an extremity. Do not subject areas of sensory deprivation or numbness to excessive pressure.

❑ With hemiparesis, the functional arm may be used to manually assist the affected limbs as prescribed by a therapist or physician. Assistance from a partner may be necessary to ensure that the participant executes movements effectively. Encourage active-assisted ROM exercises as part of a daily program on the affected side when movement is available.

❑ Be aware of signs that indicate the exercise session should be stopped immediately. At any time, if the participant's pulse becomes rapid and skin turns a dusky color or a headache, chest pain, shortness of breath, or fever occurs, all activity should immediately cease. Obtain immediate medical attention if symptoms persist. Require the individual to obtain further medical clearance before continuing with the program.

Spinal Cord Injury

The level of injury is a key factor in determining the type of flexibility program appropriate for the person with a spinal cord injury. Paraplegia, resulting from injury to the lower spinal cord region, requires minimal modification with upper body stretches. With paraplegia or quadriplegia, muscle imbalances and joint contractures may develop. Follow the recommendations for impaired sensation provided earlier. Recommend that the person independently maintain any stretching routines prescribed by a therapist or physician in addition to those offered through the fitness program. Additional specific considerations for stretching with spinal cord injury are as follows:

❑ The wheelchair can be used to maintain balance during lateral stretching by hooking one arm around the push handle or using a locked wheel or arm rest for support.

❑ People with rods or other spinal fixation devices should use twisting movements with extreme caution.

❑ When position changes are needed to execute exercises, be aware that postural changes may influence blood pressure and cause lightheadedness.

❑ Direct individuals who use a wheelchair to focus on stretching the hip flexors, knee flexors, and plantar flexors of the foot to avoid developing contractures. If active-assisted exercises can be used with any of these muscle

groups, encourage reciprocal movements. For example, hip extension movements should be done for muscle balancing with shortened hip flexors.

❑ Because of the possible presence of osteoporosis, avoid recommending positions or exercises that place excessive stress on the bones, for example, by placing extreme weight on a body part or using excessive overload during a stretch.

❑ Be aware of movements or positions that may impair the function of various appliances to deal with bladder and bowel functions.

❑ When a participant does stretching exercises out of the chair, be sure the table or floor surface is adequately padded, yet firm.

❑ Avoid recommending exercises that overstretch paralyzed back extensors because doing so may compromise upright posture and trunk stability.

❑ Never recommend stretching finger and wrist flexors simultaneously in individuals with quadriplegia who rely on tenodesis for hand function.

Spina Bifida

Most recommendations for people with spinal cord injury are also appropriate for people with spina bifida. If a shunt is in place to treat hydrocephalus, be sure that exercises will not alter the shunt's functioning. The following specific stretching modifications apply for individuals with spina bifida:

❑ Exert caution with any type of back movement because it is likely that surgery has been performed at the defect site.

❑ Joints of extremities immediately above the level of injury are a prime target for ROM exercises.

Poliomyelitis

With flaccid paralysis due to polio, gentle stretching exercises should be oriented toward reducing or preventing flexion contractures, which commonly occur in the hips, knees, and plantar flexors. Consult the individual's therapist or physician about removing braces and the presence of any immovable joints. For example, some joints may have been surgically stabilized, such as with an arthrodesis, to prevent inversion or eversion of the ankle. With lower extremity weakness, functional exercises in a pool may be an effective means of increasing ROM and flexibility. Modifications for impaired balance and muscle imbalances also may be applicable for individuals with polio.

Multiple Sclerosis

Because of the variety of symptoms and degrees of severity with multiple sclerosis, it is difficult to generalize about this condition and the use and role of flexibility exercises. Often, neurologic symptoms such as visual problems and sensory impairment cause double vision, blurred vision, and nystagmus. With these conditions, exercising from a secure and stable position is important. All the general considerations for spasticity, muscle imbalance, contractures, and impaired balance, coordination, and sensation may apply to someone with multiple sclerosis. Also consider the following additional modifications:

❑ If paralysis exists, ROM of the joint immediately above the paralyzed area is very important.
❑ A regular exercise regimen is important for the person with MS during remission. Training may have to be postponed, however, during a period of exacerbation.
❑ Participants should use periods of rest judiciously based on current health status.
❑ Exercising in a warm environment and overheating may increase the physical symptoms of MS.
❑ For some people with MS, functional flexibility exercises such as the use of a stationary bicycle may be more appropriate than standard stretching protocols.
❑ When movement becomes uncomfortable at certain stages of MS, flexibility exercises may be done in a pool. (Water temperature should not be extremely cool or warm.)
❑ Short bouts of exercise done several times a day may be more beneficial than one prolonged session.

Muscular Dystrophy

Although the role or use of resistance training exercises for people with MD is questioned by some physicians, flexibility exercises are universally accepted as beneficial and important. Range of motion exercises may help reduce the harmful effects of contractures, which are often present with MD. In the lower extremity, contractures are often associated with the Achilles tendon, hip flexors, tensor fascia latea, and hamstrings. Upper-extremity con-

tractures may be found with the forearm pronators, wrist flexors, and finger flexors. These muscles are target muscle groups for the flexibility program. General stretching modifications for contractures and impaired balance apply to individuals with muscular dystrophy. Consider also the following:

❑ Stretching exercises should be active, with emphasis upon slow movements and gentle stretching.
❑ More rest periods must be incorporated into the flexibility program as this disorder becomes more extensive.
❑ As the muscular dystrophy progresses, additional means of securing and maintaining balance may be required during the exercise program. At one stage a seat belt may be sufficient, but at a later stage a shoulder harness may also be needed.
❑ Use interesting flexibility exercises, such as functional activity stretches, when possible.
❑ Reducing the effects of gravity may become an important aspect of all flexibility exercises with muscle debilitation. Reduced-gravity exercises involve executing movements perpendicular to the pull of gravity. External support, such as sliding the forearm on a table when performing elbow flexion and extension, is often necessary.

Arthritis

Because of pain and decreased activity, weakness and muscle imbalances are often characteristic of arthritis. Flexion contractures of most major joints, especially flexors, adductors, and external rotators, are characteristic of rheumatoid arthritis. Use flexibility exercises incorporating smooth movements to emphasize extension, abduction, and internal rotation. General considerations for muscle imbalance and contractures are applicable. The following considerations may also apply to individuals with arthritis:

❑ Applying heat to affected joints before stretching may be beneficial.
❑ Some of the PNF exercises may not only improve ROM but also help develop strength to counteract the weakness often present with arthritis. Stretching protocols that include isotonic or isometric contractions, such as contract-relax and hold-relax techniques, may serve a dual function for strength and flexibility development.

❏ Develop exercise tolerance over an extended period of time.

❏ Offer functional activities such as swimming and bicycling to help develop or retain needed ROM.

❏ Recommend that flexibility exercises be performed several times a day.

❏ Keep all flexibility exercises within the participant's pain-free range especially during periods of exacerbation.

❏ Avoid maintaining stretched positions for a prolonged period (more than 20 or 30 s).

Amputation

Involve all nonamputated extremities in a standard flexibility program. An area of the body often neglected during stretching activity is the joint immediately proximal to the level of the amputation. Ironically this joint is often the joint needing more ROM exercise than any other. In many situations loss of ROM has resulted from muscle imbalances due to the amputation or as a result of positions chronically assumed to accommodate for loss of the body part. Yet the functionality of a prosthesis is to a certain extent related to the ROM present in the joint.

Stretching exercises may help reduce some of the stress and discomfort of adaptive postures resulting from the loss of all or part of a limb, and a strengthening program should accompany the stretching protocol. For example, lower limb amputees may experience low-back discomfort, but stretching the lower back and hip flexors can help reduce or prevent this problem. Developing abdominal strength should be an integral part of the stretching program. With individuals who have lower limb amputations, muscles between the shoulder blades (rhomboid and middle trapezius) may also become tight as a result of adaptive postures. In this case, the fitness program should target stretching the muscles of the shoulder girdle and strengthening the anterior shoulder muscles. Other considerations for muscle imbalances and impaired balance may apply to the individual with an amputation. Consider the following additional recommendations:

❏ Recommend removal of the prosthesis if it restricts movement and inhibits full ROM. If the participant does not wish to remove the prosthesis in a group setting, then suggest that she perform the exercise at home without the prosthesis.

❏ Address muscle imbalances in hip flexors for people who use a wheelchair.

❏ Offer exercises that focus on the shoulder girdle region, which may develop limitations in ROM over time despite considerable strength.

❏ Recommend that someone mentally exercise the amputated portion of a limb if he is experiencing phantom pain.

Summary

Modifying stretches for your clients with physical disabilities requires that you be aware of modifications both for general conditions and for specific disabilities. Conditions such as muscle imbalances, spasticity, contractures, impaired balance, impaired coordination, and impaired sensation may be common to several disabilities, and similar stretching modifications are appropriate for all of them. By considering these general recommendations, suggestions specific to the disability, and each person's needs and goals, you can develop safe and individualized flexibility programs. The next chapter applies the principles we just reviewed to develop recommendations for modifications to specific strengthening and stretching exercises.

Chapter 10

Exercises for Developing Muscular Fitness

Patrick J. DiRocco, PhD
University of Wisconsin—La Crosse

Muscular fitness involves strength, muscular endurance, and flexibility (ACSM, 1991). A comprehensive exercise program for developing muscular fitness involves all these components to achieve muscle balancing, maintain or improve postural alignment, enhance daily functioning, or improve performance in sport and recreational activities. Appropriate conditioning principles must be applied to achieve specific goals, as described in chapter 5.

This chapter describes the basic set-up for strengthening and stretching exercises, arranged in a head-to-toe format. The resistive exercises described use stretch bands (remember, however, with extreme muscle weakness, gravity alone may provide sufficient resistance), and flexibility work uses static stretches. We include modifications for specific disabling conditions when applicable.

The following set of exercises works each of the major muscle groups in the body. Many variations and different exercises for each muscle group are possible. If you are unfamiliar with the terms commonly used to describe movement in this chapter or the arrangement of each of the major muscle groups, refer to any current text on kinesiology for a review (see Recommended Readings). As an exercise leader, it is imperative that you are able to visualize the position and attachment points for each muscle and understand how they contribute to associated joint actions by lengthening or shortening.

Unless otherwise noted, exercises are from a seated position. With the resistive exercises, we describe only the concentric phase; the eccentric phase simply reverses the concentric movement. Remember to perform the eccentric phase slowly, and continue to apply pressure in the direction of the movement while returning to the starting position. We don't offer conditioning variables (such as repetitions, sets, or duration of stretch) because you must individualize these variables for each client. Also, although not described, be sure to exercise both sides of the body.

Several exercises use floor positions. Your students with lower limb impairments who use a wheelchair may be able to transfer independently or they may need assistance with a chair-to-floor transfer. Before offering to assist with a transfer, you must receive training from a qualified professional and practice until you are comfortable with the lifts. Chapter 14 describes several transfers. Be sure to plan the workout to prevent continual changes in position—if possible, group all floor exercises together to limit the need to transfer to the floor more than once.

Exercises for the Neck

Action	Major muscles
Flexion	Sternocleidomastoid
Lateral flexion	Sternocleidomastoid
	Erector spinae
	Semispinalis cervicis
	Splenius cervicis
	Splenius capitis
Rotation	Sternocleidomastoid
	Erector spinae
	Semispinalis cervicis
	Splenius capitis
Extension	Erector spinae
	Multifidus
	Rotatores
	Semispinalis cervicis
	Semispinalis capitis
	Splenius capitis

Neck Flexion

Action:

1. Assume normal alignment of the head and neck.
2. Place the heel of the hand on the forehead.
3. Apply light manual resistance for concentric and eccentric contractions of the neck flexors (see Fig. 10.1).

Tip: Partners can assist (with caution) individuals unable to independently provide manual resistance.

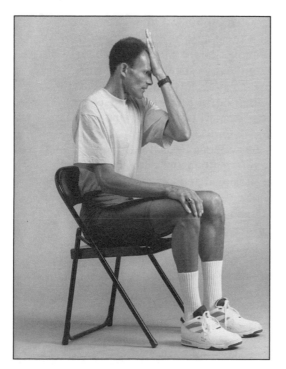

Figure 10.1 Manual resistance with neck flexion.

Lateral Neck Flexion

Action:

1. Tilt the head slightly to one side from the neutral upright position.
2. Place the heel of the hand on the upper side of the head in the direction of movement.
3. Apply light manual resistance for concentric and eccentric contractions of the lateral neck flexors.

Tip: Partners can assist (with caution) individuals unable to independently provide manual resistance.

Neck Rotation

Action:

1. Rotate the head to one side from the neutral upright position.
2. Place the heel of the hand on the side of the head in the direction of movement.
3. Apply light manual resistance for concentric and eccentric contractions of the neck rotators.

Tip: Partners can assist (with caution) individuals unable to independently provide manual resistance.

Neck Extension

Action:

1. Place the neck in a position of full flexion.
2. Place fingertips of both hands on the back of the head.
3. Apply light manual resistance for concentric and eccentric contractions of the neck extensors.
4. Do not exceed normal head-neck alignment; avoid hyperextending the neck.

Tip: Partners can assist (with caution) individuals unable to independently provide manual resistance.

Stretching—Neck Flexors

Action:

1. From "normal" upright alignment of the head and neck, retract the neck (see Fig. 10.2) by slowly pulling the chin back, creating a "double chin."
2. Keep the shoulders relaxed.

Caution: Avoid neck hyperextension, which is contraindicated for general fitness programs.

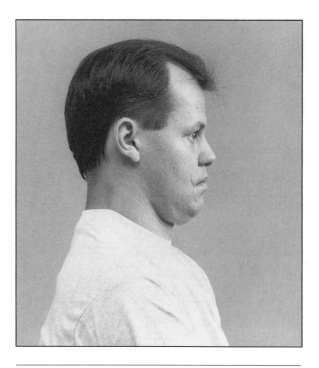

Figure 10.2 Neck retraction.

Stretching—Lateral Neck Flexors
Action:
1. Slowly lower the head to the side as if to touch the ear to the shoulder and hold.
2. Keep the shoulders relaxed (avoid shoulder elevation).

Stretching—Neck Rotators
Action:
1. Slowly rotate the head to one side and hold.
2. Keep the shoulders relaxed. (Do not move either shoulder.)

Stretching—Neck Extensors
Action:
1. Slowly drop the chin toward the chest until you feel a stretch in the back of the neck and hold.
2. Keep the shoulders relaxed.

Exercises for the Shoulder Joint

Action	Major muscles
Flexion	Anterior deltoid
	Pectoralis major
	Biceps brachii
Extension	Posterior deltoid
	Latissimus dorsi
	Teres major
	Triceps brachii
Abduction	Middle deltoid
	Supraspinatus
Adduction	Pectoralis major
	Latissimus dorsi
	Teres major
Transverse (horizontal) abduction	Posterior deltoid
Transverse (horizontal) adduction	Pectoralis major
	Anterior deltoid

Horizontal (Transverse) Shoulder Adduction (Flys)
Action:
1. Place the band around the back at mid-shoulder.
2. Grasp band with each hand, abduct shoulders 90 degrees, and flex elbows 90 degrees (see Fig. 10.3a).
3. Maintain the flexed position of the elbows and push the hands forward until they meet and cross in front of the chest (see Fig. 10.3b).
Tip: People with spastic or weak biceps may secure the band just above the elbow (avoid applying pressure to the muscle belly) and focus on pushing the elbows forward toward the midline of the body.

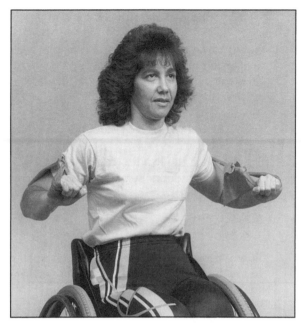
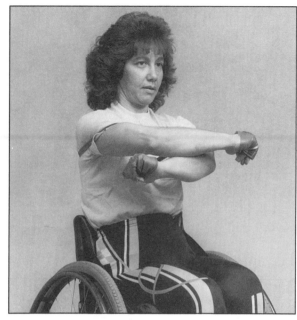

a   b

Figure 10.3 Horizontal shoulder adduction starting position (a) and end position (b).

Shoulder Flexion (Front Raise)

Action:

1. Loop the band under the seat or foot pedals of the chair and hold the ends in both hands with the palms facing toward each other at about knee height (see Fig. 10.4a).
2. Maintain elbow extension.
3. Raise the arms overhead as far as possible while maintaining elbow extension (see Fig. 10.4b).

Tips: People with impaired trunk balance may need to exercise one arm at a time. If bands provide too much resistance, then fasten one end under the chair or to foot pedals and perform the exercise by holding onto only one end of the band.

People with weak or nonfunctioning triceps can externally rotate the shoulders to have palms face the ceiling during the exercise. The resistance of gravity will maintain elbow extension.

People with spastic biceps muscles may have difficulty with this exercise. They can secure the bands at the elbows, hold hands together, and then raise the arms as high as possible. If exercising each arm separately, be sure the movement is in the sagittal plane and avoid any trunk rotation.

Shoulder Flexion-Elbow Extension (Chest Press)

Action:

1. Place the band across the upper back, underneath the arms at shoulder level.
2. Grasp the ends of the band with each hand.
3. Place hands against the chest, palms facing forward, with elbows close to the sides (see Fig. 10.5a).
4. Push the palms forward, away from the chest until they reach elbow extension and 90 degrees of shoulder flexion. In the extended position arms should be parallel to the floor (see Fig. 10.5b).

Tips: People with limited triceps strength may have difficulty with this exercise; it is therefore a good exercise for them.

It may be more beneficial to exercise one arm at a time. If the shoulders are externally rotated so the palms face the ceiling and the band is lowered down the back, the participant also may be able to work on shoulder protraction.

This is an excellent exercise for people with spasticity who have tight biceps and need to work on strengthening the triceps. If they cannot complete the movement through the full range of motion, use lighter resistance or no resistance at all. If the level of spasticity differs between the two arms, then exercise one arm at a time.

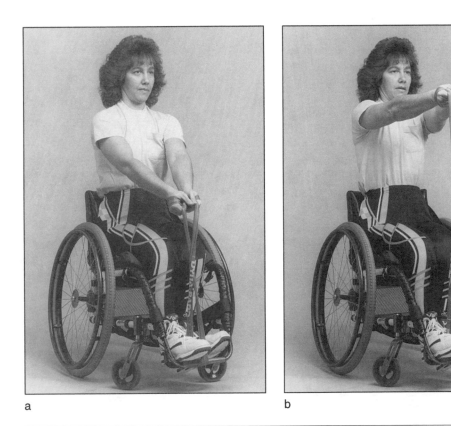

a   b

Figure 10.4 Shoulder flexion starting position (a) and end position (b).

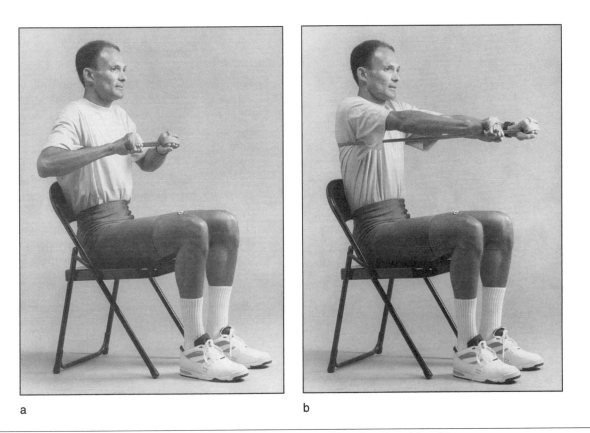

a   b

Figure 10.5 Shoulder flexion-elbow extension starting position (a) and end position (b).

Shoulder Abduction (Lateral Raise)

Action:

1. Loop the band under the seat of the chair at midthigh level and grasp each end with the palms facing inward and the arms hanging down at the sides.
2. Abduct the shoulders with the palms facing down and the elbows in extension, but not locked (see Fig. 10.6).
3. Perform this exercise in two arcs to provide resistance at both ends of the ROM.

Tips: With impaired shoulder function or trunk balance, perform the exercise unilaterally.

If weak triceps hamper the straight arm position, externally rotate the shoulder to passively lock the elbow into extension.

If maintaining straight arms is difficult due to either spasticity or weakness of the triceps, secure the band just above the elbow and focus on the movement of the arm (see Fig. 10.7).

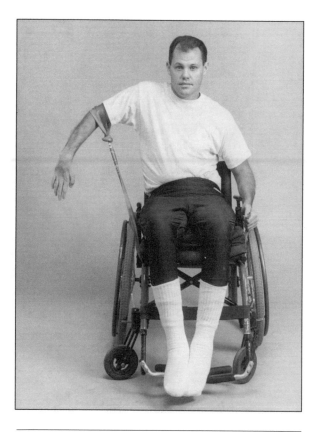

Figure 10.7 Modified attachment above the elbow for the lateral raise.

Shoulder Extension

Action:

1. Flex one shoulder while maintaining elbow extension until the hand reaches head level.
2. Grasp one end of the band and hook the other end in front of the body (or have a partner hold it) at head level (see Fig. 10.8a).
3. Keeping the buttocks in contact with the seat and the elbow extended, pull the band down and back, fully extending and hyperextending the shoulder (see Fig. 10.8b).

Tip: If triceps muscles are weak or nonfunctional, it will be difficult to keep the arms straight. In this case, the exercise can be completed with the elbow bent throughout the motion. Alternately, the band may be secured just above the elbow so the participant can concentrate on shoulder movement.

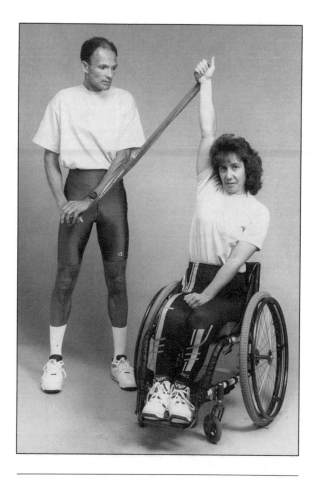

Figure 10.6 End position of the lateral raise (shoulder abduction).

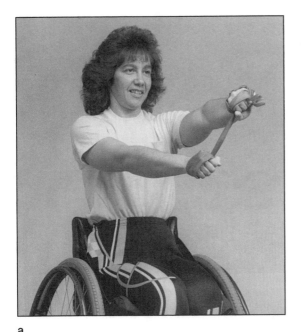 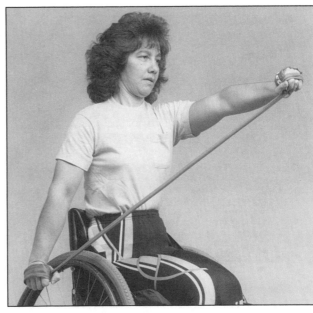

a   b

Figure 10.8 Shoulder extension starting position (a) and end position (b).

Shoulder Extension (One-Arm Rows)

Action:
1. Flex one shoulder 45 to 90 degrees with the elbow in extension and palm facing inward.
2. Fix the band at waist height or have a partner hold one end. Grasp the other end of the band at the same level (see Fig. 10.9a).
3. Hyperextend the shoulder while flexing the elbow to 90 degrees, keeping the forearm parallel to the floor (see Fig. 10.9b).

Tip: Keep the movement in the shoulder flexion-extension motion. There may be a tendency to "cheat" by outwardly rotating the shoulder.

Scapular Adduction (Retraction)

Action:
1. Abduct the shoulders 90 degrees, protract the scapula, and flex the elbows, bringing the fists several inches from the chest.
2. Wrap the band around each hand, allowing up to 6 in. between the fists (see Fig. 10.10a).
3. Push the elbows back, squeezing the scapula together, without changing the angle at the elbows. Avoid excessive horizontal shoulder abduction to isolate the action of the scapula (see Fig. 10.10b).

Tip: This exercise is important for anyone with a rounded shoulder posture caused by prolonged, poor sitting posture or muscle imbalances due to frequent wheelchair pushing.

Action	Major muscles
Retraction (adduction)	Rhomboids
	Trapezius
Protraction (abduction)	Pectoralis minor
	Serratus anterior
Elevation	Levator scapula
	Rhomboids
	Trapezius
Depression	Pectoralis minor
	Subclavius

Note. Other actions of the shoulder girdle include upward and downward rotation and upward tilt. The shoulder girdle muscles also provide important stabilization during resisted shoulder actions.

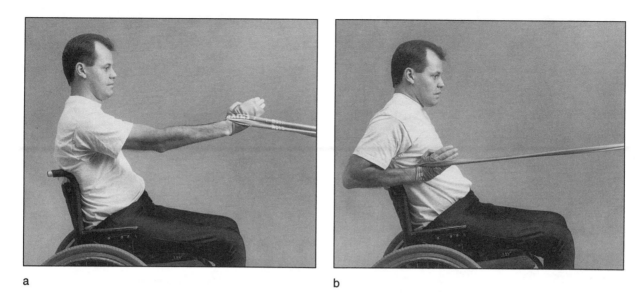

a　　　　　　　　　　　　　　　　　　　　　b

Figure 10.9 One-arm rows starting position (a) and end position (b).

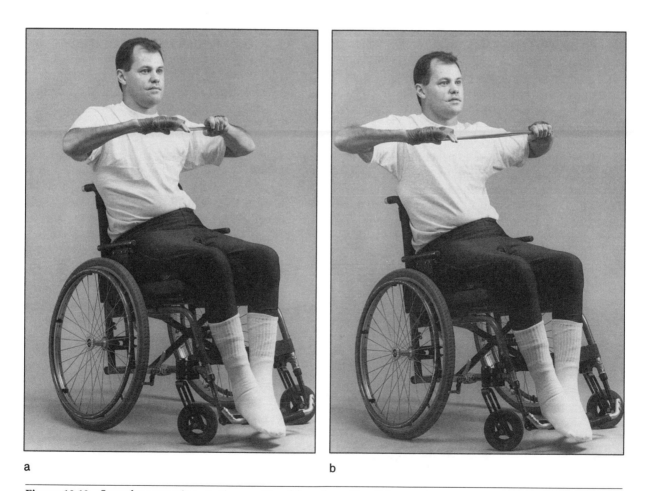

a　　　　　　　　　　　　　　　　　　　　　b

Figure 10.10 Scapular retraction starting position (a), end position (b).

126

Stretching—Shoulder Flexors, Adductors, and Elbow Flexors

Action:

1. With the elbow in extension, palm facing forward, abduct the shoulder and place the hand or forearm against that of a partner.
2. The partner applies pressure at the wrist (or elbow) and pulls the arm back (see Fig. 10.11).
3. Repeat the stretch at varying levels of shoulder abduction to stretch the pectorals at different angles.

Tips: With impaired trunk balance, hook the opposite arm around the wheelchair push handle or grasp the arm rest to maintain good seated posture.

This exercise can be done independently from a standing position with the palm placed against a wall or fixed post. Avoid excessive trunk twisting.

Stretching—Shoulder Flexors and Internal Rotators

Action:

1. From a supine position, abduct the shoulders 90 degrees, flex the elbows 90 degrees, and externally rotate the shoulders (palms will be facing the ceiling).
2. Allow gravity to pull the hands toward the floor while keeping the abdominals tight and pressing the back into the floor (see Fig. 10.12).

Tips: People with good shoulder flexibility may not feel much stretch from this exercise.

With weak or nonfunctional abdominals, a partner may be needed to maintain the posture of the lower back.

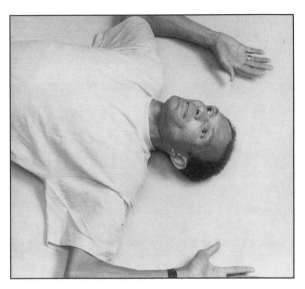

Figure 10.12 Stretching shoulder flexors and internal rotators.

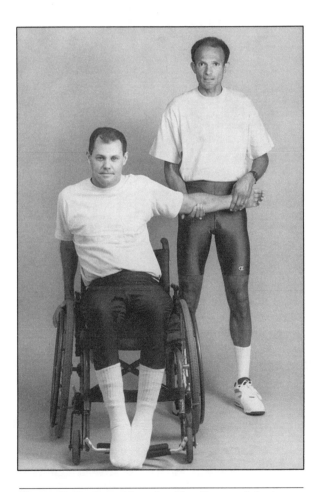

Figure 10.11 Stretching shoulder flexors, abductors, and elbow flexors.

Stretching—Posterior Shoulder and Rotator Cuff

Action:

1. With the elbows extended flex the shoulders 180 degrees.
2. Clasp the hands together with the palms crossed.
3. Pull the arms behind the head.

Tips: Participants may need assistance from a partner with positioning and holding the stretch (see Fig. 10.13).

Stay aware of balance and stability in the chair. If balance is a problem, this stretch can be performed from a supine position on the floor.

Avoid hyperextending the lower back when pulling the arms back.

Some people with impaired coordination may find it easier to perform the stretch by clasping the hands first before lifting the arms overhead.

Stretching—Posterior Shoulder and Shoulder Girdle

Action:

1. Flex one shoulder 90 degrees and grasp the elbow with the opposite hand (see Fig. 10.14).
2. Pull the arm across the midline of the chest. (Do not allow the trunk to twist in the direction of the stretch. Keep the back and buttocks stationary.)

Tips: People with limited hand function can pull the elbow with the back of the hand. The arm being stretched does not have to remain straight if triceps are weak.

People with impaired coordination can reach across the body and grasp the chair back at the level of the opposite shoulder, hold, and turn the trunk away from the hand.

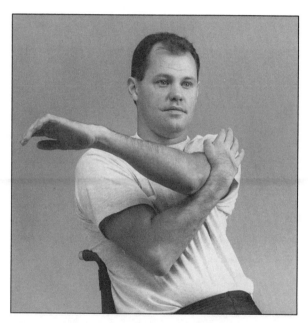

Figure 10.14 Alternate posterior shoulder and shoulder girdle stretch with limited hand function.

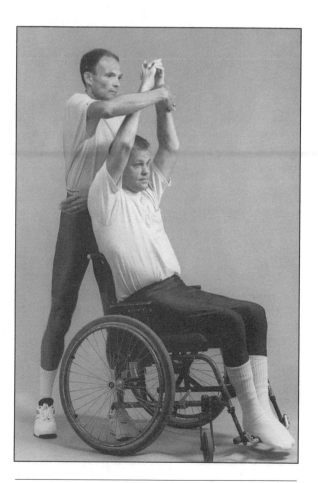

Figure 10.13 Stretching posterior shoulder and rotator cuff with partner assistance.

Exercises for the Elbow Joint

Elbow Flexion (Arm Curls)

Action:

1. Loop the band under the seat, feet, or foot rests. Grasp each end of the band allowing the arms to hang at the sides, palms facing forward.
2. Flex the elbows through the full range of motion without changing the position of the upper arm. Limit movement to the forearm only (see Fig. 10.15).

Tips: If the forearm tends to pronate during the curl, wrap the band around the hand so the resistance applies downward pressure across the thumb-side of the hand.

This exercise may not be appropriate for people with spasticity in the biceps who cannot isolate the elbow flexion movement.

If strength or ROM is not symmetrical, exercise one arm at a time.

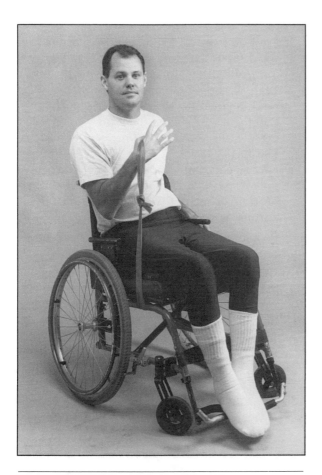

Figure 10.15 Elbow flexion, end position.

Action	Major muscles
Flexion	Biceps brachii
	Brachialis
	Brachioradialis
Extension	Triceps brachii
	Anconeus
Supination (forearm)	Biceps brachii
Pronation (forearm)	Pronator teres

Note. The biceps also stabilize the humerus in the shoulder joint.

Elbow Extension

Action:

1. Reach one hand behind the head with the shoulder in full flexion; internally rotate the other shoulder and reach the hand behind the back.
2. Grasp the band behind the back with both hands so that it runs vertically between the scapula and the back of the neck.
3. Push the band toward the ceiling and fully extend the elbow. Stabilize the shoulder and upper arm to prevent any movement (see Fig. 10.16a).

Tips: People with weak triceps may wish to use this alternate exercise: Hold the band in front of the chest with elbows fully flexed, shoulders abducted 90 degrees (arms parallel to the floor), and palms facing down. Fix one end of the band with one hand at the chest while slowly extending the other elbow (see Fig. 10.16b).

With extreme triceps weakness, perform the exercise without resistance. Do not allow external shoulder rotation as this permits "cheating" by allowing the biceps to control the action.

This exercise is important for muscle balancing with spasticity in the biceps. If spasticity or involuntary movements of the nonworking arm interfere with smooth repetition for the working arm, then secure one end of the band to a stationary object (or use a partner). If full range of motion is not possible in the overhead position, then use the modified set-up described.

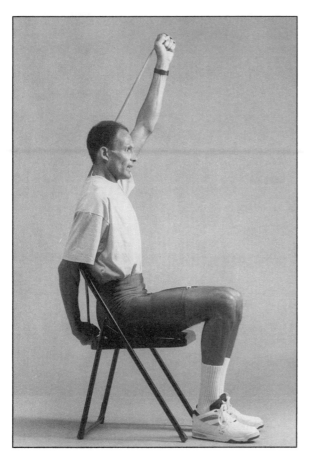

a

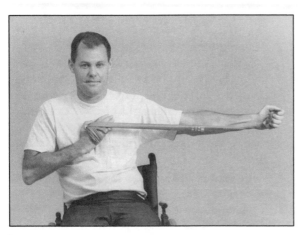

b

Figure 10.16 Elbow extension overhead (a) and with modified gravity-eliminated position (b).

Stretching—Elbow Flexors

Action:

1. Outwardly rotate and flex the shoulder about 45 degrees; support the arm of the flexed shoulder behind the elbow with the opposite hand or rest the upper arm on a table.
2. Allow the pull of gravity to pull the elbow into extension. A partner can apply additional stretch as needed if sensation is not impaired.
3. To increase the stretch, use this alternate position: Extend the elbow and outwardly rotate and hyperextend the shoulder. Place the wrist or palm on an object such as a table at the level of and behind the hips. Rotate the trunk slightly away from the extended shoulder until the stretch is felt.

Tip: This is an important stretch for people with spastic biceps muscles preceding or following resistance training (or any activity) and for limiting the development of contractures.

Stretching—Elbow Extensors and Shoulder Extensors

Action:

1. Position one arm so the elbow is pointed toward the ceiling and the palm is flat against the center of the upper back (below the neck).
2. With the opposite hand, grasp the elbow by reaching over the top of the head.
3. Pull the elbow behind the head; avoid changing the alignment of the neck and back (see Fig. 10.17).

Tips: If someone with impaired upper body function or spasticity is unable to lift the arms overhead or maintain the proper position, have a partner assist with this stretch.

People with spasticity may need to concentrate on keeping neck muscles relaxed.

People with an amputation below the elbow may especially benefit from this stretch to prevent contractures. (Remove prosthesis to do the stretch.)

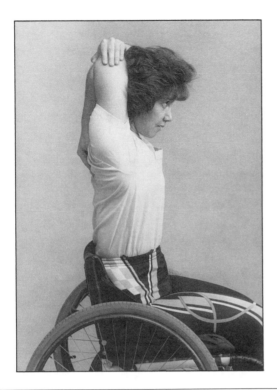

Figure 10.17 Stretching elbow extensors and shoulder extensors.

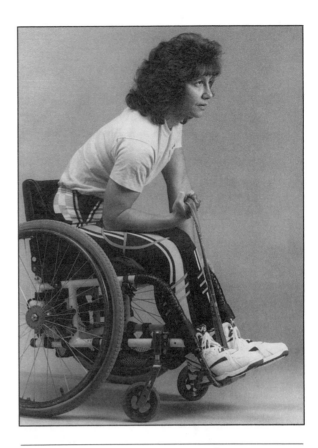

Figure 10.18 End position for wrist flexion.

Exercises for the Wrist Joint

Wrist Flexion (Wrist Curls)

Action:
1. Place one end of the band under the foot, chair, or foot rests and grasp the other end of the band with the palm facing up.
2. Rest the forearm on the thigh or arm rest with the wrist hyperextended.
3. Keeping the forearm stationary, flex the wrist through the full range (see Fig. 10.18).

Tips: The resistance of gravity alone may be adequate, depending upon muscular strength.

Stabilize the exercising forearm with the opposite hand or forearm to prevent the tendency toward elbow flexion.

This exercise is generally not recommended for people with very spastic finger and wrist flexors; instead they should concentrate on reverse wrist curls and flexor stretches.

Wrist Extension (Reverse Wrist Curls)

Action:
1. Place one end of the band under the feet or foot rests.
2. Grasp the other end of the band with the palm facing down. Allow the forearm to rest on the thigh or arm rest. (The band can be tied in a loop for gripping.)
3. Starting with the wrist fully flexed and keeping the forearm stationary, extend the wrist through the full range.

Tips: People with very weak forearm muscles may want to perform this exercise without the band, using resistance from gravity alone. You can further eliminate the pull of gravity by placing the arm on a flat surface and moving the hand in an arc perpendicular to the pull of gravity.

When spasticity is involved, do not use the band resistance unless the movement can be isolated through the full range of motion. It is very important to stabilize the forearm to prevent "cheating" on the exercise.

Stretching—Wrist Flexors

Action:

1. Pronate one forearm and rest it on the thigh or arm rest.
2. Press the palm of that hand with the opposite hand (see Fig. 10.19a), pulling the wrist and fingers into hyperextension (fingers will be pointing up).

Caution: People with quadriplegia who lack finger flexors *must* keep the fingers flexed when they are pressing the wrist into hyperextension to prevent weakening the tenodesis action they rely on for grasping.

Tip: This is an important stretch for people with spasticity and tight wrist flexors. Pressure and an outward pull at the *base* of the thumb (see Fig. 10.19b) may help relax the wrist and hand if it is extremely tight. Take care to avoid pulling the upper part of the thumb; the force should come from across the palm onto the base of the thumb. Be sure the forearm is stabilized during the stretch.

Action	Major muscles
Flexion	Flexor carpi radialis
	Flexor carpi ulnaris
Extension	Extensor carpi radialis longus and brevis
	Extensor digitorum
	Extensor carpi ulnaris
Pronation (forearm)	Pronator quadratus
Supination (forearm)	Supinator

Stretching—Wrist Extensors

Action:

1. Pronate one forearm and rest it on the thigh or arm rest.
2. Press the back of that hand with the opposite hand, pulling the wrist into flexion (fingers will be pointing down).

Tip: This exercise is not recommended for people with spastic wrist flexors.

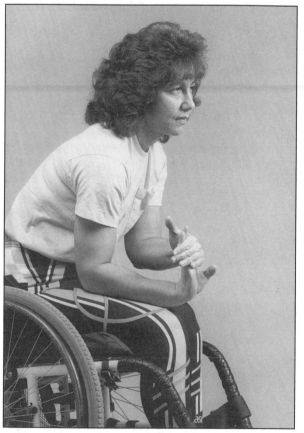

a

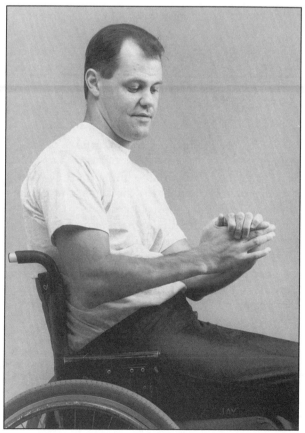

b

Figure 10.19 Wrist and finger flexor stretch (a), and modified stretch for wrist flexors only (b).

Exercises for the Trunk

Action	Major muscles
Flexion	Rectus abdominis
	External and internal abdominal obliques
Extension	Erector spinae
	Multifidus
	Rotatores
	Semispinalis thoracis and cervicis
Lateral flexion and rotation	Rectus abdominis
	External and internal abdominal obliques
	Erector spinae
	Semispinalis thoracis and cervicis
Pelvic tilt (backward)	Rectus abdominis
Pelvic tilt (forward)	Erector spinae

Note. Anterior muscles of the lower trunk also tense the abdominal wall and stabilize the lumbar spine.

Trunk Flexion (Seated Abdominal Curl)

Action:

1. Have a partner grasp both ends of the band behind the back at the level of the head. Loop the band under the arms and around the chest.
2. Cross the arms over the chest and press the elbows loosely into the sides.
3. Slowly, curl the trunk forward as far as possible; avoid use of the hip flexors (see Fig. 10.20a).

Tips: An alternate arrangement that provides more resistance is to loop the band under the chair, cross it in back, and hold the band over the shoulders (see Fig. 10.20b).

Some people with limited trunk function may only be able to perform this exercise through a limited range of motion. Placing the hands on the arm rests assists with balance.

This exercise may also be performed from the floor in a supine position (hips and knees flexed, feet flat on the floor) without band resistance.

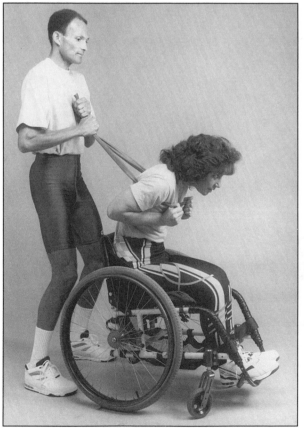

a

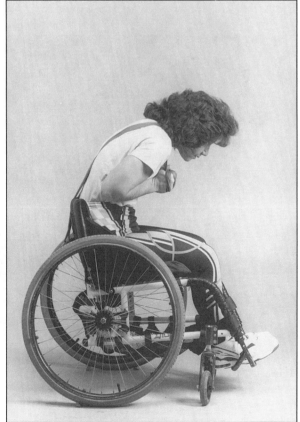

b

Figure 10.20 Trunk flexion with a partner (a) and independently with the chair-cross band position (b).

Trunk Rotation (Supine Twisting Abdominal Curl)

Action:

1. From a supine position, clasp the hands behind the head.
2. Flex the knees so the thighs are perpendicular to the floor. For additional stability, support the lower legs on a chair or with a partner.
3. Curl the shoulders off the floor while twisting to touch one elbow to the opposite knee (see Fig. 10.21). Return slowly to the starting position.

Tips: If a participant cannot touch the knee with the elbow, recommend performing the rotating movement so the elbow crosses the midline of the body toward the opposite knee.

For more stability, people with a BK amputation should support the lower leg and stump on a chair. Someone with an AK amputation can rest the unimpaired leg on a stool while pressing the stump against it to maintain a symmetrical flexed hip position. People with lower extremity amputations also can use a partner for assistance.

With adductor spasticity, it may be helpful to place an object between the knees to keep them separate.

Trunk Extension (Seated Reverse Abdominal Curl)

Action:

1. Wrap the band around the upper back and under the arms.
2. Curl the trunk forward from the waist, rolling the shoulders toward the thighs. Securely attach the ends to a stationary object in front of the body or have a partner hold the ends at about waist level.
3. Hold the band at arm level and press the elbows into the sides to prevent the band from slipping down the back (see Fig. 10.22).
4. Keep the head and spine in alignment and extend the trunk until it touches the back of the chair.

Tips: With muscle weakness, the resistance from gravity alone may be adequate.

With impaired balance, push the forearms against the thighs to assist with the movement and provide additional stability. The arm rests may also be grasped for support.

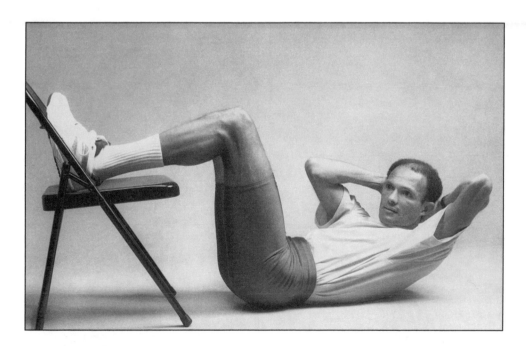

Figure 10.21 Trunk rotation.

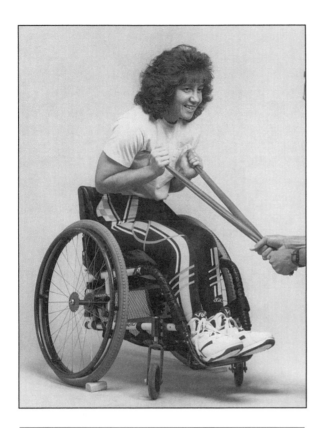

Figure 10.22 Trunk extension.

Trunk-Hip Extension—Prone

Action:
1. From the prone position, extend the arms overhead and place the forehead on the floor.
2. Simultaneously lift the right arm and left leg off the floor as high as possible (see Fig. 10.23). Hold for 5 s and return SLOWLY to the starting position.

Tips: If lower body function is impaired, do the exercise with just the arm and available trunk extensor muscles.

People with impaired balance or coordination can work only one limb at a time.

Tight hip flexors may prevent some people from performing hip extension from a prone position.

Stretching—Lateral Trunk Flexors

Action:
1. Raise one arm straight overhead and grasp the arm just below the elbow with the opposite hand.
2. Keep the buttocks stationary and laterally flex the trunk away from the extended arm (see Fig. 10.24).

Tips: Participants with impaired balance or coordination can grasp the armrest or wheel by

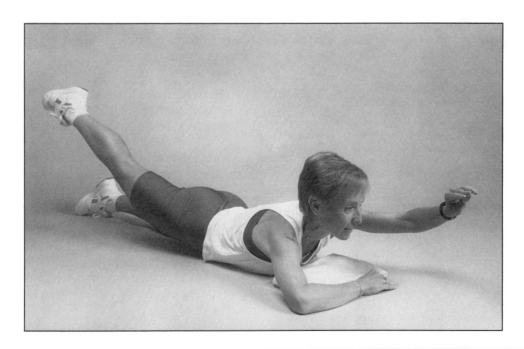

Figure 10.23 Prone trunk and hip extension.

reaching across the body, or they can rest the arm on the armrest if hand function is impaired. Raise one arm while leaning to the opposite side.

A partner can assist with lifting the arm overhead if the participant is unable to do so.

Grasping at the wrist may be easier than grasping at the elbow for some people.

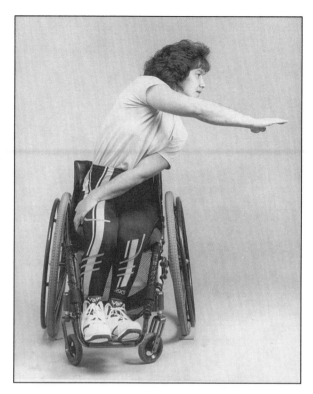

Figure 10.25 Trunk rotator stretch.

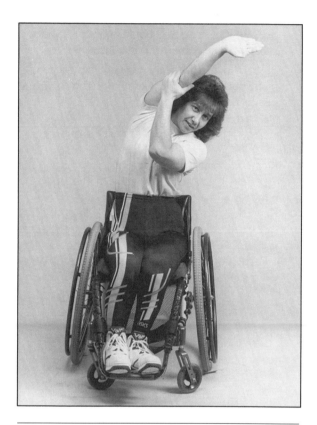

Figure 10.24 Lateral trunk flexor stretch.

Stretching—Trunk Rotators (Twists)

Action:

1. Reach across the body and grasp the chair near the opposite hip.
2. Keep the feet flat on the floor and the buttocks stationary; reach the other arm across the front of the body, twisting in the direction of the reach and looking back over the shoulder (see Fig. 10.25).

Caution: This stretch may not be appropriate for individuals with Harrington rods or any spinal fusion. Consult with the person's therapist or physician before recommending any twisting stretch.

Tip: Some people may need to adjust the exercise by hooking the arm over the push handle of the wheelchair when rotating to that direction. The opposite arm can then reach across the body to improve the stretch.

Stretching—Trunk Extensors

Action:

1. From the supine position, bend both knees, pull them to the chest, and hold (see Fig. 10.26).

Caution: If adequate flexibility is present in the lower back and hamstrings, people with impaired trunk muscles should not overemphasize this stretch. Excessive flexibility of trunk extensors might reduce functioning for these people; a rigid trunk may enhance their ability to independently transfer and maintain an upright posture.

Tips: Some people may need assistance from a partner to assume the stretch position.

People who can assume the supine stretch position may further benefit by rolling the head and shoulders up toward the knees.

People with impaired balance or a high degree of spasticity may accomplish a similar stretch by lying on one side and pulling the knees to the chest.

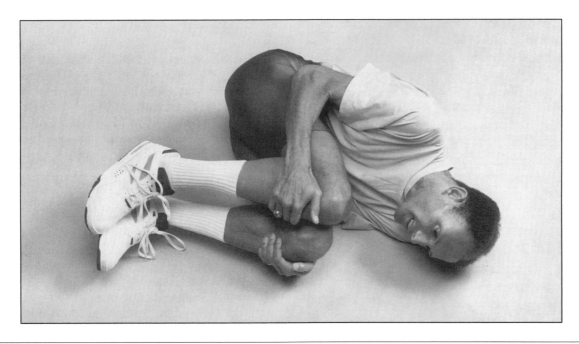

Figure 10.26 Trunk extensor stretch.

Exercises for the Hip Joint

Action	Major muscles
Flexion	Iliopsoas
	Rectus femoris
Extension	Gluteus maximus
	Biceps femoris
	Semimembranosus
	Semitendinosus
Abduction	Gluteus medius and
	minimus
Adduction	Adductor brevis, magnus,
	and longus
	Pectineus
	Gracilis
Transverse (horizontal) abduction	Gluteus maximus, medius, and minimus
	Deep lateral rotators*
Transverse (horizontal) adduction	Adductor brevis and longus
Lateral (outward) rotation	Gluteus maximus
	Iliopsoas
	Deep lateral rotators*
Medial (inward) rotation	Gracilis
	Semitendinosus
	Semimembranosus

*Deep lateral rotators are the quadratus femoris, obturator externus, obturator internus, gemellus inferior, gemellus superior, and piriformis muscles.

Hip Flexion (Seated Leg Raises)

Action:

1. Wrap the band around the thighs just above the knees, allowing enough laxity for movement.
2. Grasp both ends of the band in one hand and hold it at chair level.
3. Lift one thigh to flex the hip as much as possible (see Fig. 10.27). Perform repetitions for each leg independently or by alternating legs.

Tips: This exercise position is recommended only for people who must exercise from a chair because the seated position restricts the range of motion to a narrow arc.

People with very weak hip flexors should perform the exercise at first with resistance from gravity only.

People with high AK amputations may perform the same exercise with a cuff weight.

People with impaired coordination may exercise one leg at a time with the band looped under the chair and wrapped around only one leg.

Most people, especially those who have developed imbalances in hip and lower trunk muscles caused by seated postures for prolonged periods and people with spasticity in the hip flexors, need not emphasize this exercise.

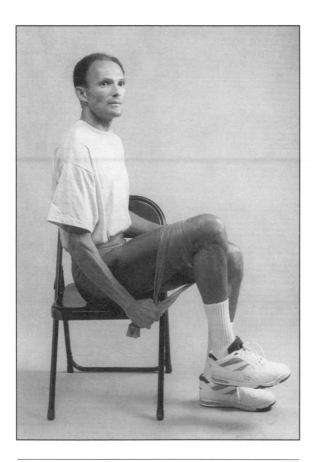

Figure 10.27 Hip flexion end position.

Knee-Hip Extension (Leg Press)

Action:
1. Flex the knee and hip. Tie the band around one ankle and foot; hold the other end with the hands at waist level in line with the hip and knee (see Fig. 10.28a).
2. Push the band forward by extending the knee and hip as far as the seated position (and balance) will allow (see Fig. 10.28b).

Hip Abduction

Action:
1. With the knees together, wrap the band around the thighs just above the knees with enough laxity to allow for movement through the full range.
2. Move one leg at a time into abduction through the full range of motion while keeping the other leg stationary (see Fig. 10.29). Keep the foot parallel to the floor by flexing slightly at the hip and lifting the foot off the ground. Avoid outward rotation of the hip.

Tips: People with weak hip abductors can use this progression: (a) perform as described above, but without any resistance from the band; (b) advance next to sitting on the floor with the knees extended, feet forward, and move the entire leg out to the side; and (c) progress to using the band as described above.

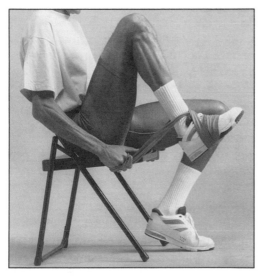

a

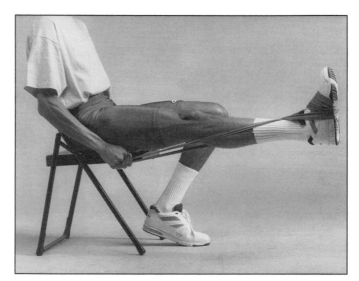

b

Figure 10.28 Knee and hip extension starting position (a) and end position (b).

If foot pedals of a wheelchair get in the way of the movement, remove them *only* if the feet can touch the ground. Do not allow the feet to dangle.

This is an excellent exercise for the person with tight adductor muscles (evidenced by a knock-kneed position and scissors gait) common with lower extremity spasticity. To isolate the movement to one leg at a time, wrap the band around only one leg and secure it by grasping the band and holding it at chair level on the opposite side.

Hip Adduction

Action:

1. Abduct one hip and loop the band around the leg just above the knee. Securely attach the other end of the band at the level of the thigh (or have a partner hold it) so resistance is felt on the inner side of the thigh (see Fig. 10.30).

2. Stabilize the nonexercising leg and slide the foot and entire leg (as a unit) to the midline of the body.

Tip: People who walk with a scissors gait or sit with knees locked together due to tight adductor muscles should use light resistance with this exercise and focus on the exercise to strengthen leg abductors.

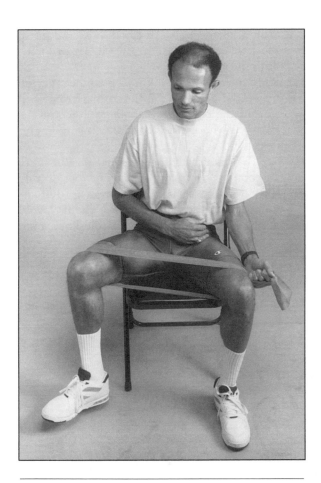

Figure 10.29 Hip abduction end position.

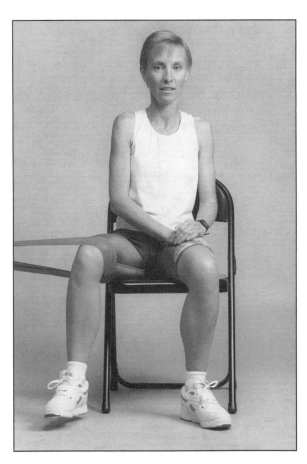

Figure 10.30 Starting position for hip adduction exercise.

Stretching—Hip Flexors

Action:

1. Assume a prone position and allow gravity to pull the hips toward the floor. To increase the stretch, elevate the knees, flex one knee, and grab at the ankle, or have a partner hold the ankle to maintain the position to increase the stretch on the rectus femoris muscle (see Fig. 10.31).

Tip: People with inadequate ROM in the hip flexors will derive the most benefit from this stretch.

Stretching—Hip Abductors

Action:

1. In a supine position with the legs and hips in full extension, flex one knee and place the heel gently on top of the other knee.
2. Grasp the outside of the flexed knee with the opposite hand.
3. Keep the foot on the extended knee and pull the flexed knee across the midline of the body toward the floor until tightness is felt in the outer hip (see Fig. 10.32).

Tips: Some people may need assistance with positioning and grasping the leg, but they may be able to independently maintain the stretch position once achieved.

This stretch may also be performed sitting erect with the foot placed on the floor outside of the extended knee to avoid putting pressure on the knee joint.

Advise caution to avoid overstretching where sensation is lacking.

People with AK amputations should grasp the stump and gently pull it toward the opposite leg to feel the stretch on the outer hip. The exercise may be done from either a sitting or lying position.

Stretching—Hip Adductors

Action:

1. Seated on the floor, flex one knee and grasp the ankle from underneath the leg with the opposite hand.
2. Keep the back as straight as possible and pull up on the ankle of the flexed leg, bringing it toward the body while pushing down on the knee with the arm on the same side until tightness is felt (see Fig. 10.33).

Caution: In this stretch, the hip is in a position very susceptible to fracture. Anyone performing this stretch, especially someone with impairment in the lower extremities, should avoid applying too much torque at the knee joint.

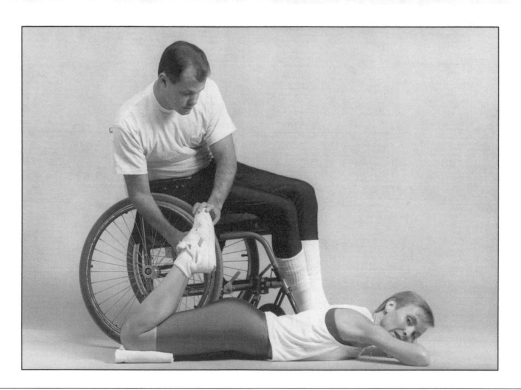

Figure 10.31 Hip flexor stretch.

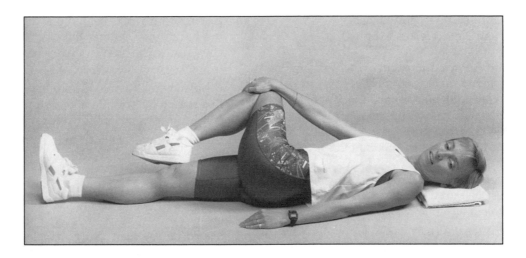

Figure 10.32 Hip abductor stretch.

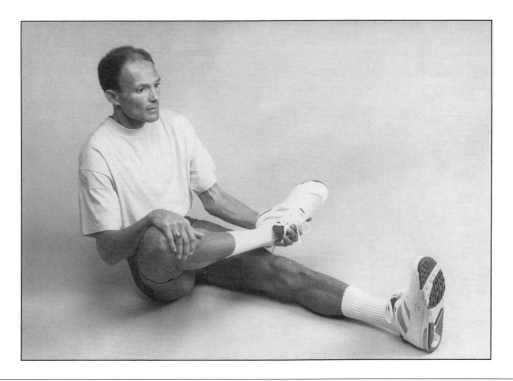

Figure 10.33 Hip adductor stretch.

Muscle weakness may impair knee joint stability, and tight passive stabilizers (ligaments and the joint capsule) may offer needed protection. With impaired sensation, overstretching this area may be difficult to avoid; therefore, for some people this stretch may be contraindicated.

Tip: This is a rather complex movement for people with impaired balance and coordination. It may also be difficult for people with AK amputations to perform depending on trunk flexibility and the length of the residual limb. Use the following alternative: Sitting erect, bend the knees until the soles of the feet are touching each other. Grasp the ankles and lean forward while trying to press the knees to the floor. This stretch may be easier to do lying down (without holding the ankles), using gravity and relaxation to accomplish the stretch. A stretch band can be used to pull the ankles toward the hips from this position. Ensure that the lower back remains flat to the floor.

Stretching—Hip Extensors and Knee Flexors (Supine)

Action:

1. From the supine position, lift one leg and grasp as close to the ankle as possible. Avoid arching the back by tightening the abdominals to press the lower back toward the floor.
2. Push the knee into extension while pulling the hip into deeper flexion until tightness is felt in the hamstrings.

Tips: The hamstring muscles cross two joints; the hip must be flexed and the knee extended to fully stretch all three muscles.

Some participants may need a partner to assist with assuming and stabilizing this position (see Fig. 10.34).

If the lower back cannot be held flat, which may be the case for people with weak abdominal and lower back muscles, then flex the knee of the opposite leg and place the foot flat on the floor.

If spasticity does not interfere, the stretch may be adapted by starting in the sitting position,

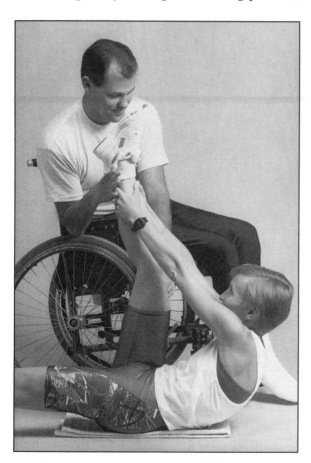

Figure 10.34 Supine hip extensor and knee flexor stretch with partner.

placing both wrists behind one thigh, and lying back while pulling the thigh toward the chest, using the biceps muscles (similar to the trunk extensor stretch).

People with BK or AK amputations can do this stretch by grasping toward the end of the residual limb and pulling it toward the head.

If balance and stability are a problem, the stretch can be performed lying on the side.

Stretching—Hip Extensors and Knee Flexors (Seated)

Action:

1. Seated on the floor, extend the legs with the feet together and ankles plantar flexed (see Fig. 10.35).
2. Keep the back flat and bend forward from the hips through the full range, placing the hands on the floor next to the knees to provide support until tension is felt. Repeat with ankles dorsiflexed.

Tips: To improve balance, stretch by sitting with the lower back against a wall.

People with a high degree of tightness, spasticity, or both may benefit by just stretching the legs out straight (without the forward lean), allowing gravity to pull the knees into extension.

Stretching—Hip Extensors and Adductors

Action:

1. Seated on the floor, straddle the legs.
2. Flex one knee, externally rotate the hip, and place the foot against the inside of the opposite thigh while pressing the knee toward the ground.
3. Keep the back straight and place the hands on the floor (for support). Flex at the hips while pressing the chest toward the knees (see Fig. 10.36).

Tips: People with an AK amputation can stretch forward with the unimpaired leg bent toward the residual limb. When stretching with the amputated leg, keep the residual limb out in a straddle position and stretch toward the straight leg, applying pressure with one hand on the residual limb to prevent it from rotating inward.

If this stretch is difficult to do with the bent knee position, assume a full straddle and bend toward each knee separately, then flex forward between both legs.

All forward flexion should come from the hips, not the trunk, to effectively stretch hip extensors and adductors.

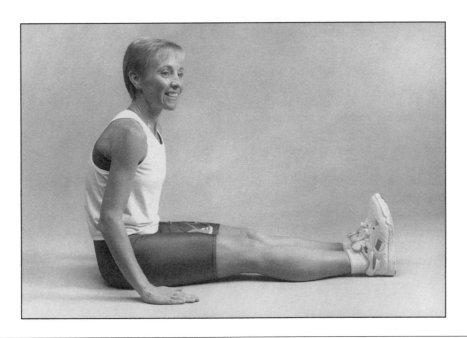

Figure 10.35 Seated hip extensor and knee flexor stretch.

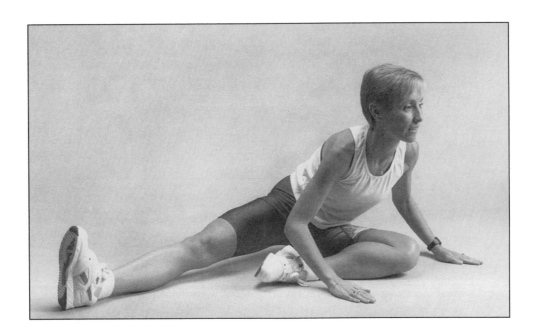

Figure 10.36 Hip extensor and adductor stretch.

Exercises for the Knee Joint

Knee Flexion (Leg Curl)

Action:

1. Attach one end of the band to a stationary object (or use a partner) about waist high in front of the body.
2. Tie the other end around the ankle (see Fig. 10.37a) with the knee in full extension and the hip at 90 degrees of flexion (the leg will be parallel to the floor).
3. Keeping the other foot on the ground, flex the knee as far as the seated position will allow (see Fig. 10.37b).

Tips: The following progression is recommended for weak knee flexors: (a) from a prone position on the floor, flex the knee toward the buttocks through the full range, keeping the hips and thighs on the floor; (b) add Velcro cuff weights around the ankles and follow the previous step; and, as strength increases, (c) perform the exercise from the seated position as described earlier.

People with excessive tone in lower extremity knee flexors should use light resistance for this exercise and emphasize quadriceps strengthening instead.

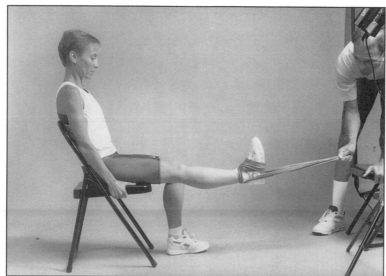

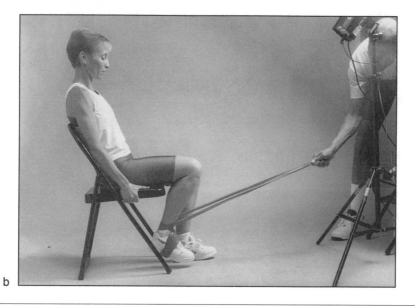

Figure 10.37 Knee flexion with partner starting position (a) and end position (b).

Action	Major muscles
Flexion	Biceps femoris
	Semitendinosus
	Semimembranosus
Extension	Rectus femoris
	Vastus intermedius, medialis, and lateralis
Inward rotation (leg)	Sartorius

Knee Extension

Action:
1. Flex one knee and tie one end of the band around the foot and ankle. (See Fig. 10.38 for suggested wrap.)
2. With the hand on the same side, secure the loose ends of the band at the seat next to the hip (see Fig. 10.39).
3. Slowly extend the knee.

Tips: People with weak knee extensors should perform the exercise without any resistance at first.

People with a BK amputation should attach a Velcro cuff weight on the stump to work the amputated side.

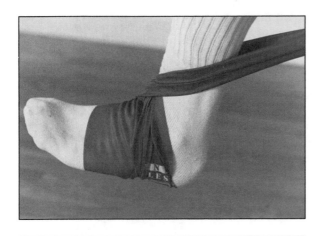

Figure 10.38   Ankle wrap for knee extension.

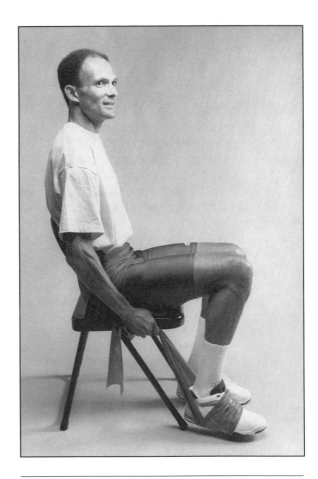

Figure 10.39   Knee extension, flexed position.

Stretching—Knee Flexors

See Supine and Seated Hip Extensors and Knee Flexors stretches (Figures 10.34 and 10.35).
Action:
1. Dorsiflex the ankles to increase the stretch on knee flexors.

Stretching—Knee Extensors

See Prone Hip Flexor Stretch (Figure 10.31).
Action:
1. To increase the stretch on knee extensors, pull the ankle toward the buttocks in line with the thigh.

Caution: Avoid overstretching connective tissues of the knee joint, which may compromise joint stability.

Exercises for the Ankle Joint

Ankle Dorsiflexion

Action:

1. Attach one end of the band to a stationary object, or have a partner hold it in front of the body at knee level.
2. Wrap the other end of the band around the foot and ankle; the resistance should pull the foot into plantar flexion without the band slipping off the foot.
3. Fully extend the knee and support the leg on a chair (see Fig. 10.40).
4. Dorsiflex the ankle through the full range, avoiding eversion or inversion of the foot.

Tip: This is an important exercise for people with tight plantar flexors who have problems with "toe walking."

Action	Major muscle
Dorsiflexion	Tibialis anterior
	Extensor digitorum longus
	Extensor hallucis longus
Plantar flexion	Gastrocnemius
	Soleus
	Tibialis posterior
	Flexor digitorum longus
	Flexor hallucis longus
Inversion	Tibialis anterior
	Tibialis posterior
	Flexor hallucis longus
	Flexor digitorum longus
	Extensor hallucis longus
Eversion	Extensor digitorum longus
	Peroneus brevis and longus

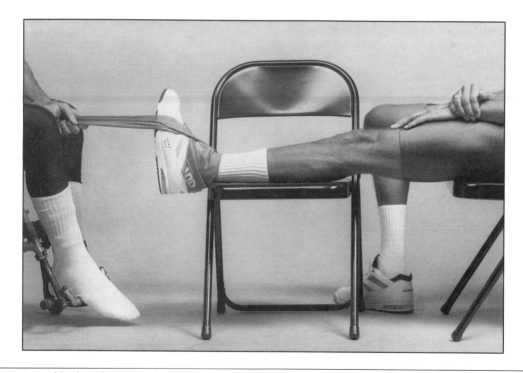

Figure 10.40 Ankle dorsiflexion with partner.

Plantar Flexion

Action:

1. With the knee in full extension and the leg supported on a chair, wrap the band around the instep of one foot. Dorsiflex the ankle and hold the ends of the bands.
2. Maintaining knee extension, plantar flex the ankle against the resistance.

Tips: Avoid curling the toes to prevent cramping in the foot.

People with weak plantar flexors can do this exercise without the band from the prone position. Flex one knee and plantar flex the ankle against the resistance of gravity.

People with tight plantar flexors should perform the exercise with light resistance or gravity alone. They should focus instead on strengthening dorsiflexors and stretching plantar flexors.

Stretching—Ankle Dorsiflexors

Action:

1. Cross one leg over the opposite knee and grasp the heel or ankle with one hand to stabilize the position. Pull the ankle into plantar flexion with the other hand, avoiding inversion or eversion at the ankle (see Fig. 10.41).

Stretching—Plantar Flexors

Action:

1. Assume the starting position for strengthening the plantar flexors. Use the band to pull the ankle to stretch the plantar flexors.

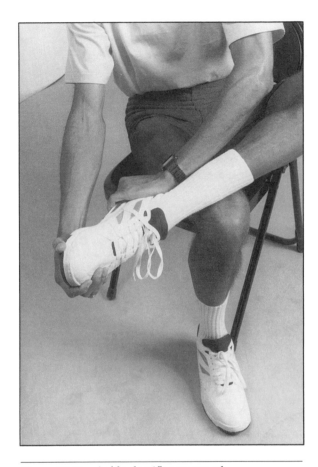

Figure 10.41 Ankle dorsiflexors stretch.

Chapter 11

Aerobic Dance Exercise

Kathy F. Normansell, MEd
Ohio University of Zanesville and Muskingum Area Technical College

Almost everybody, regardless of ability, can derive physical, social, or psychological benefits by participating in an aerobic dance exercise program. Just as you would not expect a beginner to safely enjoy an advanced aerobics class, you should not expect a person with a disability to participate in a general class without having appropriate movement modifications. Your challenge as an exercise leader is to offer modifications that individualize instruction in a group setting while maintaining the value of the program for all participants, with or without disabilities.

This chapter reviews the benefits of group aerobic conditioning programs and their importance for people with physical disabilities. It provides a set of core aerobic dance movement patterns that you can modify in a variety of ways to meet individual needs. And, finally, this chapter offers a system for categorizing conditions associated with disability to enable you to modify core moves and make your aerobic dance program safe, effective, and appropriate for participants with physical disabilities. Chapter 12 provides general suggestions for managing group exercise programs.

Do not assume that someone with a physical disability will inherently know how to adapt your routines to meet his needs and abilities. Your guidance is essential to prevent students with disabilities from becoming frustrated and dropping out of the program. Though many of the guidelines in this chapter appear to be common sense, failure to consider them can mean the difference between a positive and a negative experience or a successful and unsuccessful workout for the participant with a disability. Your skill at modifying aerobic dance routines depends upon your basic knowledge of the general characteristics and exercise implications associated with physical disabilities (chapter 2) and your knowledge of each participant's physical status.

This chapter assumes that you are somewhat knowledgeable and experienced in leading aerobic dance exercise. For a review of basic principles of leading aerobic dance, refer to one of the texts listed in the Recommended Readings. If you are a novice, but wish to develop an adapted program, you should participate in an aerobic dance class and work closely with an experienced instructor. Although nothing can replace experience, nothing can better prepare you for a successful first experience than study and practice. After studying the modifications presented in this chapter, practice teaching (even if you're just teaching yourself in a mirror!) using the suggested guidelines.

Benefits of Aerobic Dance Exercise

For many people, aerobic dance is an enjoyable way to condition the cardiorespiratory system. Exercising to music in a group setting removes some of the drudgery that many people experience in trying to maintain an exercise program alone. For some, the social nature of the aerobics class becomes the primary incentive to continue with a regular program of exercise.

Aerobic dance may offer other important benefits for people with physical disabilities. Chapter 4 reviewed these benefits (see p. 52). It is not uncommon to find that some people with physical disabilities have limited recreational interaction with the nondisabled community because of either self-imposed exclusion or physical and social barriers imposed by society. By providing an accessible aerobics class, you can open new doors as well as educate your nondisabled clients about the abilities and rights of people with disabilities.

Selecting Movement Alternatives

As an aerobics instructor you face the challenge of providing a workout for individuals with a variety of movement abilities, fitness levels, and personal goals. To meet this challenge, you must develop basic routines and build a repertoire of alternatives to meet diverse needs. Selecting exercise modifications for anyone, especially for people with disabilities, must always be guided by three important questions:

- Are the movements *safe*?
- Will the modifications be *effective* for delivering an appropriate training effect?
- Are the movement modifications *appropriate* given the person's abilities, level of conditioning, and movement characteristics?

To answer these questions for participants in your program, you must be knowledgeable of their disabilities and associated movement restrictions. Preliminary assessment and screening highlight areas of concern. If possible, it is also helpful to run through a brief set of core moves and alternatives with each participant to determine which movements are *safe*, *effective*, and *appropriate* for that person. Overall, you must also evaluate whether your program is *enjoyable*.

Before teaching an adapted class, try taking a "regular" class while sitting in a chair to experience which movements feel awkward and which provide the most intensity. You can also impose other limitations on your movements, such as limiting reach to shoulder height or exercising with only one side of your body. These experiments give you insight into what it is like to have a disability and also highlight considerations you should address when leading a class. For example, many arm movements are easy to perform when standing, but armrests may get in the way when performed seated.

Modifying Core Moves

Adapting your aerobics classes to make them accessible for people with disabilities does not mean that you have to change all your movement patterns and routines. By following a few simple guidelines, you can modify the basic or core moves that you combine for the workout. Throughout this chapter, we will discuss selected core moves in terms of their appropriateness or adaptability for conditions associated with various physical disabilities. These moves can be roughly categorized as arm patterns and low-impact or no-impact leg movements:

Basic Arm Patterns

Cross and pull
Press/punch/reach and pull
Swings
Curls
Swimming/backstroke/breaststroke

Low-Impact Leg Moves

March (knee lifts)
Kicks
Lateral step and touch/kick
Toe and heel taps
Hamstring curls

No-Impact Leg Moves

Lunge/hip rock
Pliés/knee bends/squats
Stationary ball-change

This list of core moves is by no means exhaustive; you can use the principles for modifying basic movements described in this chapter with your personal style and repertoire to achieve the same results.

Most people who participate in your aerobic dance classes can exercise with the upper body. Some participants with physical disabilities may also be able to incorporate lower body movements (from either a standing or sitting position), whereas others will be unable to use the lower body for exercise because of paralysis, amputation, or extreme limitations in coordination and balance. People who can exercise from a standing position but who have impaired balance, coordination, or joint function may be limited to low- or no-impact leg moves (i.e., moves that eliminate jumping or hopping). Any modifications you can incorporate into the routine that utilize leg muscles despite limitations with impact and traveling will likely increase the aerobic demand over that imposed by arm and upper body movements alone. With all these considerations in mind, much of your focus should be directed toward developing and varying dynamic upper body moves in an adapted class. You may want to redesign some of your routines that primarily require traveling moves to avoid discouraging participants who use wheelchairs or who have difficulty with locomotion. By using the right music, appropriate intensity, and movement variety, you can create stationary routines that are still challenging, vigorous, and fun.

Varying Intensity

You can vary core moves, as needed, to change the intensity of the action. Incorporate lower intensity movements for warm-up and cool-down and for people restricted by health problems that contraindicate high-intensity exercise. Some disabilities, such as MS or postpolio syndrome, cause early fatigue with exertion. Other conditions that limit the available muscle mass for exercise also cause fatigue. The following techniques for decreasing exercise intensity can be taught to enable your participants to independently modify their workouts, as needed, while still enjoying a full class without debilitating fatigue.

❏ Use lower arm movements: overhead arm movements are more demanding than movements below shoulder level.
❏ Use unilateral movements: bilateral moves incorporate more muscle mass and are therefore more intense. Perform arm patterns on one side of the body and then repeat them on the other side, or alternate between left and right sides for an entire pattern.

❏ Decrease the lever-arm length of a movement: movements with a shorter lever arm are less intense (see Figure 11.1).
❏ Decrease the range of motion: swinging, pressing, or reaching through a partial range decreases the intensity of the effort.
❏ Decrease the speed of the movement: avoid double-time moves and use half-tempo movements as needed.

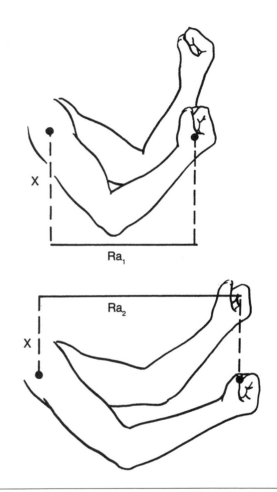

Figure 11.1 Greater force is required to move a limb against gravity when the lever-arm length is increased. X = axis of rotation at the shoulder joint, Ra_1 = lever arm of the resistance with 90 degrees of elbow flexion, Ra_2 = lever arm of the resistance with the elbow at 120 degrees of flexion.

Seated Aerobic Dance Exercise

Individuals in an aerobics class may exercise from a seated position for a variety of reasons. Impaired mobility can prevent standing exercise. Impaired balance or coordination, impaired joint function, or lower limb muscle dysfunction may make working out from a seated position more satisfactory. Some people choose seated exercise because they are very deconditioned. In general, seated exercise employs fewer muscle groups than standing exercise and thereby lessens the aerobic demand of the workout. In fact, the heart rate response with seated aerobic dance exercise may be an exaggerated indicator of the aerobic demand ($\dot{V}O_2$), especially when compared with leg exercise. This is also true in low-impact aerobic dance that emphasizes arm movements (Parker, Hurley, Hanlon, and Vaccaro, 1989). Unless seated exercise is required because of a limitation, encourage a standing workout to provide greater aerobic benefits. The choice, however, is that of the participant.

Nonambulatory participants most likely prefer to exercise in their wheelchairs. Brakes may be locked to prevent the wheelchair from moving. The power should be turned off on a power chair. You should have sturdy, armless chairs available for ambulatory individuals who wish to work out from a sitting position. Chapter 14 provides further general guidelines for any type of exercise from a wheelchair (see p. 184).

Seated Alignment and Exercise Form

Good sitting posture (Figure 11.2) will help maintain proper diaphragmatic breathing during exercise and provide additional support for vigorous movement. People who maintain habitual sitting positions often have poor posture with rounded shoulders and overstretched posterior shoulder and shoulder girdle muscles. To counteract poor sitting posture, incorporate additional backward shoulder movements and movements that "open" the chest during the workout. Arm actions that stretch anterior shoulder muscles and require use of posterior upper body muscles are effective for this purpose. Backstroke, backward arm circles, and reverse "flys" emphasizing a posterior "squeeze" are examples of movements useful for counteracting poor sitting posture.

With seated exercise the base of support becomes narrower and is limited by the surface area of the body in contact with the seat or the floor. This base of support is further reduced if the contacting surfaces are nonfunctional muscles. During lateral stretches or movements outside of the base of support, the participant can use the side of the wheelchair or chair for support either by leaning on one armrest or wheel while stretching the opposite side, or by crossing an arm to the opposite wheel

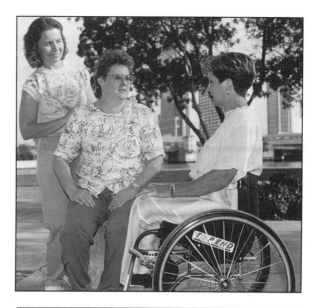

Figure 11.2   Good sitting alignment.

or armrest while reaching with the other arm (see Figure 11.3 a and b). Chest straps can allow the seated participant with impaired balance more freedom to perform vigorous upper body movements. If participants with limited trunk musculature choose not to use chest straps, they may have more upper body movement freedom in a seated position leaning slightly backward. Although this is not ideal seated postural alignment, it is an accepted alternative if it allows for more vigorous arm activity.

To prevent injury and loss of balance, it is helpful to continually reinforce control of arm movements, especially with large movements that tend to encourage "flinging." Remind your students never to lock their elbows or force the shoulders into hyperextension. A slower tempo (less than 150 beats per minute) should be used to allow full range of motion without use of momentum and undue stress on the joints.

Recommend that people with spasticity or who maintain reflexes such as the extensor thrust consider leg and hip strapping to increase hip and knee flexion.

Emphasizing Upper Body Moves

To provide an adequate seated workout, focus on providing conditioning through upper body movements. Low-impact choreography is usually the easiest to modify for seated exercise because the routine generally involves greater focus on upper body activity than high-impact aerobic dance. Low-impact classes generally use a slower tempo,

Kicks, alternating heel and toe taps, marching, or side-stepping are examples of simple leg movements that can be used with seated exercise. If attempting to incorporate leg movements lowers the overall aerobic intensity of the workout, then eliminate lower body work.

Choreography for classes that include seated exercisers should not rely excessively on traveling moves. Although wheeling long distances is an excellent form of aerobic exercise, moving forward and backward four "steps" in a wheelchair does not create much aerobic demand. Instead, the seated participant can use the same arm movements as ambulatory class members during traveling. Even if you present alternatives, classes that incorporate excessive traveling can make seated participants feel as if they are in the way and don't belong.

Because the muscle groups preparing for or recovering from vigorous aerobic activity should receive additional emphasis during the warm-up and cool-down, people exercising from a seated position should focus predominantly on upper body muscle groups. Always suggest alternative upper body movements when other class participants are exercising the lower body during the warm-up and cool-down.

Remaining seated for stretching during the cool-down may be most comfortable for some people, provided there is adequate back support. The advantage of stretching from the floor, however, is that it reduces the vertical distance between the feet and heart, lessening the relative work for the heart. Hip flexors are also more easily stretched from a lying position.

Be sure to include stretches for the legs during the cool-down, even if they were not exercised during the workout. Encourage nonambulatory people to transfer to the floor to do these stretches, or demonstrate stretches that can be done at home. Many people will not feel comfortable transferring to the floor during a class and should not be forced to do so. If the nonambulatory participant does not transfer out of the wheelchair during the cool-down, she can repeat arm stretches while the other class participants perform lower body stretches.

Hand and Wrist Weights

Some people who exercise from a seated position may wish to increase the intensity of the workout by using hand and wrist weights. Although use of hand weights has been shown to increase the heart rate during low-impact aerobic dance exercise, it has not definitively been shown to increase

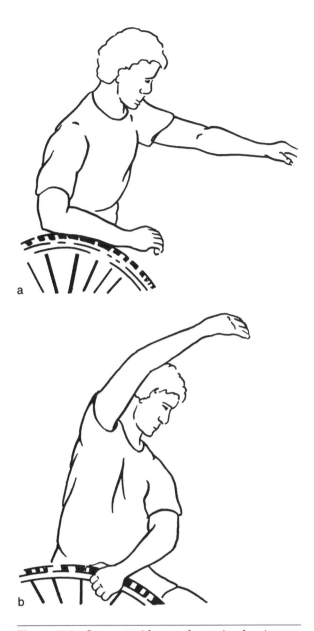

Figure 11.3 Support with seated exercise: leaning on the wheelchair (a), and cross grasp with overhead reach (b).

which allows easier incorporation of large arm movements. Low-impact choreography, however, uses a lot of movement in the vertical plane, and you should not encourage the seated exerciser to imitate these standing movements by repeatedly flexing and extending the trunk.

With forethought, you can find creative alternatives for most leg movements. Replace a kick with an arm swing, a "rock" with alternating arm punches. The possibilities are unlimited.

Incorporate leg movements into a seated exercise routine whenever possible if such efforts do not interfere with the intensity of the workout.

aerobic demand (Carroll, Otto, & Wygand, 1991). Because of the nature of the large, exaggerated arm movements in the adapted aerobics class, use of weights could place unwanted stress on the joints and connective tissues. Additionally, the use of hand weights may increase local muscular fatigue, making the workout anaerobic and defeating the purpose of the aerobic workout. In most cases, the risk of using hand weights will outweigh the benefits, and their use should be discouraged.

The nearby box summarizes considerations for the seated exerciser.

Conditions Requiring Modifications

A physical disability may have associated conditions that require movement modifications to allow benefits from aerobic dance. A system of categorizing general conditions has been developed to ease the task of modifying aerobic dance routines for people with physical disabilities. These categories are not offered as a system for classifying disabilities because a disability may involve one or more of the conditions identified. For example, cerebral palsy involving upper body spasticity may impair balance and coordination, requiring modifications to address both of these conditions. Most participants' needs can be addressed by a creative, problem-solving approach to movement challenges combined with a basic knowledge of disability characteristics and principles of aerobic conditioning.

Impaired Balance

Impairments resulting from injury to or disease of the nervous system (cerebral palsy, head injury, or multiple sclerosis) or disabilities that result in structural changes in the body, such as amputation, may affect balance. Asymmetrical function in muscles and limbs, as with hemiplegia, may also impair balance. Regardless of the cause of impaired balance, preliminary observation of simple movement capabilities should guide your recommendations for appropriate modifications.

Of primary importance when selecting moves for people with impaired balance is to prevent or minimize falls. Secondarily, movements must not cause the participant to focus exclusively on maintaining balance at the expense of exercising vigorously, which would defeat the purpose of aerobic training. Ambulatory persons with severe balance impairments may receive a better workout sitting than standing.

Base of Support and Center of Gravity

Balance generally increases during standing exercise with a widened base of support and lowered center of gravity. Position the feet slightly wider than shoulder width and keep the knees slightly bent throughout the workout. This strategy is beneficial for all except people with lower limb amputations who might feel more comfortable with a narrower base or a staggered foot position. Many prosthetic knees are less likely to buckle if they are kept locked in a toe-in position. People with hypertonic hip adductors (common with spastic CP) or hemiplegia also may need to try a variety of positions to maximize balance with foot positioning. By experimenting with several alternatives you will be able to determine what works best for each participant.

Recommend that people with impaired balance keep their center of gravity over the base of support. Side to side double arm movements with presses or swings cause rapid shifts in the center of gravity from outside the base of support, so these actions are generally contraindicated for people with impaired balance. A preferable alternative is to use bilateral, symmetrical arm actions such as jumping-jack arms, crosses, punches, and presses within the base of support.

ADAPTING AEROBIC DANCE FOR SEATED EXERCISE

- Encourage good sitting posture, alignment, and movement form.
- Offer a chair for support to maintain balance, if needed.
- Use slower tempo music (under 150 beats per minute).
- Limit use of traveling moves or provide movement alternatives.
- Focus on upper body movements during peak activity.
- Emphasize upper body movements and stretches during the warm-up and cool-down.
- Incorporate leg stretches in the cool-down.
- Encourage trunk and leg movement when possible.
- Discourage the use of hand and wrist weights.

Leg movements that shift support entirely to one leg, such as pendulum rocks, also bring the center of gravity to the limits of the support base and compromise balance. If leg and arm movements are coordinated to keep the center of gravity over the base of support, balance can be maintained with a variety of combinations.

Complex and highly coordinated leg patterns and dance steps are more likely to compromise balance and should also be avoided. For example, grapevine or cross-over steps are not recommended. Single-step touches in place may be less challenging than patterned-step touches in one direction.

If one or both feet leave the floor during leg movements, the likelihood of falling increases. A conservative approach with impaired balance is to offer movement patterns that leave both feet firmly planted on the floor, such as knee bends, hip rocks, or lunges. People with less severe balance problems can safely perform marching steps, heel or toe taps, step-together-step patterns, or alternating step-touches. Examples of leg movements likely to be too difficult for people with impaired balance are slides, skipping, pendulum rocks, high knee lifts or kicks, and one-legged hopping.

In general, balance is more likely to be maintained throughout the aerobics workout if you emphasize vigorous upper body movements coordinated with very simple leg movements. The result will be a more effective workout because participants can pay attention to maintaining the proper exercise intensity instead of maintaining balance.

Directional Changes

Momentum is generated when the body or a body part travels rapidly in one direction. A sudden change in direction is difficult for people with impaired balance. When using traveling moves, incorporate a brief period of stationary movement between changes in direction—for example, use a four-count forward march, four-count march in place, and four-count backward march—to prevent participants from losing balance.

Additional Support

Even when a person with impaired balance wants to exercise while standing, provide a chair, table, or ballet barre to grab for support as needed. In addition, everyone should have a chair available for sitting if standing begins to interfere with the workout or causes excessive fatigue (see Figure 11.4). If the individual with impaired balance

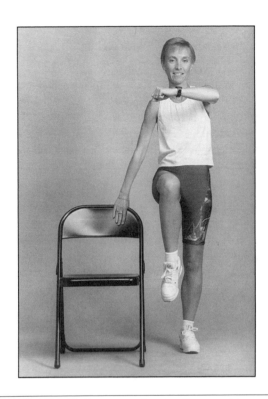

Figure 11.4 Chair support for standing aerobic dance.

chooses to exercise from a seated position, refer to pages 151-154 for modifications on seated exercise. Use the chair for support during lateral stretches and movements, and avoid movements in which both arms move to one side of the body, outside the center of balance.

The nearby box summarizes recommendations for modifying aerobic dance for people with impaired balance.

Considerations for People With Amputations

People with lower limb amputations have unique challenges affecting balance that require additional consideration. Low-back problems are often associated with lower limb amputation because of improper postural alignment with gait changes caused by use of a prosthesis. Often, the person with an amputation places more weight on the unimpaired leg, causing undesirable hip and low-back postures. During standing exercise, direct the person with an amputation to keep the hips level with the floor and avoid tilting or twisting actions. This participant also must pay extra attention to keeping the abdominal muscles firm and the lower back flat throughout the workout.

Discourage people with lower extremity amputations from hopping on one leg for an extended

---

ADAPTING FOR IMPAIRED BALANCE

- Select postures that enhance balance.
- Offer movements that maintain the center of gravity within the base of support.
- Avoid complex leg patterns.
- Choreograph routines that focus on upper body work.
- Use leg movements that maintain contact with the floor.

- Provide props for extra support, such as a chair, table, ballet barre.
- Avoid unsupported lateral stretches and movements.
- Avoid quick changes in direction or rapid alternating side-to-side movements.

---

period of time (more than eight counts). Permit hopping only for people with above-average fitness, no evidence of knee, ankle, or hip problems, and the ability to maintain good pelvic alignment while hopping. Use hopping in intervals, alternating it with low-impact standing or sitting movements. A sturdy chair, table top, or wall must be available for additional support when needed.

Direct your participants with lower limb amputations to monitor the residual limb for rubbing and irritation during the exercise session. Recommend that participants who use a stump sock have an extra one available as a replacement after exercising. Stump socks soaked with perspiration can cause painful and unnecessary skin irritations.

Because the muscles of the residual limb are also exercised during aerobics, be sure to include limbering and stretching exercises for these muscles during the warm-up and cool-down.

Some people may have a fuller range of motion during exercise when the residual limb is not restricted by a prosthesis. People with above-the-elbow amputations who use a shoulder harness prosthesis probably prefer to exercise without it because the straps may restrict movement and become abrasive. Below-elbow prostheses tend to be less restrictive and can be removed according to individual comfort and need.

Pay special attention to proper body alignment and control if a lower limb prosthesis is removed during exercise. Maintaining balance without the prosthesis can be quite difficult during an aerobics workout and may overstress the muscles of the supporting leg. For this reason, it is usually recommended that if the prosthesis is removed, the individual should remain seated during the peak phase of the workout.

Some prostheses are designed for use with a specific style of shoe (such as a dress heel) and may cause leg heights to differ when an aerobics shoe is worn. If the difference is slight, a wedge in the heel of the shoe may help. If the difference is too great, causing uneven hip alignment, then standing leg movement is contraindicated with the prosthesis. Someone with such a problem may, over time, choose to purchase a sports prosthesis. The immediate solution, however, is to exercise from a seated position.

Remember that the decision to wear or remove the prosthesis must always be left to the exerciser. It is your responsibility, however, to make appropriate recommendations and to ensure that proper precautions are followed once a decision has been made.

The nearby box summarizes modifications appropriate for people with amputations.

Impaired Coordination

When motor control is impaired as a result of injury to or disease of the brain (such as with CP, stroke, head injury, MS, etc.) coordinating movement patterns can become challenging. These challenges are further complicated with spasticity, which causes abnormal co-contraction of agonist and antagonist muscles during voluntary movement. For a review of other forms of movement incoordination, refer to chapter 2.

Two considerations in leading aerobic dance exercise for people with impaired coordination are to simplify movements and to avoid eliciting undesirable movement patterns when possible. Attempting to follow a routine in which one arm does something different from the other while the legs do something else entirely becomes frustrating at best for people with impaired coordination. Simplifying body movements should not be confused with simplifying verbal instructions, however. Unless a receptive communication disorder or cognitive impairment is present, offer instructions just as you would to any other class participant.

In participants with spasticity, you also must avoid causing significant increases in muscle tone during the workout. Incorporate relaxation techniques, breathing drills, and prolonged stretching during the warm-up to help prevent an increase in tone with exercise. During the cool-down these techniques may help reduce tension and spasticity

MOVEMENT CONSIDERATIONS FOR PEOPLE WITH AMPUTATIONS

- Prevent excessive stress to the lower back by focusing on proper alignment.
- Prevent excessive strain to the unimpaired supporting leg; discourage excessive hopping on one leg with a lower-extremity amputation.
- Exercise and stretch the residual limb.
- Recommend seated exercise during peak phases if the prosthesis is removed.
- Consider modifications for impaired balance.

that increase as a result of the workout. Always keep in mind that static stretching is best performed after warming up the muscles with loose, rhythmic, limbering movements. After vigorous exercise, the heart rate must be lowered before beginning static stretching. You should never halt vigorous exercise abruptly for stretching just as you should never initiate vigorous activity after stretching unless you have first gradually increased the heart rate to the target range.

Prolonging the warm-up and incorporating a more gradual increase in heart rate will be most beneficial for people with impaired coordination due to CP. Stretching for an extended period can be effective for increasing ROM in preparation for vigorous exercise. This approach also allows the person with impaired coordination plenty of time to assume the desired stretching position. However, be conscious that the "warm-up effect" can be lost with prolonged stretching. Ballistic stretching or pulsing during a stretch is contraindicated in most circumstances, especially with spastic muscles.

Slow and Simple

In general, participants with impaired coordination feel more success with large, fluid movements rather than specific stylized moves throughout the aerobics workout. Excessive use of small, rapid, tense movements is not recommended, especially for people with spasticity. This type of movement may increase tone in spastic muscles, which reduces ROM. Attempting to perform abrupt actions probably will frustrate people who normally function with slow, deliberate movements. If you do use fast, tight movements, follow them with an extended set of slower, large movements.

Some people are unable to maintain the pace you set in a traditional aerobics class. By offering half-tempo alternatives that can be repeated once for every two moves that other class members are using, you may prevent these individuals from experiencing the frustration that may otherwise occur as a result of trying to maintain a quick pace. Likewise, avoid continuous counting of moves,

which can frustrate participants who cannot keep tempo. You can also decrease the music tempo to accommodate slower large movements. Continually encourage participants with impaired coordination to keep moving even if they are unable to stay with the beat or precisely simulate your movements.

Combinations that are relatively simple for a person without a disability may be difficult for a person with impaired coordination. For example, heel or toe taps combined with arm presses may cause some people with impaired coordination a great deal of frustration. Recommend that these participants focus on either upper body or lower body movements independently and do what they can to keep the intensity up to the intended level.

When you introduce new movements into a routine, do so for only the upper or lower body instead of initiating new arm and leg patterns simultaneously. Give participants with impaired coordination an extended opportunity to repeat a single pattern before adding additional movements or variations in another part of the body. If you introduce complex arm movements, restrict leg movement to simple marching, rocking, lunging, or pliés. Movement patterns that require intense concentration from people with impaired coordination may lessen the intensity of the overall effort and reduce the aerobic training effect of the workout.

Limit Variety

Within a single exercise session, limit the number of arm, leg, and combination patterns to decrease the amount of concentration devoted to mastering a movement and increase the participant's feeling of success.

A typical aerobics class may include four-count or eight-count movement patterns, or it may incorporate a descending set, such as transitions from eight-count to four-count to two-count, and alternating single movements. This type of choreography is inappropriate for most people with impaired coordination. Repetitions for a minimum of 12 to 16 counts are preferable.

With disabilities such as spastic CP, symmetrical movements may be easier to perform because some asymmetrical moves of the head, neck, and spine may elicit reflexes that inhibit further movement or range of motion. Although you needn't concentrate exclusively on avoiding eliciting primitive reflexes when choreographing routines, knowledge of their characteristics and effects with movement is valuable for making some movement choices. Chapter 2 includes a discussion of primitive reflexes.

With spastic CP, excessive flexion and adduction tends to predominate, often affecting wrists, elbows, shoulders, hips, knees, and ankles. Excessive use of moves that reinforce these positions, such as biceps curls, is not recommended. Movements that require use of extensors and abductors should be encouraged.

Directional Changes

Rapid changes in direction with traveling or arm movements are difficult to coordinate and are not recommended for people with impaired coordination. When these participants attempt rapid changes in direction, they often find themselves traveling in the opposite direction of everyone else in the class. As recommended with impaired balance, incorporate a holding pattern between traveling moves.

Exercise Intensity

People with some disabilities that impair coordination, such as CP, experience an exaggerated heart rate response to exercise due to extraneous movements or efforts to counteract unintended movement. People with impaired coordination may also have difficulty taking their own pulse. The RPE scale is a useful alternative for assessing exercise intensity with these conditions. Chapter 5 provided two RPE scales.

To delay the onset of fatigue with people likely to experience a rapid rise in heart rate or people who may begin exercise with an elevated heart rate (athetoid CP), use a prolonged and gradual warm-up. During peak activity, an interval system of work and recovery may be useful for controlling exercise intensity. *Recovery* does not necessarily mean *rest*; it may refer to a period of less intense movement during which the heart rate is allowed to lower slightly. Seated exercise can also be used as a recovery period, alternated with standing exercise.

Form and Alignment

People with spasticity may be unable to assume proper postural alignment and will not move all joints through the full range of motion during exercise. At times, proper postural alignment may be sacrificed to achieve greater aerobic benefits during the workout. For example, with some forms of CP, the Achilles tendons may be tight, preventing full dorsiflexion and resulting in tip-toe walking. This tendency is exaggerated with aerobic dance. Although bouncing up and down on the toes is usually contraindicated because it is stressful to the shins, this caution may be overlooked to a degree because walking on the toes may be considered normal for participants with this condition. Follow the aerobic workout with thorough stretching of the lower-leg muscles. Don't ignore contraindicated movements or unsafe postural alignment, but recognize differences in what may be "normal" for each individual. Carefully weigh the advantages and disadvantages of exercising and achieving an aerobic workout versus maintaining proper alignment. Your overall objective with the workout should be to enable your clients to achieve aerobic benefits without becoming injured or experiencing a decline in function after exercise.

The nearby box includes considerations for aerobic dance exercise for people with impaired coordination.

Limited Upper Body Function

During exercise, the amount of exercising muscle and oxygen consumption are directly related. The more exercising muscle mass, the greater the potential for obtaining an aerobic training effect. With a limited muscle mass, it is difficult to create a demand large enough to stress the aerobic systems (lungs, heart, circulation, and muscle). When a small muscle mass becomes the limiting factor in exercise, a greater percent of energy is derived from anaerobic metabolism, which drives up the heart rate, rendering it a less accurate indicator of the aerobic work being performed. With this principle in mind, encourage your students to utilize as much functional muscle as possible during an exercise session, within the limits of safety and tolerance, to increase the demand on the cardiorespiratory systems.

A decrease in trainable muscle may be due to paralysis or paresis such as with spinal cord injury, spina bifida, hemiplegia, MS, MD, or polio. It also may be due to conditions that limit joint ROM such as arthritis, arthrogryposis, or spastic CP. With restricted ROM, the limitations are imposed not so much by lack of functional muscle as by conditions that prevent full use of the muscle groups.

ADAPTING FOR IMPAIRED COORDINATION

- Avoid movements that cause excessive increases in muscle tone and spasticity.
- Emphasize movements that work muscle groups opposing spastic muscles.
- Emphasize large, fluid arm movements; avoid "stylized" moves.
- Offer half-tempo alternatives.
- Simplify or eliminate choreographed upper and lower body combinations; do not change arm and leg patterns simultaneously.
- Limit the variety of movement patterns you introduce in each class.

- Maintain each movement pattern for a prolonged period (12 to 16 repetitions).
- Avoid rapid changes in direction; maintain movements in one direction for an extended period before changing directions.
- Use a subjective RPE scale to assess intensity if pulse monitoring is difficult.
- Accept modified alignment and form but consider its impact on safety and potential injury.
- Minimize counting.

Exercising with limited or small muscle groups increases the potential for developing early fatigue because a greater demand is placed on fewer muscle fibers. Aerobic dance for people with decreased trainable muscle mass, therefore, should incorporate a wide variety of moves and use shortened sets of pattern repeats and intervals. In addition, provide adequate opportunity during the warm-up to prepare the muscles for activity, such as with ROM work, stretching, or relaxation drills, so maximum benefits can be derived during peak efforts.

Safety Checks

Before beginning an exercise class, run a brief series of safety checks to help you and the participant with decreased muscle function identify potential problem areas that may affect the outcome of the class or possibly jeopardize safety. Check balance, stability, and tolerance for twisting, and be aware of areas that lack sensation and of the participant's ability to tolerate heat.

Most participants know their limits regarding trunk stability, but you may wish to run through a set of core moves before beginning class to identify what works and what can be modified if necessary. Often, as participants progress with the workout, they find they can stretch their balance point beyond its initial limits.

Although everyone should control spinal twisting, it can be especially dangerous for people who have Harrington or Luque rods or similar types of vertebrae fusion. The Harrington rod fuses portions of the vertebrae together to provide more stability to the spinal cord. Joint movement is obviously compromised at the fusion site. Excessive twisting can damage the spine at the vertebral

joints adjacent to the fused joints and should thus be avoided.

Also advise your aerobics students to routinely check body areas that lack sensation for abrasions that may occur due to movement or rubbing against the chair back, wheels, or seat.

The autonomic nervous system (ANS) regulates heart rate, blood pressure, and thermoregulatory responses to exercise. When the ANS is impaired, generally with spinal cord injury at or above the T5 to T1 level (Mathers, 1985) or possibly with multiple sclerosis, heart rate cannot be increased above approximately 100 to 120 beats per minute. People with this condition must use an RPE scale to monitor exercise intensity (see Table 5.4 on p. 73)

Exercise Intensity

With lower extremity dysfunction, upper body work creates the aerobic demand during exercise. Encourage maximum use of trunk muscles, within safe limits of balance and stability, to increase the conditioning effect of the workout. For example, when punching the arms forward, have participants reach with the whole side of the body. When crossing and uncrossing the arms, rock the trunk forward and backward. In general, large arm movements that require full range of motion and reaching offer the greatest potential for aerobic training.

If leg function permits, recommend that your students who exercise from a seated position further increase the aerobic demand of the workout by including simple leg movements such as kicks, alternating heel taps and toe taps, marching, or side stepping.

People with hemiplegic involvement may derive more aerobic benefit from a workout by exercising primarily the noninvolved side because more caution is required when exercising paretic limbs. Movements are generally slower and less coordinated on the involved side, and in many cases movements should not be performed rigorously. Attempting to incorporate movement of paretic limbs during the peak aerobic phases may reduce the intensity of the overall workout. However, during warm-up or cool-down, a participant may use the unimpaired side to help with range of motion limbering exercises on the weak side. Movements that require holding and moving the arms and hands together further facilitate use of both sides of the body during warm-up or cool-down. Although an aerobics class is not intended to be a therapy session, there is no reason why some therapeutic aspects cannot be incorporated into the less vigorous components of the workout.

Delaying Fatigue

When a limited amount of muscle mass is available to contribute to aerobic work, the individual tends to fatigue quickly with any type of exercise. In this case, you can delay fatigue and prolong exercise by modifying arm movements (to reduce intensity and eliminate anaerobic work) and by using interval systems.

With participants who have limited muscle function, choreograph routines to avoid excessive use of narrow range and intense arm movements (such as rapid pulsing or small arm circles). Static contractions cause rapid buildup of lactic acid in the muscle, inducing quick fatigue and inhibiting aerobic development. Increases in oxygen consumption do not parallel increases in heart rate with this type of action, which is generally used to anaerobically work the muscles and increase muscular endurance. Incorporate any intense armwork after the full aerobic phase of the workout to avoid decreasing the potential for aerobic conditioning.

Aerobics classes often use eight-count movement repetitions. People with decreased muscle function better tolerate fewer repetitions of each movement pattern. In particular, avoid overtaxing the middle deltoids, which may fatigue quickly in new aerobics students.

You can also delay fatigue by simply reducing exercise intensity. This can be done with nearly any basic movement to change the intensity of the effort. Specific techniques for modifying movement patterns to decrease intensity are reviewed on page 151.

An effective technique for delaying fatigue is to employ an interval system of work/recovery or work/rest. Due to the demand placed on a small exercising muscle mass, much of the "aerobic routine" for some people with decreased muscle function will actually be anaerobic. Frequent changes in movement patterns will allow alternating muscle groups to recover. Work/recovery intervals can include alternating between movements that are fast and slow, large and small, overhead and below the shoulders, or unilateral and bilateral.

You can also incorporate intervals of work and rest as needed. Limit the duration of the rest period to prevent a significant drop in heart rate, which decreases the overall conditioning potential of the workout. Individual needs determine the length of the rest period or work/recovery interval. The RPE scale can help participants judge interval periods. Table 11.1 summarizes techniques for delaying fatigue during upper body exercise.

Table 11.1 Techniques for Delaying Fatigue With Upper Body Exercise

Movement patterns	Increase variety
	Decrease pattern repetitions (maximum: 8 counts)
Intensity	Reduce length of lever arm
	Decrease ROM
	Decrease speed of movements
	Limit static contractions
Interval systems	Incorporate work/rest intervals
	Incorporate work/recovery intervals:
	Fast/slow
	Large/small
	Overhead/below shoulder
	Bilateral/unilateral
	Regular tempo/half tempo

Warm-Up and Cool-Down

Movements that require raising both arms over the head simultaneously are too strenuous to be considered a warm-up or cool-down for people with decreased muscle function, particularly people with quadriplegia. Therefore, keep warm-up and cool-down arm movements below shoulder level. A slower tempo allows movement to be completed through the full range of motion. During the warm-up, keep movements slow, simple, flowing, and relatively small in the beginning and progress to larger, "open" moves that stretch chest and upper back muscles. An appropriate sequence of arm movements might be shoulder raises, alternating shoulder rolls, large shoulder rolls led with the elbows, and backstroke arm circles. You can reverse this type of sequence for the cool-down.

Keep intensity changes during the warm-up and cool-down gradual for people with limited muscle function. You may want to experiment with prolonging the warm-up and cool-down for an extended period at a lower intensity. Normally, muscular contractions from leg movements during the cool-down act as a venous pump to return blood to the heart and assist with removal of waste products that accumulate with exercise. With lower limb paralysis, this muscle pumping action is absent, resulting in a tendency for blood and fluids to pool in the lower extremities. Maintaining upper body movement is an important alternative to lower limb work to help keep an even flow of blood circulating with less strain on the heart. Delay static stretching until all participants have had adequate time to cool down appropriately. As with any group, never stop exercise abruptly.

If decreased muscular strength prevents participants from assuming or maintaining positions for stretching during the cool-down, have partners assist. Remind your students to be cautious and maintain communication throughout partner stretches to prevent injury. Never permit partner stretching of muscle groups where sensation is lacking unless the partner is trained and qualified to perform passive stretching. Also, discourage bouncing or pulsing to the music during partner stretches.

People with limited upper body function may experience increased tension in neck and shoulder muscles following a workout. Emphasize neck relaxation and stretching exercises during the cool-down to relieve any tension that may have developed. Include movements such as head semicircles, neck rotation, lateral neck stretches, and neck flexion and retraction. Neck hyperextension is contraindicated. The box nearby includes modifications for people with limited muscle function.

Impaired Joint Function

With conditions that decrease range of motion due to an impairment in the structures of the joint, such as arthritis, it is essential that exercise training does not decrease functioning or increase pain. An exchange may have to be made in favor of "gentle" conditioning over higher intensity exercise that may cause excessive stress to joint structures. Avoid training during periods of exacerbation or flare-up. Discontinue exercise if it causes increased pain.

Impact and Stress on Joint Structures

People with impaired joint function should use smaller, slower, well-controlled movements during aerobic dance. Movements that are large and fast tend to be ballistic, and it is difficult to control the end-points in the movement range. Reducing the lever-arm length of arm movements also reduces the level of stress imposed on joints. If the participant is exercising from a standing position, use no-impact leg moves, including gentle swaying, lunging, rocking, and pliés. To boost the conditioning potential of the aerobic workout, however, be sure to incorporate the large muscle groups.

Warm-Up and Cool-Down

As with routines for people with decreased muscle function, prolong the warm-up and cool-down for people with impaired joint function. Take additional time for static stretching. Slow movements that emphasize the full range of motion are good

---

ADAPTING FOR LIMITED MUSCLE FUNCTION

- Conduct safety checks: balance, stability, twisting limitations, abrasions with impaired sensation, temperature regulation.
- Accept modified postural alignment within safety limits.
- Recommend chest strapping for balance or lower limb strapping to prevent interference from spastic muscles.
- Encourage use of all functional muscles.
- With hemiplegia, do not encourage involvement from paretic limbs during peak activity if it reduces exercise intensity.

- Delay fatigue of arm muscles (see Table 11.1).
- Use a subjective RPE scale with subnormal HR responses to exercise.
- Employ a prolonged, gradual, low-intensity warm-up and cool-down.
- Use partners for active-assisted stretching as needed during the warm-up and cool-down.
- Incorporate additional neck stretching and relaxation.

ADAPTING FOR IMPAIRED JOINT FUNCTION

- Emphasize fluid movements with controlled endpoints.
- Reduce the speed and length of the lever arm with upper body movements.
- Recommend seated or no-impact standing exercise.

- Offer a prolonged, low-intensity warm-up and cool-down, incorporating slow, full ROM movements.
- Emphasize prolonged static stretching (45 to 60 s) during the warm-up and cool-down.
- Discontinue exercise with pain.

---

limbering moves. Include static stretching of all major joints for 30 s or more in the cool-down (see the above box).

Decreased Exercise Tolerance and Progressive Conditions

Several disabilities are associated with a low tolerance to exercise and chronic fatigue. For example, progressive disorders such as multiple sclerosis and muscular dystrophy may gradually decrease an individual's tolerance to exercise. People who have had a stroke also may be restricted to lower exercise intensities as a precaution against developing recurring symptoms of a CVA. People with postpolio syndrome who have received approval from their physician for exercise also may become easily fatigued and must reduce the intensity of their workouts. And finally, low fitness levels common to all conditions that impair mobility require that new exercise programs be initiated slowly with very gradual increases in exercise intensity.

As an exercise leader, you must continually communicate with your students with low tolerance to exercise about postexercise fatigue to ensure that the program is not decreasing their ability to function. If exercise has a negative impact on function, increase modifications to further reduce exercise intensity and discourage participation during periods of exacerbation.

In addition to the techniques suggested in Table 11.1 for delaying local muscle fatigue during exercise, consider the following measures:

- Conduct more frequent intensity checks using the HR method or the RPE scale. Make sure all students know what their limits should be and understand how to adjust exercise intensity when necessary.

- Pay close attention to the temperature of your exercise space. Because warm and humid environments can cause rapid and excessive fatigue, particularly with MS and quadriplegia, you may want to discourage participants with impaired tempera-

ture regulation from exercising under these conditions or recommend that they further reduce exercise intensity.

- Have equipment to check blood pressure and someone qualified to perform the check available for clients with a history of stroke.

Some people with extremely low tolerance to exercise or with progressive conditions may not actually be able to increase cardiorespiratory fitness by participating in aerobic dance classes. Regular exercise, however, may delay complications associated with inactivity, especially with progressive conditions. Often, these people also benefit from the social interaction afforded by group exercise programs.

Visual Impairment

Although visual impairment is not generally considered a physical disability, this condition presents challenges to movement in an aerobics class. Hegey and Aceves (1991) offer the following ideas for introducing new movement patterns to people with impaired vision.

Verbal Cues

Consistent, simple, and direct verbal cues are an effective means of referring to movement patterns that have already been learned and labeled. They can also be used to direct new actions, if the description or movement is not overly complex. It is very important that you always use the same verbal cue to describe a specific movement or exercise. If the participant doesn't appear to catch on, expanding the cue may be helpful. Build movement patterns with verbal cues by isolating an action and then adding additional movements or positions after the participant understands the initial instructions.

With some forethought, many exercise movements can be described in terms of other common actions. Understanding some cues, however, depends on whether the individual has actually seen the object or action being described. Someone with congenital blindness may not be able to understand cues such as "Move your arms like windshield wipers." Once participants do understand the explanation, you can substitute shorter phrases or codes to simplify future instructions.

When cuing persons who are visually impaired, try not to correct every movement. Praise the person even when the movement is partially correct (as long as the movement is safe and effective). Constant corrections may cause frustration.

Manual Guidance

Occasionally, verbal cues are not effective for describing complex movement patterns. It may be helpful in this situation to manually guide the person into the desired position or through an intended action. Consider the following guidelines when offering manual guidance to a person with a visual impairment:

- Always request permission before touching someone.
- Indicate exactly how and where you intend to touch the person.
- Use a gentle touch.
- Reinforce physical demonstrations with constant and consistent verbal cues.

Two techniques have been devised for offering manual guidance that can be used with aerobic dance instruction. The "braille-me" method is the less invasive of the two because it allows the participant to feel your movements.

Braille-Me Method. With this method, you demonstrate an action while the participant feels your movements (see Figure 11.5). For example, you can stand in front of the participant while performing alternating lateral lunges. The participant can put his hands on your waist or legs to "feel" the movement of your entire body. You may need to guide the participant's hands to place them in a location that allows her to best feel the action you are demonstrating.

Hands-On Method. In this method, after requesting permission, you guide the participant through an action by grasping his arms, legs, or waist and moving them through the desired movements (see Figure 11.6).

Wandering

People with a visual impairment may tend to wander from their designated spot during an aerobics class. Some people may prefer to use a chair that

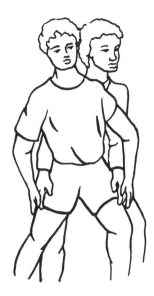

Figure 11.5 The braille-me instructional technique for people with visual impairment.

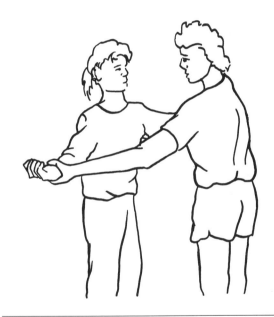

Figure 11.6 The hands-on instructional technique for people with visual impairment.

they can touch as a "base" to keep them in place. An assistant can help participants return to their areas using the following means:

1. Verbally instruct the individual how to return (forward, back, to your right, etc.).
2. Direct the person to move toward the voice that is in the appropriate location.
3. Provide physical assistance by allowing the individual to take an arm and be guided to the appropriate spot.

Team Teaching

Teaching an adapted exercise class that includes people of all abilities can be very challenging, especially if the ability levels of the participants vary dramatically. Team teaching is an effective tool for accommodating different needs in a group setting without sacrificing the quality of the program. Effective team teaching involves planning, compatibility, and mutual respect. If you are working with another instructor, be sure to clearly develop an instructional team strategy before leading your classes. Be sure the class knows who to look for as the lead instructor. Table 11.2 lists several methods for working with a partner in a team teaching situation.

Table 11.2 Strategies for Team Teaching

1. Standing/sitting	Each instructor teaches the routine and modifications from either a standing or seated position
2. Full/half tempo	One instructor demonstrates movements at full tempo; one demonstrates modified tempo as needed
3. Stationary/roving	One instructor maintains the routine from a position in front of the class; one roams through the class to offer individual assistance as needed
4. Standard/modified	One instructor leads the routine without modifications; one demonstrates a variety of modifications

Summary

Aerobic dance exercise is a wonderful way to combine both effective cardiorespiratory training and enjoyment in a social environment. As an instructor, your task is to ensure that the program is safe, effective, appropriately modified, and enjoyable for all participants. Your ability to effectively modify routines and movement patterns must be combined with a basic knowledge of each participant's disability and general medical and health history. Regular and direct communication with each person is also invaluable in developing a successful program.

Part IV

Managing Accessible Fitness Programs

●

Managing the fitness program that includes participants with physical disabilities requires more than knowledge of disability and exercise modifications. The development of new programs requires careful planning and effective promotion to attract and retain exercise clients with physical disabilities. You also must have the skills and knowledge to educate clients with disabilities about fitness and exercise modifications, accommodate different learning styles, and motivate clients of all abilities to stick with their exercise programs. In addition, you must be knowledgeable of medical conditions commonly associated with physical disabilities, and you must be prepared to respond appropriately to prevent or manage medical emergencies. Finally, because many clients with disabilities use wheelchairs, you must know how and when to provide assistance with maneuvering or transferring an individual to or from the wheelchair, as requested by the user.

Chapter 12 addresses overall program and class management concerns of fitness directors and instructors. Chapter 13 highlights common medical conditions associated with physical disabilities as well as how to recognize and respond to possible medical emergencies. Chapter 14 familiarizes you with the components of a wheelchair and several different types commonly used today. It also introduces you to techniques for assisting individuals who use wheelchairs with maneuvers and transfers.

Recommended Readings

American College of Sports Medicine. (1991). *Guidelines for exercise testing and prescription* (4th ed.). Philadelphia: Lea & Febiger.

American College of Sports Medicine, Sol, N., & Foster, C., (Eds.) (1992). *Health/fitness facility standards and guidelines*. Champaign, IL: Human Kinetics.

Berg, K.E. (1986). *Diabetic's guide to health and fitness*. Champaign, IL: Human Kinetics.

Braddom, R.L., & Rocco, J.F. (1991). Autonomic dysreflexia: A survey of current treatment. *American Journal of Physical Medicine and Rehabilitation*, **70**, 5, 234-239.

Bruyn, G.W., & Vinken, P.J. (Eds.) (1986). *Handbook of clinical neurology: Part 2*. Amsterdam: Northland.

Girdano, D.A., & Dusek, D.E. (1988). *Changing health behavior*. Scottsdale, AZ: Gorsuch Scarisbrick.

Gumnit, R.J. (Ed.) (1981). *Epilepsy: A handbook* (4th ed.). St. Paul: University of Minnesota.

Kazdin, A.E. (1980). *Behavior modification in applied settings*. Homewood, IL: Dorsey Press.

Kozak, G.P. (1982). *Clinical diabetes mellitus*. Philadelphia: W.B. Saunders.

Nixon, V. (1985). Spinal cord injury: A guide to functional outcomes in physical therapy management. Rockville, MD: Aspen.

Whaley, D.L., & Malott, R.W. (1971). *Elementary principles of behavior*. New York: Appleton-Century-Crofts.

Wilkens, E.W. (Ed.) (1989). *Emergency medicine: Scientific foundations and current practice* (3rd ed.). Baltimore: Williams & Wilkins.

Chapter 12

Administration Guidelines

Kimberly D. Hardin, PT

Operating a successful fitness program that is accessible to people with physical disabilities extends beyond mere knowledge of disability, exercise science, and technique modifications. Attempting to attract people with disabilities to participate in your classes, particularly if you operate in a community facility, may create an additional set of unique challenges. These challenges are best met by the skilled program director with a solid plan for promotion and program development. Once you succeed at encouraging people with disabilities to join your programs, the challenge extends to the exercise leader, who must not only deliver an effective program but also maintain the interest of each new client.

This chapter offers suggestions for developing, promoting, and managing accessible fitness programs and includes instructional and motivational strategies you can apply to group programs.

Program Development

Developing a successful adapted exercise program depends on the skill and efforts of the program director, who must invest the time to plan and promote accessible classes well in advance of their availability. In addition to evaluating transportation resources, scheduling restrictions, facility accessibility, and equipment needs, the program director must also develop an effective plan for promoting the program to ensure participation by members of the community with disabilities. Qualified exercise leaders must be selected. Volunteers and class assistants should be recruited to provide support for program administrative duties and class activities. And finally, registration and assessment procedures must be developed to ensure the safety and effectiveness of the program for all participants.

General Planning

Once the decision has been made to actively promote a facility or specific class as being accessible to people with physical disabilities, the program director must identify the specific program goals and objectives, evaluate transportation resources, and examine scheduling options.

Despite your good intentions to promote your classes as being accessible to all, don't expect a sudden flood of new members with disabilities. Many people with physical impairments do not feel comfortable with the idea of exercising in a setting that has traditionally served able-bodied people. You may have more success introducing people with disabilities to your programs initially by promoting a particular class as being accessible or by encouraging individuals with a certain disability to register for a specific program. Make these decisions in advance so you can develop a successful promotional plan.

Program Objectives

An exercise class can include a variety of components intended to suit many purposes. The program director and exercise leaders must collaborate in advance to determine the specific objectives of the exercise class before proceeding to develop the program. First, consider which components of physical fitness you will address, and identify the intended outcome of the program. Is the exercise class intended for improving aerobic fitness, strength, flexibility? Is this program for general health enhancement, improving sport performance, providing a socially integrative experience for people with

disabilities? Next, predict the abilities and needs of the expected clientele. You will promote and manage an existing exercise class that you expect will attract a few people with disabilities differently than a class you expect to be attended by people with extensive physical impairments.

Transportation Resources

For many people with disabilities, inaccessible transportation is a barrier to participation in community-based programs. Contact public and private transportation systems in your area to determine what accessible systems are available and what their schedules, reservation requirements, and costs are. This information may affect decisions you make about when to schedule a particular class. If accessible public transportation is unavailable, plan for alternatives, such as volunteer assistance or car pools among class members. Include transportation information in the registration information given to prospective class participants.

Scheduling Concerns

If you decide to offer an accessible program and promote it as such, consider the population you intend to serve before selecting an appropriate time. Employed people generally prefer evenings, and retired people generally prefer early afternoons. On the other hand, people with multiple sclerosis may want to avoid early afternoon classes because they may experience greater fatigue at that time.

The objectives of the program will dictate the length of the exercise class. A comprehensive fitness program that addresses aerobic and muscular conditioning may require 90 min of class time and, ideally, should be offered a minimum of two to three times per week. Also consider the duration of the program. Will it be ongoing or will it last a specified number of weeks? The intended structure and progression of the class determine your decision about duration. In some geographic regions it may also be important to consider what time of year might be most attractive to your intended audience. If attendance is normally affected by weather, community events, and holiday or vacation seasons, select a time to start your program that will ensure the greatest opportunity for success.

Facility Accessibility

Evaluate your exercise facility in advance for accessibility and amenities. A facility is not fully accessible if someone in a wheelchair cannot enter the building from a parking area, use the bathrooms or locker rooms, or get to the exercise class area. Water fountains and telephones also should be accessible from a wheelchair. A telephone for emergencies must be immediately accessible.

Evaluate the exercise area for lighting, acoustics, ventilation, heating and cooling, and flooring. For example, a room with poor lighting and acoustics poses challenges for someone with a visual impairment who relies on residual vision and verbal information for guidance. Poor acoustics can prevent the person with impaired hearing from obtaining verbal instructions. Floors that are slippery may be unsafe for people with impaired balance.

Evaluating Equipment Needs

Group exercise programs that are accessible to people with disabilities may require additional equipment or modifications to existing equipment. Be sure to assess equipment needs several months in advance of the scheduled program to allow adequate time for ordering special equipment or for making and testing items such as modified cuff weights, Velcro handles and attachments, devices for securing stretch bands to walls and ceilings, and the like. In addition to the usual equipment needed for an exercise class, you'll find it useful to have the following items available in the adapted program:

- Sandbags or blocks to immobilize wheelchairs
- Additional exercise mats for people with impaired balance
- Sturdy armless chairs with nonslip bases for seated exercise or for additional support with standing exercise
- Adaptable resistive exercise equipment such as resistive bands or surgical tubing
- Belts or wraps to secure people in their wheelchairs as needed
- Velcro strips to be used as makeshift handles
- Water, cups, and straws
- Paper towels or hand towels for spills or personal accidents
- Disposable gloves for personal accidents

Selecting Program Staff

Many people may be involved in developing and conducting an exercise program for people with disabilities, including program directors, exercise leaders, exercise specialists, fitness and medical consultants, an advisory board, assistants, and vol-

unteers. A comprehensive team of experts and energetic individuals will ensure the success and safety of the program. In many cases, one person may be qualified to assume several roles to guide the development of the program.

Exercise Leaders

Selecting qualified instructors can mean the difference between an effective, enjoyable, and safe program versus one that is mediocre and possibly dangerous. A qualified exercise leader is skilled at leading group exercise and knowledgeable of basic exercise principles of conditioning. Many reputable organizations offer certification to recognize competence among aerobics and fitness instructors. Exercise leaders should maintain current CPR certification and be trained in first aid. Additionally, the adapted exercise leader has experience and training with physical disability. If one person is not available with all the necessary qualifications, team teaching by instructors with a combination of expertise may be an effective alternative. For example, a physical therapist and an aerobics instructor can work together to develop routines that are both safe and effective.

Exercise Specialists

To ensure the safety of your exercise programs, require all participants to undergo preparticipation health screening to help you identify people who may be at risk in a group exercise program. An exercise specialist qualified to approve or disapprove participation by each potential program participant should evaluate the completed screening forms (described in a subsequent section). This process may require the support of a physical therapist or physician who can recognize disability-related conditions that may be of concern. These fitness and medical consultants may also help develop individual exercise prescriptions and fitness assessments.

Advisory Board

Establish an advisory board to assist with the management and design of the accessible exercise program. Advisory board members not only may provide technical assistance but also may contribute significantly to developing promotions, identifying participants, and securing funding. You may wish to invite people with the following qualifications or affiliations to participate on your program board:

- Medical and health care professionals
- Qualified area fitness leaders

- Adapted physical educators
- Exercise specialists
- Media and marketing professionals
- Financial sponsors
- People with disabilities
- Representatives from local disability organizations

Volunteers and Class Assistants

Good support staff members are an invaluable part of the accessible group exercise program. Knowing how to recruit, train, and utilize assistants greatly enhances the smooth operation of the program. Depending on their qualifications, volunteers can assist with program registration, screening and evaluation, transportation, and actual class activities. Volunteers need to be well recognized for their work and encouraged to become an integral part of the program's development and success to secure their continued support. Time spent training volunteers and assistants ensures effective use of this valuable resource.

Volunteers can be recruited from a variety of sources, limited only by the creativity and initiative of the program director. Examples of sources include volunteer organizations, support groups, senior citizen and youth groups (scouts, 4-H clubs, etc.), family members and friends, university adapted physical education students, other exercise class members (able-bodied and disabled), and church organizations. Professionals for tasks requiring specific expertise can be recruited from health clubs, wellness centers, sports medicine clinics, and rehabilitation or therapy centers.

Volunteers who assist with the exercise class may assume any of several roles, including assistance with positioning during stretching or resistance training, equipment use, and intensity assessment (HR or RPE) and monitoring participants to ensure their safe and effective participation in the class. Volunteers can also assist by providing water or cleaning up any spills or personal accidents that may occur. Any support provided by the class assistant frees the primary instructor to focus on leading exercise and running a smooth program.

Strongly encourage all class volunteers to actively participate in the exercise classes in addition to assisting. Therefore, they should submit all registration and screening materials before participating. Class assistants that help class members with disabilities but do not participate in the activities may present a negative image that this exercise is only for people with special needs.

Staff Training and Orientation

Plan one or more orientation meetings for all staff and volunteers who will participate in some phase of the adapted fitness program. At these meetings you can review program objectives, administrative and emergency procedures, and information about disability and exercise. Clearly define the specific role of each staff member and volunteer during this orientation. Continually stress the value and importance of the volunteers' contribution to the program and encourage their feedback to secure their continued interest in developing the project. Give program staff and volunteers a manual or notebook that includes important information and procedures.

To supplement staff training, consider offering a disability awareness seminar to highlight psychological and social issues associated with physical disability. You could ask people with physical disabilities from the community to attend this seminar and participate in a panel presentation and discussion to stimulate sensitivity among program staff. All instructors, volunteers, and other facility or program personnel should attend the disability awareness session.

During orientation, briefly review the principles of fitness conditioning and exercise implications associated with physical disabilities for staff who will assist with actual class activities. In addition, staff training could include actual techniques and modifications for fitness development, proper body alignment, adapting exercise equipment, handling wheelchairs, performing transfers, and partnering skills for assisting clients with sensory or cognitive impairments. Videotapes of an adapted exercise class may also be helpful. You can include CPR training for staff assistants who would like to become certified.

Registration and Screening

Everyone, disabled or able-bodied, should complete registration forms and participate in a general health screening before participating in any exercise class. The information you get from this process highlights the needs and abilities of class members and indicates potential risks that may be associated with vigorous exercise. You may wish to establish procedures in advance to accommodate individuals who want to join the class after it has begun.

In addition to standard health and fitness checks (heart rate, blood pressure, and general health and fitness assessment), include a consent form with registration materials if you plan to photograph your classes for possible media promotions. Also consider conducting personal interviews with an exercise specialist present, which will enable you to offer an individualized approach within the context of a group setting. During this interview, you can assess movement capabilities and limitations and identify or formulate personal goals.

A checklist of forms and assessment procedures to include in the registration process follows. Appendix B includes several sample forms.

Registration Forms

Health appraisal and general medical history
General registration and participant profile
Physician referral (as needed)
Waiver and consent forms
    Insurance and liability (as required by the facility)
    Participating in an exercise program
    Photo consent

Preparticipation Assessment

Resting heart rate and blood pressure
Baseline fitness assessment
Health and risk assessment (physician or exercise specialist directed)
Personal Interview

An exercise specialist or certified fitness instructor who is knowledgeable of both physical disability and risk factors that may affect participation in an exercise class should evaluate the preparticipation materials. A team of professionals with appropriate expertise may be necessary for a thorough evaluation. Communicate information derived from registration materials, assessments, health appraisals, and interviews with the exercise instructors to highlight areas of need or concern. Such professionals are qualified to determine whether registrants need clearance from a physician before participation or whether health restrictions require that participation be denied.

Promoting the Accessible Program

Attracting people with disabilities to a community-based group exercise class can be extremely challenging. An effective promotional plan is essential. As part of the plan, you must develop appropriate promotional materials to advertise the goals of the program and to attract the intended audience. The extent of your promotional efforts is limited only by the time, money, and creativity you have available for the promotional package.

Developing a Promotional Plan

Maintain a clear focus on the program goals and intended audience to develop an effective promotional plan. Attempts to attract participants to the accessible exercise class will be most successful if you first map out a comprehensive strategy, based on available resources, before developing any single component of the plan. Possible avenues for attracting interest include distributing fliers, program brochures, and posters; obtaining media coverage; making outreach efforts and presentations to interested groups; and performing demonstrations at large gatherings, health fairs, shopping malls, and athletic facilities or events.

Preparing Promotional Materials

Once you have mapped out the promotional strategy, you'll need to produce fliers, posters, news releases, and public service announcements. All promotional items should express the specific goals of the program and should include role models whenever possible. If a prominent disabled athlete or disabled fitness professional is available, support from that person may provide additional visibility for your program and attract people with disabilities to join it.

Distribute media materials to all local newspapers, city magazines, radio stations, and TV stations. Recruit volunteers with expertise in acquiring media coverage to help you access this very important promotional tool. Also consider recruiting someone with creative writing skills to write a human interest story about the program and submit it to the local newspapers.

Program Outreach

Initiate your outreach campaign by contacting all local groups and professionals with a potential interest in exercise programs for people with disabilities. You can formulate an extensive list by checking resources at the library and in the phone book. Some organizations may be willing to share their mailing lists or offer to print a program announcement in their newsletters. Contact organizations both to attract participants and to recruit volunteers for program administration. You may want to address your outreach to the following organizations (Appendix C lists national groups):

- Disability organizations and associations
- Disabled sports associations
- Young Men's Christian Associations (YMCAs), Young Women's Christian Associations (YWCAs), and Jewish Community Centers (JCCs)
- Hospitals and rehabilitation centers
- City or county park and recreation departments
- Health care professionals: therapeutic recreation specialists, occupational therapists, physical therapists
- Health clubs and wellness centers
- Universities (physical education and adapted physical education departments)
- Public and private schools
- Civic organizations (Kiwanis, Rotary Clubs, etc.)

Class Management

Instructing a group exercise program, whether it be aerobics, group resistance training, stretching, or some other mode of exercise, requires that you have knowledge of exercise conditioning principles and techniques and that you also have skills in managing a diverse group while maintaining group cohesiveness. The task of working with a "mixed group" inherent with the adapted exercise program is extremely challenging for even the most seasoned instructor. When people with disabilities participate in the program, you must not only address the need for modifications with various disabilities, but also provide instruction appropriate for the skill and fitness level of each participant. Your success in accommodating a variety of individual abilities will be measured, in part, by your students' adherence to your exercise program.

Advance Preparation

Leading an adapted exercise class should always be preceded by advance planning and practice. This preplanning may involve experimenting with choreography modifications or developing a plan for offering alternative techniques and exercises. You are well advised to actually try out any modifications you intend to recommend to your students or practice teaching them to a friend. Also consider the progression of the overall program from class

to class in your preplanning, particularly if the program is composed of a fixed number of classes per session.

If you are team teaching the exercise class, rehearse routines, instructional roles, and strategies with your partner. It is also essential that you work with any class volunteers and assistants in advance to clearly delineate their roles. For example, you may wish to assign some volunteers the task of assisting with exercise intensity checks or with equipment modifications for specific students. You also may wish to assign the tasks of cleaning up personal accidents or calling for assistance in the case of an emergency.

Participant Education

As a fitness instructor, you should assume the dual roles of exercise leader and educator (within the limits of your knowledge) to teach each participant something about the importance of exercise and how to set and reach individual goals. Opportunities to educate your clients are available during registration, interviews, and health screening; during first-day orientation and preclass instructions; and on an ongoing basis during each exercise session. To supplement the exercise class experience, you also may wish to provide additional educational experiences directed toward improving health, such as seminars on nutrition, stress management, and smoking cessation.

Shaping Attitudes

Part of your role as educator also extends to shaping attitudes about the rightful place an individual with a disability has in the community exercise program. Your role may include dispelling ideas the nondisabled members of your class may harbor about disability and inability. This challenge is often met by simply providing integrated classes and structuring activities in a way that fosters social integration between all members of your programs. You can also help shape acceptable attitudes by setting an appropriate example in the way you personally interact with and refer to people with disabilities. For a review of these considerations, refer to chapter 1.

Your actions will also help some people with disabilities overcome doubts they may have about their rightful participation in community-based group programs. The integrated situation may initially be intimidating or even frightening for a person with a lowered self-concept or negative body image. Without focusing directly on the issue, providing an enjoyable group exercise class for everyone will likely educate both the able-bodied and disabled class members about the abilities, needs, and rights of people with disabilities.

Fitness Principles

Discuss the overall goals and objectives of the exercise class with each class participant. You may also need to educate some participants about the importance of physical fitness and provide realistic expectations about the therapeutic benefits of an exercise class. Although balance, coordination, and functioning may improve as a result of participating in the program, rehabilitation is generally not the primary focus. The primary goal of any fitness class is to enhance physical and psychological well-being through participation in an exercise program designed to improve aerobic capacity and muscular fitness.

Educating your exercise clients about conditioning principles and technique modifications can ease your task of individualizing instruction in a group setting. Typically, a group exercise class includes people with a wide range of abilities and fitness levels. Though difficult for the instructor, a successful program caters to all levels, providing enough but not too much challenge to yield benefits for all. When your students are able to individually modify the exercises or routines, you are freer to concentrate on maintaining the flow, unity, and fun of the class.

Educating class members about exercise basics should be an ongoing process. Always cover principles of conditioning, self-pacing, the importance of a proper warm-up and cool-down, assessing exercise intensity, and proper body mechanics and postural alignment. This education not only gives participants greater independence in your class, but also allows them to carry the knowledge and skills to other settings, further enhancing their independence.

Personal Responsibility

Once you have provided students with a foundation of basic information, encourage them to assume responsibility for their own fitness and safety. Suggest that the students maintain their training if they are unable to attend your class. Teach them to recognize warning signs that indicate possible health or medical problems. Encourage them to adopt and maintain other healthy lifestyle habits, and provide them with resources for further self-education about fitness. Note, however, that participant education does not relieve you of responsibility for students' safety or for providing an effective exercise program. Further-

more, some participants with memory or other cognitive impairments may be less able to assume personal responsibility than others and may require extended attention from you or an assistant.

Preclass Instruction

Take advantage of the time just before the class begins for important reminders about the exercise session, such as reminders about self-pacing, signs of overexertion or possible medical problems, and the importance of hydration. You can also use this opportunity to review general techniques for modifying routines or exercises.

You also may wish to provide some students with private reminders about managing personal functions. Most people routinely deal with these concerns and do not need or desire your input. For example, although most participants with bowel and bladder dysfunction routinely empty their leg or bladder bags (urine collection devices), some may need an additional reminder prior to class. Should an accident occur, support staff should be prepared to discreetly escort the person to the restroom and quietly clean up the accident.

Teaching Strategies for Group Programs

You can employ many teaching strategies to accommodate people with varying abilities in a group setting and still maintain the safety and effectiveness of the program. Your most effective tool is educating your students to enable them to individualize modifications independently. With group programs, you also must be able to maintain a wide visual field and group cohesiveness in addition to individualizing instruction. Developing a useful system for modifying exercises and employing instructional approaches for people with different learning styles also eases your task with this challenging situation.

Visual Field

You must maintain a wide visual field during group program instruction while simultaneously focusing on individual needs. You should be able to spot someone having difficulty with the routine and momentarily offer the necessary modifications without disrupting the flow of the general class. The ideal method of accomplishing this split task is to use team teaching or employ qualified volunteers and assistants. Several strategies for team teaching are discussed on page 164.

To provide individual modifications without detracting from a group workout, use eye contact and body language. You can lean toward an individual and temporarily exaggerate your movements so that it is obvious to the other class members that your movements are a modification and not a change in the routine. A nod of the head or a thumbs-up signal can acknowledge that the person has successfully adopted the modification.

Categorizing Modifications

Although it is important to avoid applying stereotypes to people with like physical attributes (e.g., all people with spinal cord injury are the same), it is efficient to mentally group modifications according to the needs of people with similar conditions, movement patterns, or skill levels. For a review of modification "systems," refer to the chapters in Part III. From these generalized patterns, more individualized movements can be incorporated as needed.

One method for teaching to a group of people with mixed abilities is to isolate or focus on one particular need or modification for a segment of the workout until the participants can independently apply the appropriate adaptations as needed. Another segment of the workout can then be devoted to a different type of modification. This strategy requires that you invest time in advance preparation and that you know your students and their abilities. Do *not* actually group individuals with like disabilities in specific locations (e.g., all people using wheelchairs on the right side of the class, all people with strokes on the left, etc.), despite the ease it may afford you in offering exercise modifications. This strategy is a form of stereotyping and denies people the right to choose their own space.

Teaching to Different Learning Styles

Learning is a change in behavior brought about by experience (Whaley & Malott, 1971). Physical learning styles refer to the way people obtain and process information from physical experiences. Four types of learning styles have been identified: visual, auditory, tactile, and kinesthetic (Winnick, 1990). Although many people use all of these styles, they tend to favor one in physical learning situations such as exercise. In a person with a physical impairment, one or all of the learning styles may be affected, depending on the disability. As an instructor, you should be proficient at teaching people with a variety of learning styles. Table 12.1 summarizes the four learning styles.

Table 12.1 Four Styles of Learning

Style (sensory mode)	Instructional considerations
Visual (sight)	Visual cues: pointing, gesturing, counting with hands/fingers Written directions Visual aids Wear attire that enables you to clearly demonstrate movements Preferred by most sighted people, also people with memory dysfunction Difficult with impaired body awareness, ataxia
Auditory (hearing)	Concise explanations Oral directions Student can talk self through movements Difficult for individuals with hearing impairment, receptive aphasia
Tactile (touch)	Student feels instructor's movements Useful for individuals with impaired vision
Kinesthetic (movement)	Experimentation with movement trials Manual guidance Useful for individuals with visual impairment and some cognitive impairments

Teaching Movement to People With Visual Impairments

The challenge of leading an exercise class for people with visual impairments is not so much due to their movement limitations as to the necessity for modifying instructional methods. When someone with a visual impairment participates in your exercise classes, take additional time to check the exercise area and to provide a thorough orientation to the program and facility. Chapters 7 and 11 offer specific suggestions for resistance training and aerobic dance programs. Also consider the following general suggestions, offered by Hegey and Aceves (1991), to create a welcoming, enjoyable, and safe experience.

❏ Provide a thorough orientation to the program and facility. Offer a tour of the facility and indicate the location of restrooms, phones, water, tables, chairs, and other amenities. Show people with guide dogs a safe place for securing their dogs during the class.

❏ Before beginning a program, introduce yourself to each participant individually. Spend a few minutes learning about the person and his needs and abilities.

❏ Introduce new people to each other. In a group program, be sure everyone knows who they are positioned next to and how far away they are from them.

❏ Assign a skilled partner or assistant to work with your clients with visual impairment to help them with equipment or exercises. Provide the assistant with basic information about visual impairment and methods for providing assistance.

❏ Be sure the exercise area is cleared of all unnecessary and removable obstacles. Keep doorways and hallways clear. Leave doors entirely closed or open.

❏ Make sure each person knows where her towel, water bottle, and other personal items are located and do not move them to another location without indicating that you are making a change.

❏ Suggest a particular area or space for exercising that will be safe and that enables the participant to move without fear of restrictions. Offer to direct the person to a specific location that you recommend. Request that the person move around slowly in the space with arms spread to be sure the space is adequate.

❏ People with visual impairments may tend to wander from a designated spot during an aerobics class. Redirect the person verbally or, with permission, provide manual guidance.

❏ Always provide adequate explanations about each class or routine and maintain a continual verbal dialogue with the class. Keep students informed of what is happening. For example, indicate when you are moving to another area of the room and explain the actions of another person that may have brought laughter to the rest of the group.

❏ Offer simple and concise verbal cues for all movements. Once movement patterns or exercises have been learned, assign specific labels to each action to avoid having to reteach movements repeatedly. To prevent overwhelming new students, limit the number of labels introduced during each class.

❏ Reassure your clients with visual impair-

ments that, with time, they will learn the routines and that it is normal for all newcomers to feel awkward with unfamiliar movements.

❏ Provide feedback frequently and offer plenty of verbal praise. Avoid overcorrecting movements as long as safety is not an issue and remain sensitive to each participant's frustration level. Offer assistance if someone appears to be having difficulty.

❏ Before attempting to teach a class that includes people with visual impairments, practice by teaching a group of blindfolded friends. Teaching an entire class highlights the full challenge of the task. In addition, you may wish to attend a class blindfolded to appreciate the perspective of the person with a visual impairment.

Summary

This chapter presented ideas for developing and managing accessible fitness programs. When establishing a new program, the director must clearly identify appropriate objectives and evaluate facility and equipment needs before scheduling classes or developing a promotional plan. She must also select qualified exercise leaders and support staff and can form an advisory board to help shape and direct the program. Auxiliary personnel who are unaccustomed to working with individuals with disabilities may need additional training. In addition, the program director must develop useful registration materials and provide adequate preparticipation screening.

Managing the day-to-day operation of the accessible fitness program is generally the responsibility of the exercise leader, who must have knowledge and skills beyond simply delivering a safe and effective exercise class. The well-qualified instructor also has a variety of instructional and motivational strategies suited not only for individuals with disabilities, but also for group programs comprised of people with diverse needs and abilities. You must provide both preliminary and ongoing education for class participants about topics such as exercise principles, program objectives, exercise modifications, and personal safety. And, just as with exercise and technique modifications, effectively managing the exercise class requires that you individualize your approach to meet the needs of each student.

Chapter 13

Medical Conditions Associated With Physical Disabilities: Intervention and Emergency Procedures

Chrys Kub, MPT
Charlotte Rehabilitation Institute

This chapter reviews several common medical conditions that may be associated with physical disability and that may have an impact on a client's participation in an exercise class. For each identified medical condition, we will describe the condition and type of disability it may be associated with, explain the symptoms that should alert you to intervene, and describe appropriate action to take. It is essential that you be familiar with this information to ensure the safety of the participants in your exercise programs.

Before leading any type of fitness or exercise program, be sure to obtain or update your CPR certification. You also should be trained in basic first aid. This training can be obtained through a local chapter of the American Red Cross.

Epilepsy

Epilepsy is a medical condition characterized by seizures and convulsions. It can occur in the general population and in people with a disability due to brain damage, such as occurs with cerebral palsy, head injury, and stroke.

Grand Mal Seizure

A person experiencing a grand mal seizure may lose consciousness and postural control, fall, stiffen, and make jerky movements. The skin may appear pale or bluish, secondary to difficulty with breathing.

You can take several steps to help prevent an individual from sustaining an injury during a seizure. Do not, however, try to restrain the individual because a seizure cannot be stopped.

❑ Attempt to assist the client into a reclining position and place something soft under the head.
❑ Place the person on his side to minimize aspiration of food or secretions. Do not attempt this if it requires a struggle.
❑ Clear the area of hard or sharp objects.
❑ Do not force anything into the person's mouth.

Occasionally, a person may have an internal sensation called an "aura" that indicates a seizure is coming. If someone feels this sensation, you may be able to help her prepare for the seizure by doing the following:

❑ Help the person to the ground or onto a flat, uncluttered surface.
❑ Clear the area of hard or sharp objects.

Following a grand mal seizure the following steps are appropriate:

❑ If the individual is not already on his side, turn him onto his side to allow the saliva to drain from his mouth.
❑ The individual may be confused or disoriented after regaining consciousness and should not be left alone until fully alert. Arrange to have someone stay with her until she is fully alert.
❑ Do not offer the individual anything to eat or drink until he is fully awake because food or liquids could be aspirated.
❑ Most people feel exhausted after a grand mal seizure and probably should not continue exercising that day.

It is usually not necessary to activate the emergency medical service except in these cases:

• The individual does not start breathing after a seizure. (Begin rescue breathing immediately.)
• The individual is injured.
• The individual requests an ambulance.

Petit Mal or Partial Seizure

The petit mal seizure is a mild form of seizure. Someone experiencing this type of seizure stops participating in the activity and may have a glassy stare. He may not respond to questioning or may give an inappropriate response. He may sit, stand, or walk aimlessly, fidget with his clothes, or appear drunk, drugged, or psychotic. There is an 80% chance that the person will also exhibit incidental movements such as blinking, facial twitches, or chewing.

Petit mal seizures usually last less than 20 s and generally involve no loss of postural control. It may be advisable to help the person standing to sit down so he does not lose his balance. The following intervention procedures are recommended:

❑ Do not try to stop or restrain the individual.
❑ Try to remove harmful objects from the individual's pathway or coax him away from them.

Following the petit mal seizure, the individual may continue participating in the exercise activity as before. Further intervention is only required with the following circumstances:

• The individual is injured.
• The individual stops breathing. (Begin rescue breathing immediately.)
• The individual requests an ambulance.

Diabetes

Diabetes is a metabolic disorder resulting from an insufficient production of insulin or an inability to use available insulin. Diabetes is not more prevalent with any certain disability. A person with diabetes can suffer from adverse effects during exercise if his insulin level is not matched with his blood sugar and activity levels. Therefore, people who change their daily activity levels should consult with their physicians to adjust medical or dietary treatments.

Type I diabetes, known as juvenile diabetes, appears during childhood. This condition usually involves insufficient insulin and requires insulin injections daily. Type II diabetes (adult onset) generally manifests itself in later adulthood. In many cases, someone with Type II diabetes does not need to supplement with insulin but can control the condition with a proper diet.

Ketoacidosis

Ketoacidosis refers to a severe imbalance in the blood sugar level and is an emergency situation. A person experiencing this condition complains of increased thirst, drowsiness, headache, and shortness of breath. The skin may appear dry, hot, and flushed. In severe cases, the person may lose consciousness. Ketoacidosis is a medical emergency and assistance should be summoned immediately.

Hypoglycemia

Hypoglycemia occurs when a person has an extremely low blood sugar level. A person with this condition may exhibit confusion and loss of coordination. She may experience weakness and dizziness. The diabetic usually recognizes the symptoms of hypoglycemia, but you should discuss symptoms with the client before beginning the program and ask the client to let you know if they occur.

The following steps are recommended if someone with diabetes exhibits symptoms of hypoglycemia.

❏ Offer the person a sugary snack or a high-carbohydrate food that is quickly digested. Examples of appropriate foods are candy, oranges, sodas, or fruit juices.
❏ The person should consume the sugary snack immediately and only continue exercising once the symptoms disappear.

The incidence of hypoglycemia can be decreased if the participant learns to eat prior to physical exercise to prepare for the upcoming increased demand for blood sugar. Advise the participant not to inject insulin into a muscle that will be extensively exercised during a workout because the muscle absorbs the insulin quickly and the anticipated timing of insulin release will be affected. Those clients on insulin and beta blockers may have masked hypoglycemic symptoms and should be sure to adequately prepare for exercise by increasing their intake of readily digestible sugars or carbohydrates prior to the exercise session.

Emergency assistance need not be requested for someone with symptoms of hypoglycemia unless the symptoms persist or worsen.

Autonomic Dysreflexia

Autonomic dysreflexia is an uninhibited reflex response to a noxious stimulus (often from the bladder or bowel). The noxious stimulus initiates a reflex action of the autonomic nervous system, resulting in total body vasoconstriction that cannot be overcome by the body's normal compensatory mechanisms. This condition is very dangerous and can result in cerebral hemorrhage, damaged blood vessels, and heart failure. It is most prevalent in people with spinal cord injury, particularly with autonomic nervous system impairment due to injuries at or above the T1 to T5 level. Autonomic dysreflexia can also occur in people with other disabilities involving the central nervous system, although the incidence is much smaller.

The symptoms of autonomic dysreflexia include a pounding, severe headache caused by increased blood pressure. You may note flushed skin above the level of the injury and pallor below, with shivering and goose pimples initially, then profuse sweating above the level of the injury. The participant may also have a fast, pounding pulse.

People prone to dysreflexia usually can identify the cause. You can help relieve the symptoms as follows:

❏ Create postural hypotension (decreased blood pressure) by having the person assume a sitting position (if he has been lying down).
❏ Relieve the noxious stimulus: (a) check the catheter and tubing for plugging or kinks, (b) empty the leg bag if it is full, and (c) check for skin irritation.
❏ Call for emergency assistance if symptoms do not immediately subside.

Impaired Temperature Regulation

Disruption of the autonomic nervous system (ANS) may be associated with impaired temperature regulation, occurring most commonly in people with spinal cord injuries, especially above the T5 level. Impaired temperature regulation may also occur in other people with central nervous system (CNS) dysfunction, which causes them to be more vulnerable to heat exhaustion or heatstroke.

Heat Exhaustion

The symptoms of heat exhaustion resulting from overheating include dizziness with nausea, headache, and muscle cramps.

If symptoms persist beyond 1 to 2 hr, you should summon emergency assistance. Before you reach that point, attempt the following to relieve symptoms of heat exhaustion:

❏ Get the person to a cool environment and begin rehydration with oral fluids.
❏ Spray the person with alcohol solutions and expose her to cold air with a fan to increase evaporation. A solution can be made from two parts water and one part rubbing alcohol and applied with a spray bottle.

Heatstroke

Someone experiencing heatstroke will have such signs of CNS disturbance as stupor, seizures, or coma. The person will also exhibit an absence of sweating, and the skin will be hot and dry to the touch.

Heatstroke requires immediate emergency assistance. You should attempt to lower the individual's body temperature while awaiting assistance.

Postural and Exercise Hypotension

Peripheral pooling of blood in the extremities due to a loss of vascular muscle tone causes hypotension. In postural hypotension a change to a more vertical position causes increased pooling of blood in the lower extremities and decreased venous return of blood to the heart. Postural hypotension may occur in persons with spinal cord injury or poor circulation and in persons who are very sedentary.

Hypotension during exercise occurs for reasons similar to postural hypotension. An increase in heart rate increases the flow of blood through the body; however, if an individual cannot activate lower body skeletal muscles during upper body exercise, blood may pool in the lower extremities. This occurs with quadriplegia and with ANS impairment, which prevents blood from being redistributed appropriately during exercise.

An individual with hypotension might complain of dizziness and feel faint. His blood pressure and heart rate will decrease.

❏ Tilt the individual back or place him in a position to lower the head and increase blood flow to it.
❏ Request that the individual maintain the position until the dizziness abates.
❏ If symptoms do not disappear with intervention, call for emergency assistance.

Summary

Table 13.1 summarizes the medical conditions discussed in this chapter, their symptoms, and recommended interventions.

As an exercise leader, you must remain aware of possible medical complications in each of your clients that may arise during an exercise class. A person with a physical disability may be more susceptible to certain medical problems secondary to the specific disability. Careful preparticipation screening of all clients provides you with this information. Consult the participant's physician or therapist if you have any questions about the effect a specific condition may have during vigorous exercise. If you are trained in CPR and basic first aid and you are familiar with the appropriate intervention for the medical problems this chapter discusses, you will be more effective in leading a safe exercise program for all your clients.

Table 13.1 Medical Considerations During Exercise for People With Disabilities

Condition	Associated disabilities	Symptoms	Intervention/emergency procedures
Grand mal seizure	Epilepsy, head injury, CP	Loss of postural control, convulsions	Place soft object under head; clear area of all obstacles; call 911 if client stops breathing, is injured, or requests an ambulance
Petit mal seizure	Epilepsy, head injury, CP	Glassy stare, no response to stimulation or questions	Remove harmful objects from area, call 911 if symptoms of grand mal seizure develop
Ketoacidosis	Diabetes	Increased thirst, drowsiness, headache, shortness of breath	Medical emergency, call 911
Hypoglycemia	Diabetes	Confusion, dizziness, weakness, loss of coordination	Provide sugary snack or drink and if symptoms persist, call 911
Autonomic dysreflexia	Spinal cord injury, some head injury	Severe headache, increased blood pressure, flushing, goose bumps, fast pulse	Position to reduce blood pressure (sitting), relieve noxious stimulus, call 911 if symptoms persist
Heat exhaustion	Spinal cord injury; any person in hot, humid conditions	Dizziness, nausea, headache, muscle cramps	Get person to cool environment, spray with water, give oral fluids, and if symptoms persist more than 1 to 2 hr, call 911
Heatstroke	Spinal cord injury; any peron in hot, humid conditions	Stupor, seizure, or coma, lack of sweating	Medical emergency, call 911
Postural and exercise hypotension	Spinal cord injury, other CNS impairment	Dizziness, decreased blood pressure, increased heart rate, fainting	Lower head to heart level to decrease blood pressure and if symptoms persist, call 911

Chapter 14

Wheelchairs and Transfers

Diane Huss, MSEd, PT
Woodrow Wilson Rehabilitation Center, Fishersville, VA

Many people with physical disabilities who participate in an exercise class may move about with the use of a wheelchair or other assistive device. As an exercise leader, you should be familiar with the basic design of the equipment, be prepared to offer recommendations about exercise from a wheelchair, and be able to assist the person as needed. You may need to push the wheelchair to overcome physical obstacles or assist with a transfer from the chair to the floor or other surface. With these skills, you can increase the accessibility of your exercise classes and provide everyone with the opportunity for participation.

Wheelchairs

Wheelchair design continues to advance to meet the needs of the people who use wheelchairs. A large variety of styles has been developed for general use and specific purposes. Next we describe features common to most chairs as well as the various types of chairs available.

Components of a Wheelchair

Depending on the purpose of the chair, it may include a variety of components. Generally, all chairs have drive wheels and hand rims, casters, hubs and axles, seat upholstery, a backrest, and footplates or footrests. Some wheelchairs also have armrests, push handles, brakes, tipping levers, and antitip bars. Figure 14.1 illustrates these basic features. Wheels, footrests, and armrests may be removable with push-button, lever, or hook devices.

As an exercise leader, you should be familiar with the basic components of several types of wheelchairs and know how to operate them. Practice removing and assembling detachable parts, locking brakes, and folding different types of chairs. Check with a local hospital or medical supply store to see if you can practice on their equip-

ment or arrange for a variety of wheelchairs to be brought to your facility as part of a training session for staff and volunteers.

Types of Wheelchairs

Chairs can be roughly categorized into two groups: chairs designed for general locomotion and chairs designed for performance. Wheelchairs designed primarily for general locomotion, stability, and comfort include the standard or "hospital" chair, lightweight chair, and motorized chair. Performance wheelchairs include sports chairs and racing chairs. Some people also use motorized chairs for sporting events. Figure 14.2 illustrates four basic wheelchair designs.

Chairs for General Locomotion

The standard wheelchair, often referred to as the hospital chair, has been available for more than 50 years. It is the original design on which other chairs are based. This chair typically has brakes, armrests, footrests, removable seat cushions, push handles, and a high back. It can be folded and is relatively heavy. The standard chair is designed primarily for comfort and durability. Adjustable, lightweight wheelchairs are also designed for general locomo-

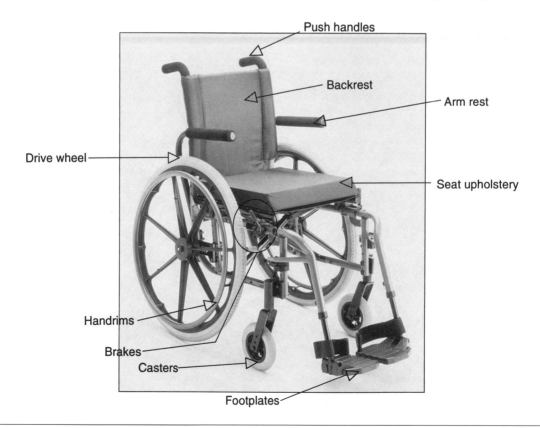

Figure 14.1 Components of a wheelchair. Photo courtesy of Top End by Action.

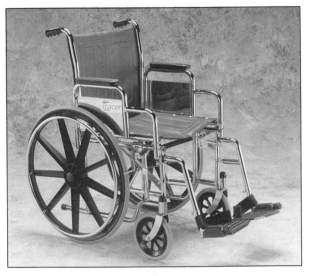

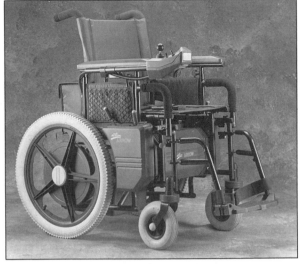

a

b

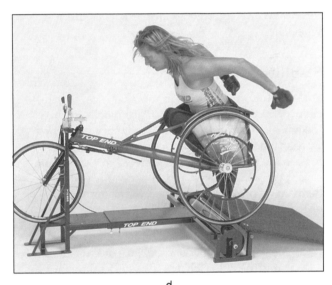

c

d

Figure 14.2 Four types of wheelchairs: standard (a), motorized (b), sports chair (c), and track chair for racing (d). Photos a and b courtesy of Action by Invacare; photos c and d courtesy of Top End by Action.

tion but have features to meet more specific needs. They are made of lightweight materials and have the rear axle positioned closer to the user's center of gravity. This adjustment allows greater maneuverability and propulsion speed. These chairs are also easier to lift, which helps when loading into and out of a car. The motorized wheelchair (inappropriately labeled the "electric" chair) is a heavy, battery-powered chair used to provide locomotion for people with more severe disabilities. This chair is typically nonfolding and is controlled by the hand, mouth, or head, depending on the user's functional abilities.

Chairs for Performance

The newest and most rapidly changing designs are in wheelchairs made for athletic performance. A variety of chairs have been marketed to meet needs in specific sporting events. Primarily, these chairs offer greater maneuverability and are much lighter than standard wheelchairs. They often have lower backs and may not have push handles, armrests, or brakes. Many have rigid frames and do not fold, although they have quick-release wheels to ease transport. Some people choose to use a sports chair for general locomotion as well as for sporting events.

Track chairs, used only for wheelchair racing, are designed for generating maximum speed. The positions of the wheels, hand rims, and seating are modified to decrease wind resistance and enhance body position for maximum propulsion efficiency.

Exercising in a Wheelchair

General fitness exercise can be vigorous, enjoyable, and beneficial from a wheelchair. By offering a few commonsense guidelines to your clients who use wheelchairs, you can ensure that their workouts are both safe and effective. Remember that wheelchairs are personal items considered by many who use them as an extension of the body. Respect this relationship and never push or maneuver a chair without permission. Normansell (1986) developed the following guidelines for exercise from a wheelchair.

Stability

For maximum stability, immobilize the wheelchair. If brakes do not hold, place blocks against the wheels. To prevent the chair from tipping backwards, place sandbags or other weights on the footrests, if needed. Some wheelchairs are not equipped with brakes and the people who use them may prefer not to have the chair fixed to one spot. As always, consult the individual before taking an action.

❑ Check the stability and balance of the person using the wheelchair *before* beginning exercise. Request that the person try different movements slowly with arms overhead, in front, and to the sides. If he loses balance, be sure he can regain a seated position.

❑ You may want to recommend that participants with trunk impairment use a chest or waist belt to increase stability. Be sure the belt does not overly restrict movement or reduce circulation—the belt material should have some stretch. Some people view strapping as a loss of freedom or independence. Although the choice of using a support belt is up to the individual, you might point out that chest straps can actually increase a person's freedom to perform exercises that might otherwise be impossible because of the inability to maintain balance with certain types of moves. With aerobics, a chest or waist belt may enable the individual to increase the overall conditioning effect of the workout because it

allows more vigorous upper body movements, eliminating the fear of falling.

❑ If excessive spasticity in the legs interferes with exercise (particularly with extensor tone), you could secure a flexible cord around the legs. Experiment with seating positions. For example, deepen hip and knee flexion by raising the footrest to reduce the incidence of extensor thrust (see Table 2.2).

Postural Alignment

Encourage good sitting alignment during exercise according to each participant's available trunk support. With minimally impaired upper body function, the trunk and head should be erect to maintain good alignment of the spine. Shoulders should be comfortably pressed down and rolled back.

For some people, however, modified alignment may be appropriate. With impaired trunk support, leaning backward for support from the chair back may improve balance and allow more freedom of movement. Leaning backward should not cause excessive forward flexion of the neck, however. Use of chest straps may improve alignment and movement freedom for some people who must modify alignment during exercise.

Personal and Safety Concerns

Participants should empty their bladder or leg bags before exercise to prevent accidents. Consider this equipment when designing exercise positions and movements to avoid obstructing its function or causing spills.

People with Harrington rods or any fusion or fixation devices between the vertebrae should use extreme caution in twisting movements.

Remind people who lack sensation to periodically check for any abrasion to the skin due to rubbing against the chair. These participants should wear a long T-shirt that will stay tucked in. Encourage frequent push-ups off the seat because people with paralysis and poor circulation are especially susceptible to pressure sores, which can be debilitating.

General Exercise Considerations

In a group exercise setting, encourage the person in a wheelchair to assume a location in the class where the view of the instructor is not obstructed by standing class members. You should avoid designating an assigned area for individuals who use wheelchairs, however.

The participant should remove all unnecessary items (backpacks, purses, wallets, or keys) from the wheelchair to allow maximum freedom of movement. Consult the person before beginning exercise to determine if wheelchair parts can be removed, and keep these items near the participant but not where they can cause tripping. People with good trunk control may want to remove armrests to allow added lateral movement. Footrests can be removed or repositioned to allow leg movement, as long as the feet can rest on the floor and do not dangle.

Wheelchair Assistance

People who use a wheelchair and participate in a fitness program may or may not have the strength and endurance to independently push their wheelchairs. Occasionally, they may request assistance in challenging situations. It is appropriate to offer assistance to a person who suddenly encounters an obstacle or who is having difficulty overcoming one. A few commonsense principles about providing assistance with the wheelchair include these:

❑ Always communicate with the person in the wheelchair to identify his needs and desires before providing assistance.
❑ Never approach a wheelchair from behind and maneuver someone without warning.
❑ Avoid sudden acceleration or deceleration.
❑ Do not allow a battery-powered wheelchair to tip because battery acid could spill.

To appreciate the perspective of the person who uses a wheelchair, try maneuvering a wheelchair independently or with assistance. Arrange to spend a day performing daily activities from a chair to experience some of the challenges and barriers that may not be immediately obvious to you.

Rough Terrain

Grass, gravel, and rock make wheelchair travel significantly more difficult, and the person in a wheelchair may be unable to cross such surfaces independently. To assist a person over rough terrain, tip the wheelchair back approximately 30 degrees into a "wheelie" position and push with straight arms (see Figure 14.3). This position prevents the casters from catching on obstacles and

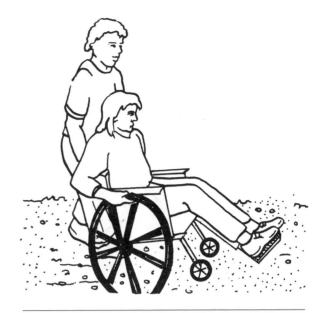

Figure 14.3 The wheelie to provide assistance over rough terrain.

reduces the likelihood that the movement will be suddenly halted, causing the individual and assistant to be thrown forward.

Inclines

Inclines require strength and muscular endurance to ascend or descend and may be too challenging for some participants, depending on their strength or the grade of the slope. Provide assistance for ascending inclines from behind so that both you and the seated person face up the hill. When descending inclines, back down the slope (see Figure 14.4).

Stairs

Ascending and descending stairs in a wheelchair generally requires assistance, preferably from two people for safety. The approach to stairs is opposite to that for ascending and descending inclines. With two people available for assistance, the stronger person should be to the back of the wheelchair. Both assistants should maintain good body mechanics throughout the maneuver. The person in back of the chair should maintain a lowered center of gravity and turn slightly to keep the load as close to the body as possible. The assistant in front should be sure to grasp a fixed component of the chair, not removable parts such as footrests or armrests. If antitip casters on the back of the chair prevent rolling over stairs, remove them or you

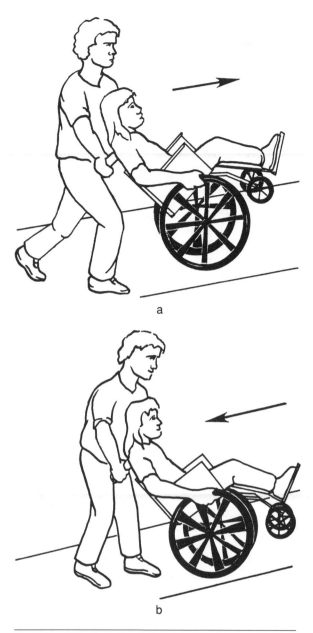

Figure 14.4 Assistance with an incline ascent (a) and descent (b).

To assist someone descending stairs, face the direction of the movement and remain one step away from the wheel of the chair. Tilt the chair back to clear the front casters and gradually lower it to each step. An assistant in front can push against the chair to reduce the pull of gravity that the person behind must resist (see Figure 14.5b).

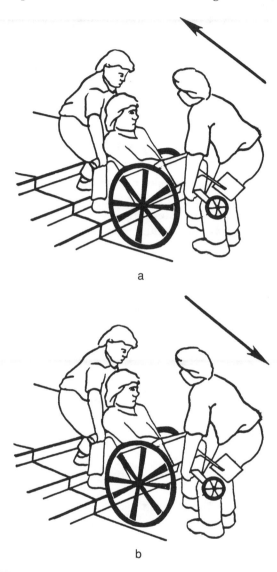

Figure 14.5 Assistance during stair ascent (a) and descent (b).

may have to lift the entire chair. For sport chairs without push handles, you'll have to maneuver the chair by grasping the frame of the seat back.

Stair ascent is the reverse of the descent—pull the wheelchair up the stairs backward (see Figure 14.5a). Pull the tilted chair from behind with straight arms using leg (not back) muscles. An assistant in front can lift the lower part of the chair from the front to reduce the strain of pulling the chair on the person in back. Maintain adequate backward tilt to keep the weight on the rear wheels and keep the chair balanced backward.

Curbs

All curb maneuvers should be approached perpendicular to the line of the curb to prevent lateral tipping. To ascend a curb, push down with the foot on the tipping lever to raise the front casters off the ground and tilt the wheelchair back. Then push the chair forward until the back wheels make contact with the curb. Ease the casters down onto the surface. Then, turn one hip into the back of the chair, bend the knees, and lift up on the push handles to ease the rear wheels over the curb.

Curbs are descended with the same technique used for descending stairs. See the previous section for a description of this technique. Figure 14.6 illustrates the technique for providing wheelchair assistance over curbs.

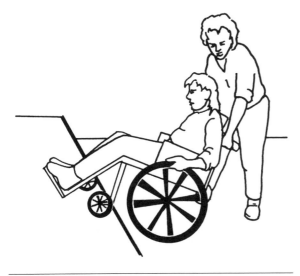

Figure 14.6 Positioning is the same when providing assistance with ascending and descending a curb.

Transfers

In a fitness class, some exercises may be more easily accomplished from the floor. Many people who use a wheelchair are capable of independently transferring to the floor, whereas others need assistance. To become competent at assisting with a transfer, you need both training from an appropriate professional and practice with subjects of a variety of sizes and weights.

Body Mechanics for Manual Lifting

With any type of lift, good body mechanics must be practiced to prevent injury to the lower back. The following principles for safe lifting apply whether the object you are lifting is heavy or light.

❏ Keep the lower back in normal alignment. This is the position of strength for the low back and is especially important for lifting.
❏ Use the legs to support as much of the load being lifted as possible by bending at the knees instead of the waist.

❏ Maintain a firm grip on the load, keeping it close to the body while it is being lifted or lowered.
❏ Place the feet to maintain a wide base of support—they should be at least shoulder-width apart with one foot ahead of the other.
❏ Avoid twisting the trunk while turning—turn with the entire body by side-stepping the feet toward the direction of the movement. This action avoids excessive muscle strain that twisting at the waist can create.
❏ Tense the abdominal muscles during a lift to increase the pressure within the abdominal cavity and relieve some of the pressure on the spine. This maneuver also serves to "set" the muscles to prepare for the strenuous activity.
❏ Keep the head and shoulders upright to maintain proper alignment in the neck and low back.
❏ Whenever possible, move an object with forces derived from body weight and controlled momentum, rather than with strength provided from isolated muscle groups. Lift gradually, without quick, jerky motions.
❏ Avoid reaching to move a load. Use a stepladder or step stool to reach high places.

Principles for Performing a Safe Transfer

In addition to practicing good body mechanics with lifting, several general principles for performing safe transfers from one surface to another should also be applied, regardless of the technique used to perform the transfer.

❏ Communicate with everyone involved in the transfer (the person in the chair and assistants) to establish a plan before beginning. Explain the steps in the procedure to the person being transferred. Inform the person before touching him. Identify what signal will be used to begin the maneuver (such as "one, two, three, lift") and who will be giving the command.
❏ Allow the person being transferred to control the situation. Use the type of transfer preferred by the wheelchair user if it differs from the one you prefer.
❏ Stabilize the chair by locking the brakes or by having an assistant hold it. Remove footrests or move them out of the way. Some transfers are easier if the armrests are removed.

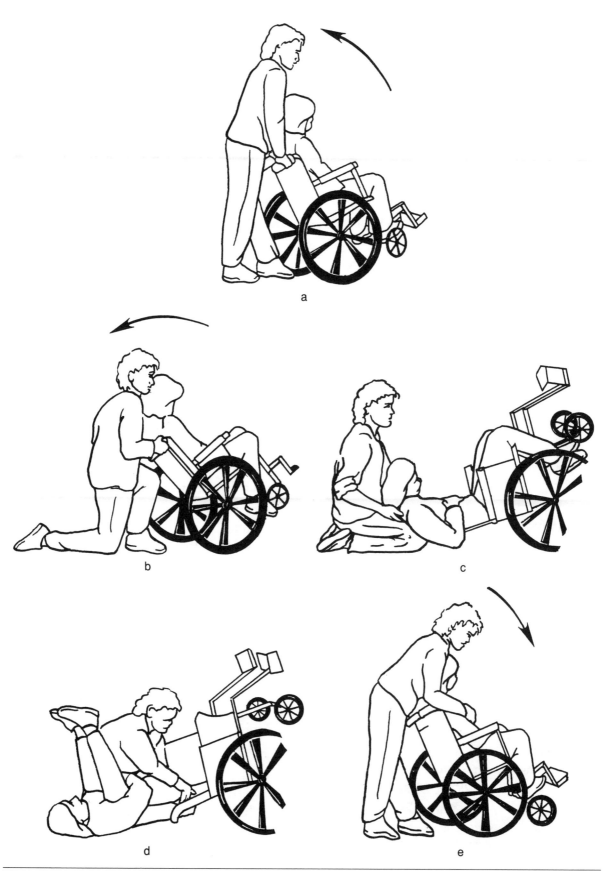

Figure 14.7 Steps for performing a one-person scoop transfer: support during the descent (a), pause and balance on one knee (b), cradle the neck (c), lift the buttocks (d), and support the chest on the return to upright (e).

❏ Ensure that the weight of the individual can be managed by those assisting with the transfer and will not jeopardize anyone's safety.

Types of Transfers

Transfers may be performed by one, two, or more assistants. You should only perform a transfer independently if you are certain you have sufficient strength to undertake the maneuver safely. Generally, two or three people should lift heavier people.

The Scoop Transfer—A One-Person Lift

A one-person transfer is difficult and potentially dangerous to perform unless the person being transferred is of significantly less weight than the person providing the assistance. The "scoop" transfer was designed to remedy this situation with a maneuver that never involves actually lifting the individual out of the chair (Ford & Duckworth, 1974). To perform this transfer, you will tip the chair back while supporting the person with body contact. After lowering the individual backward in the chair to the floor, you will slide the chair out from underneath the buttocks. To transfer the individual from the floor to the chair again, you will reverse the steps and "scoop" the person back into the chair. This transfer is not appropriate for use with a motorized wheelchair because the battery acids may spill when the chair is tipped.

A more detailed outline of the procedure for performing the scoop transfer follows, and Figure 14.7 illustrates the steps. Before using this transfer, practice all steps several times with a small, lightweight person and have an assistant review the technique as you practice. Then practice with a heavier individual.

1. Lock the brakes on the wheelchair and remove the footrests.
2. Push down on the tipping lever and push handles to tilt the wheelchair backward while pressing the hip and side of the body against the back of the chair to control the movement.
3. During the descent, slowly drop to one knee and shift the point of contact and support (between you and the person in the chair) to your arms and chest while maintaining an erect upper body.
4. Lower the back of the chair to the floor, cradling the individual's head between the forearms, taking care not to cause excessive neck flexion. Ease the person's head to the floor.
5. Release the brakes.
6. With the knees in flexion, pull the individual's hips into deeper flexion. The person being transferred can assist by wrapping her arms behind her knees. This is possible even if she does not have functional use of her hands because the force of gravity on her legs will keep her arms tucked in behind her knees.
7. Position yourself to the side of the wheelchair and lift the buttocks off the back of the chair with one hand, curling the trunk. Slide the chair out and away with your other hand.
8. Extend the knees and trunk and lower the legs to the floor.

To reverse the scoop transfer (floor to chair), take these steps:

1. With the brakes unlocked and seat cushion removed, tip the wheelchair back to place the push handles on the floor.
2. With the person in a supine position, pull the individual's knees and hips into flexion until the knees are resting on the chest. To maintain this position, the person being transferred can hold the legs in position by securing his arms behind the knees.
3. By placing one hand under the buttocks, curl the trunk into flexion using the free hand to scoop the chair under the person's back. This process may have to be repeated in stages until the buttocks are close to the seat of the chair.
4. At this phase, lock the brakes and put the seat cushion in place. Place the legs over the front edge of the wheelchair seat.
5. Grasp the push handles by sliding your arms under the head and shoulders, which can rest in your lap.
6. Begin to bring the chair upright while keeping close body contact with the individual and maintaining an erect posture. Use leg strength for lifting.
7. Stop halfway to reposition the legs and rest, as needed.
8. At the completion of the lift, stabilize the individual's upper body by placing one arm across the chest. Watch the legs to ensure that they do not become caught under the chair as you lower it.

Two-Person Transfer

When two assistants are available to perform a transfer, the risk of injury is lessened because the load is distributed between two persons. One assistant should direct the maneuver and provide the verbal commands. One person controls the legs

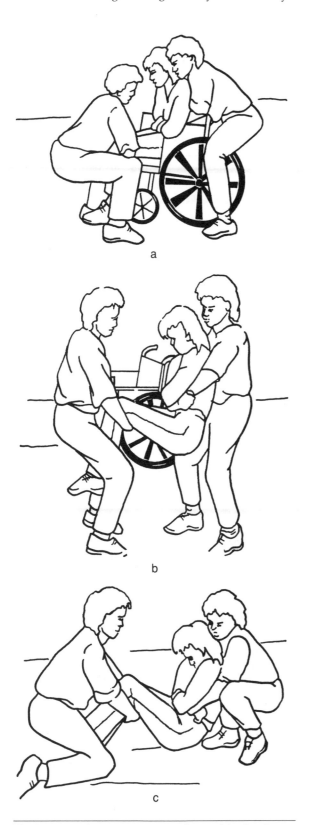

Figure 14.8 A two-person transfer: positioning before the lift (a), lateral movement after the lift (b), and lowering the person to the floor (c).

and one controls the body. A third person can be added at the hips for very large people. The person being transferred should keep the knees bent during the entire transfer to ease the process. Figure 14.8 illustrates steps for a two-person lift.

❏ Lock the chair before beginning the transfer and determine the direction of the transfer before beginning.
❏ The assistant controlling the legs should grasp them as close to the hips as possible.
❏ The assistant who controls the body should be positioned at the head and should wrap his arms around the person's chest. Perform the lift by putting pressure on the chest, not by pulling up on the armpits, to avoid placing excessive pressure on the shoulder girdle. The person being transferred can support this maneuver by holding onto the assistant's arms.
❏ To perform the move, both assistants should lift simultaneously on the count of three. Lifting should precede lateral movements to prevent rubbing the person's back across the tire of the wheelchair or other surface.
❏ When lowering the individual be sure to keep the back straight and bend the legs when squatting down to the floor.
❏ The assistants assume the same position to reverse the transfer from the surface to the chair. The lift is made straight up, using the leg muscles. Complete the transfer by moving the person over and into the chair.

Summary

The wheelchair may be the primary form of locomotion for some people with physical disabilities who participate in your fitness classes. It is important that you know how chairs function, safety considerations for exercise from a wheelchair, and how to provide assistance with maneuvering a chair if someone requests your help. You should also be skilled at performing transfers, as needed, to enable all your students to exercise from the floor or with other equipment as desired. Your skills will allow each individual the opportunity for maximum participation in your fitness programs.

Appendix A

Pharmacologic Agents: Effects on Heart Rate and Blood Pressure During Rest and Exercise

Key

Possible effects in therapeutic doses:

+	increase
–	decrease
0	no change
RHR	resting heart rate
EHR	exercise heart rate
RBP	resting blood pressure
EBP	exercise blood pressure

Note: Lower case notation refers to actions of a specific drug only. Drugs may also exert no effect. Absence of information indicates unknown or no known effect.

Exercise precautions

DE	dehydration
DI	dizziness or lightheadedness
EH	exercise or postexercise hypotension
HI	heat intolerance
MI	muscular incoordination
OE	overexertion

OH	orthostatic hypotension
UN	unsteadiness
VI	vision disturbances
WE	weakness

The following information summarizes general effects that specific classes of drugs may have on cardiovascular function at rest and during exercise (if known) as well as precautions with their use. Remember that in addition to causing different responses among individuals, pharmacologic agents induce dose-related responses. Furthermore, within each major class of drugs, specific agents may have differing or even opposite effects.

This is not intended to be a comprehensive list of pharmacologic agents. A discussion of the specific effects of each available drug is beyond the scope of this text. It is essential that you discuss any medications used by your clients with their physicians to determine the safe limits for exercise and expected responses with exercise.

Angina, arrhythmia, hypertension

Drug		Possible cardiovascular effects	Exercise precautions
Generic name	Brand name		
Ace inhibitors		R/EBP –	DE, DI, HI
Benazepril	Lotensin		
Captopril	Capoten, Capozide*		
Enalapril	Vasotec, Vaseretic*		
Fosinopril	Monopril		
Lisinopril	Prinivil, Prinzide*, Zestril, Zestoretic*		
Quinapril	Accupril		
Ramipril	Altace		

(continued)

(Continued)

Drug		Possible cardiovascular effects	Exercise precautions
Generic name	Brand name		
Alpha-adrenergic blockers		R/EHR +/0	DI, EH, OH
Prazosin	Minipress, Minizide*	R/EBP –	HI
Terazosin	Hytrin		
Antiadrenergic agents		R/EHR –/0	DI, EH, OH, HI
Centrally or peripherally acting:		R/EBP –	
Clonidine	Catapres, Combipres*		
Doxazosin	Cardura		
Guanabenz	Wytensin		
Guanadrel	Hylorel		
Guanethidines	Ismelin, Esimil*		
Guanfacine	Tenex		
Methyldopa	Aldomet, Aldoril*		
Reserpines	Diupres, Regrotan, Hydropres, Salutensin		
Antiarrhythmic agents (Class I)			
Disopyramide	Norpace	r/ehr +/0 rbp +/0	DI, HI, OH, VI
Procainamide	Procan, Promine, Pronestyl	rhr +	DI
Quinidines	Cardioquin, Quinidex	r/ehr +/0 rbp +/0	DI
Beta adrenergic blockers		R/EHR –	DI, OE, HI
Acebutolol	Sectral	R/EBP –	
Atenolols	Tenormin, Tenoretic*		
Betaxolol	Kerlone		
Bisoprolol	Zebeta, Ziac*		
Carteolol	Cartrol		
Labetalol	Normodyne, Trandate, Normozides*, Trandate HCT*		
Metoprolol	Lopressor, Toprol XL		
Nadolol	Corgard, Corzide*		
Penbutolol	Levatol		
Pindolols	Visken		
Propranolols	Inderal, Inderide*		
Timolol	Blocadren, Timolide*		
Calcium channel blockers		R/EHR +/–	OE
Amlodipine	Norvasc	R/EBP –	
Bepridil	Bepadin, Vascor		
Diltiazem	Cardizem, Dilacor XR	r/ehr –	
Felodipine	Plendil		
Isradipine	DynaCirc		
Nicardipine	Cardene		
Nifedipine	Adalat, Procardia	r/ehr +	
Verapamil	Calan, Isoptin, Verelan	r/ehr –	
Digitalis glycosides			
Digitoxin	Crystodigin		
Digoxin	Lanoxin, Lanoxicaps		

Drug		Possible cardiovascular effects	Exercise precautions
Generic name	Brand name		
Nitrates		RHR +	EH, OH
Erythrityl tet-ranitrate	Cardilate	EHR +/0 RBP −	
Isosorbide dinitrate	Dilatrate, Isordil, Sorbitrate	EBP −/0	
Nitroglycerine	Nitrogard, Nitrol, Nitr-Dur, Nitrocap, Nitrolin		
Pentaerythri-tol tetrani-trate	Duotrate, Peritrate, Pentritol		
Vasodilators		RHR +	
Hydralazine	Apresoline, Apresazide	EHR +/0	
Minoxidil	Loniten	R/EBP −	

*diuretic

Anxiety, depression, psychotic disorders

Drug		Possible cardiovascular effects	Exercise precautions
Generic name	Brand name		
Benzodiazepines			DI, MI, UN
Alprazolam	Xanax		
Chlordiaze-poxide	Librium, Libritabs		
Clorazepate	Tranxene		
Diazepam	Valium, Valrelease	ehr/bp −	
Halazepam	Paxipam		
Lorazepam	Ativan		
Oxazepam	Serax		
Prazepam	Centrax		
MAO inhibitors		RBP −/0	DI, OH
Phenelyzine	Nardil		

(continued)

(Continued)

Drug		Possible cardiovascular effects	Exercise precautions
Generic name	Brand name		
Phenothiazines		EHR +	DI, HI, OH, VI
Chlorproma-zine	Thorazine	EBP −	
Fluphenazine	Permitil		
Perphenazine	Trilafon		
Prochlorpera-zine	Compazine		
Thioridazine	Mellaril		
Trifluopera-zine	Stelazine		
Seratonin uptake inhibitors			DI, MI, OH,
Fluoxetine	Prozac		impaired
Paroxetine	Paxil		judgement
Sertraline	Zoloft		
Velafaxine	Effexor		
Tricyclic antidepressants		R/EHR +/0	DI, OH
Amitriphyline/ Chlordiazi-poxide	Limbitrol	R/EBP −/0	
Amitriphyline/ Perphena-zine	Triavil		
Amitriptyline	Elavil, Endep		
Amoxapine	Asendin		
Clomipramine	Anafranil		
Desipramine	Norpramin		
Doxepin	Sinequan		
Imipramine	Tofranil		
Nortriptyline	Aventyle, Pamelor		
Protriptyline	Vivactil		
Trimipramine	Surmontil		
Others			
Bupropion	Wellbutrin	RHR+	DI
Buspirone	BuSpar	RHR+	DI
Chlormeza-none	Trancopal		DI
Clozapine	Clozaril	R/EHR+ R/EBP−/0/+	DI, OH, VI
Maprotiline	Ludiomil		DI, OH, WE
Meprobamate	Equanil, Miltown		DI, MI, UN
Trazodone	Desyrel	RHR +/− RBP −	DI, OH

Asthma, bronchospasms, pulmonary disease

Drug		Possible cardiovascular effects	Exercise precautions
Generic name	Brand name		
Antihistamines			
Astemizole	Hismanal		
Loratadine	Claritin		
Terfanadine	Seldane		
Bronchodilators—adrenergic		R/EHR +/0	
Albuterol	Proventil, Ventolin, Volmax	R/EBP +/0/−	
Bitolterol	Tornalate		
Isoetharine	Bronkosol		
Isoproterenol	Isuprel	ehr/bp +	
Metaprotere-nol	Alupent, Metaprel		
Pirbuterol	Maxair		
Terbutaline	Brethair, Brethine, Bricanyl		
Bronchodilators—xanthine derivatives		R/EHR +/0	
Aminophyl-line	Somophyllin	R/EBP +/0	
Dyphylline	Dilor, Lufyllin		
Oxtriphylline	Choledyl		
Theophylline	Aerolate, Bronkodyl, Slo-bid, Theo-bid, Theo-Dur, Uniphyl		
Corticosteroids			
Beclometha-sone	Vanceril, Beclovent		
Flunisolide	AeroBid		
Triamcinolone	Azmacort		
Others			
Cromolyn	Intal		
Isoproterenol and phenyl-ephrine	Duo-Medihaler		

Convulsions, seizures, epilepsy

Generic name	Brand name	Possible cardiovascular effects	Exercise precautions
Barbiturates			For all classes: DI, WE, MI, OH, UN
Mephobarbital	Mebaral		
Benzodiazepines			
Clonazepam	Klonopin		
Clorazepate	Tranxene		
Diazepam	Valrelease, Valium	ehr/bp −	
Lorazepam	Ativan		
Carbonic anhydrase inhibitors			
Acetazolamide	Diamox		
Hydantoins			
Phenytoin	Dilantin		
Others			
Carbamazepine	Tegretol		
Felbamate	Felbatol		
Gabapentin	Neurontin		
Primidones	Mysoline		
Valproic acid	Depakene, Depakote		

Inflammation, pain with arthritis

Generic name	Brand name	Possible cardiovascular effects	Exercise precautions
Nonsteroidal anti-inflammatory drugs			DI, VI
Diclofenac	Voltaren		
Diflunisal	Dolobid		
Etodolac	Lodine		
Fenoprofen	Nalfon		
Flurbiprofen	Ansaid		
Ibuprofen	Advil, Motrin, Nuprin		
Indomethacin	Indocin		
Ketoprofen	Orudis, Oruvail		
Nabumetone	Relafen		
Naproxen	Aleve, Naprosyn, Anaprox		
Oxaprozin	Dapro		
Phenylbutazone	Butazolidin		
Piroxicam	Feldene		
Sulindac	Clinoril		
Tolmetin	Tolectin		

Drug		Possible cardiovascular effects	Exercise precautions
Generic name	Brand name		
Corticosteroids, cortiocotropins			
Betamethasone	Celestone		
Cortisone	Cortone Acetate		
Dexamethasone	Decadron, Haxadrol		
Hydrocortisone	Cortef		
Methylprednisolone	Medrol		
Prednisolone	Prelone		
Prednisone	Deltasone, Meticorten, Orasone		
Triamcinolone	Aristocort, Kenacort		
Gold compounds			
Auranofin	Ridaura		
Salicylates			
Aspirin	many brands		
Choline Salicylate	Athropan		
Choline and Magnesium Salicylates	Trilisate, Tricosal		
Magnesium Salicylates	Magan, Mobidin		
Salsalate	Amigesic, Disalcid		
Others			
Capsaicin	Zostrix (cream)		Heat and sweating may increase stinging on skin
Hydroxychloroquine	Plaquenil		
Methotrexate	Rheumatrex		Bruising or injury may occur from contact sports
Penicillamine	Cuprimine, Depen		

Spasticity, muscle spasms

Drug		Possible cardiovascular effects	Exercise precautions
Generic name	Brand name		
Benzodiazepines			
Diazepam	Valrelease, Valium	ehr/bp –	For all classes:
Lorazepam	Ativan		DI, MI, WE UN, VI
Skeletal muscle relaxants			
Carisoprodol	Soma	RHR +	
Chlorzoxazone	Paraflex		
Metaxalone	Skelaxin		
Methocarbamol	Robaxin, Robaxisal		
Orphenadrine Citrate	Norflex, Norgesic		
Others			
Baclofen	Lioresal		
Cyclobenzaprine	Flexeril		
Dantrolene	Dantrium		▽

Resources

The United States Pharmacopeial Convention. (1993). *Drug information for the health care professional* (13th ed.). Rockville, MD: Author.

American College of Sports Medicine. (1991). Medications relative to exercise testing and training. In R.R. Pate, S.N. Blair, J.L. Durstine, D.O. Eddy, P. Hanson, P. Painter, L.K. Smith, & L.A. Wolfe (Eds.), *Guidelines for exercise testing and prescription* (pp. 273-279) (4th ed.). Philadelphia: Lea & Febiger.

Appendix B

Sample Registration Forms

General Registration Form

Name _____ Age _____ M   F

Address _____
City/State   Zip

Phone (day) _____ (eve) _____ Education _____

Occupation _____ Employer _____

In an emergency, who should we contact? (Indicate name and phone):

Friend/Relative _____ Phone _____

Physician _____ Phone _____

What are your short-term and long-term fitness goals? _____

_____

_____

What type of exercise/physical activity do you enjoy the most? _____

_____

_____

What do you consider to be the greatest barrier to your *regular* participation in an exercise program?

_____

_____

What are your concerns regarding participation in an exercise program? _____

_____

_____

Health Appraisal and Medical History Questionnaire

Name _____ Date _____

Age _____ Height _____ Weight _____ Resting BP _____ Resting HR _____

Please complete this form carefully. All information will be treated as strictly confidential.

When were you last seen by a physician? _____

Reason? _____

May we call him/her? **YES NO** Has your physician ever advised you against exercise? **YES NO**

If you have a physical disability, please provide the following information:

Disability: _____ Years disabled: _____

Assistive devices: _____

Movement limitations: _____

Medical precautions: _____

Are you presently receiving physical therapy? **YES NO** If yes, therapist's name and phone number?

_____

Reason for therapy? _____

May we call him/her? **YES NO** Has your therapist ever advised you against exercise? **YES NO**

FAMILY HISTORY

Is your father living? **YES NO** If not, age and cause of death: _____

Is your mother living? **YES NO** If not, age and cause of death: _____

Have your parents, grandparents, or siblings had any of the following (indicate who):

❑ Hypertension _____ ❑ Heart attack _____
                                            (at age 50 or younger)
❑ Stroke _____ ❑ Heart Attack _____
                                            (over age 50)
❑ Diabetes _____ ❑ Other _____
❑ Cardiovascular disease _____

MEDICAL HISTORY

Have you ever had, or do you currently have, any of the following:

❑ Cardiac disorder   ❑ Asthma   ❑ Emphysema
❑ Cancer   ❑ Chest pains   ❑ Fainting
❑ Dizziness   ❑ Phlebitis   ❑ Shortness of breath
❑ Diabetes   ❑ Hernia   ❑ Gout
❑ Abnormal EKG   ❑ Anemia   ❑ High blood pressure
❑ Heart medications   ❑ Hypoglycemia   ❑ Epilepsy
❑ Irregular heart beats   ❑ Embolism   ❑ Kidney problems
❑ Numbness or tingling in   ❑ Respiratory infections   ❑ Pulmonary disorder
  arms, hands, legs   ❑ High cholesterol   ❑ Arthritis

Health Appraisal and Medical History Questionnaire (*continued*)

❏ High triglycerides   ❏ Nerve damage   ❏ Bone fracture
❏ Thyroid condition   ❏ Surgery   ❏ Other medical
❏ Low back pain

Injury to: ❏ hip or pelvis   ❏ ankle/foot   ❏ arm/elbow   ❏ shoulder   ❏ face
           ❏ knee/thigh   ❏ back   ❏ wrist/hand   ❏ clavicle

Please explain any items checked above: _____

_____

Please list any other medical conditions or chronic illnesses you have or have had: _____

_____

Please list any medications you are currently taking: _____

_____

Do you have any conditions that limit the range of motion at any joint or in part of your body and that might be aggravated by exercise? **YES NO** Please describe if "yes": _____

_____

HEALTH HABITS HISTORY

Do you regard yourself as being:

❏ Overweight   ❏ Underweight   ❏ Optimal weight
❏ Sedentary   ❏ Moderately active   ❏ Very active
❏ Unfit   ❏ Moderately fit   ❏ Very fit
❏ Very stressed   ❏ Moderately stressed   ❏ Without stress
❏ Unhealthy   ❏ Moderately healthy   ❏ Very healthy
❏ Always fatigued   ❏ Occasionally fatigued   ❏ Energetic

Do you currently, or have you ever smoked cigarettes? **YES NO**

If yes, how many packs per day? _____.

If you have stopped smoking, what was the approximate date? _____.

Do you smoke cigars or pipes? **YES NO**

How many times/week do you currently engage in physical activity of at least 20 min duration? _____ What type of activity?

_____

(*continued*)

Describe physical activity (exercise/sports) during the past 12 months:

Type of activity	Dates of participation	Frequency (days/week)	Intensity (mild/moderate/intense)

I have answered the preceding questions to the best of my ability. I further understand that thorough and honest responses to these questions are essential to my safety and for prudent recommendations and guidance from the exercise leaders at this facility.

Signature _____ Date _____

Physician Recommendation for Participation in Exercise Classes

Date: _____

Physician's name: _____ Phone: _____

_____ has registered to participate in exercise classes at
(Participant)

_____

A description of the class is provided below:
(Include duration, frequency, intensity, and mode of activity.)

Is this individual currently taking any medication(s) that will affect his/her participation or exercise responses in this program? If yes, please identify the medication(s) and describe the effects.

_____

_____

Please indicate your recommendations for this individual's participation in the exercise class described above:

❑ I recommend participation without limitation.

❑ I recommend participation with the following limitations:

_____

_____

❑ I do not recommend participation.

❑ Please call me for specific recommendations.

_____   _____
Physician signature   Date

Please return this form to:

    (name of program facility and director)

Appendix C

Resources

National/International Disability Organizations

American Amputee Foundation
Box 55218
Little Rock, AR 72225
501-666-2523

American Foundation for the Blind
1615 M Street NW, Ste. 250
Washington, DC 20036
202-457-1487

The Arthritis Foundation
1314 Spring Street, NW
Atlanta, GA 30309
800-283-7800 or 404-872-7100

Disabled American Veterans (DAV)
P.O. Box 14301
Cincinnati, OH 45250
606-441-7300

Epilepsy Foundation of America
4351 Garden City Dr.
Landover, MD 20785
800-332-1000 or 301-459-3700

Muscular Dystrophy Association
3300 E. Sunrise Dr.
Tucson, AZ 85718
800-572-1717 or 602-529-5300

National Amputee Foundation
73 Church Street
Malverne, NY 11565
516-887-3600

National Easter Seal Society
70 E. Lake St.
Chicago, IL 60601
312-726-6200

National Head Injury Foundation, Inc.
1776 Massachusetts Ave.
Washington, DC 20036
800-444-NHIF or 202-296-6443

National Multiple Sclerosis Society
733 3rd Ave.
New York, NY 10017
800-532-7667 or 212-986-3240

National Rehabilitation Information Center
(NARIC)
8455 Colesville Rd., Ste. 935
Silver Spring, MD 20910-3319
800-346-2742

National Stroke Association
300 E. Hampden Ave., Ste. 240
Englewood, CO 80110
303-762-9922

Paralyzed Veterans of America
801 Eighteenth Street, NW
Washington, DC 20006
800-424-8200 or 202-872-1300

Spina Bifida Association of America
4590 MacArthur Blvd., NW
Washington, DC 20007
800-621-3141

Spinal Cord Injury Network
250 Hungerford Dr., Ste. 115
Rockville, MD 20850
301-424-8335

United Disability Services
326 Locust Street
Akron, OH 44302
216-762-9755

National and International Disabled Sports Organizations

Canadian Amputee Sports Association
18 Hale Dr.
Georgetown, ON
Canada L7G 4C2

Canadian Blind Sports Association (CBSA)
333 River Rd.
Ottawa, ON
Canada K1L 8H9

Canadian Wheelchair Sports Association
1600 James Naismith Drive
Glouchester, ON
Canada K1B 5N4
613-748-5685

Cerebral Palsy-International Sports and
  Recreation Association (CP-ISRA)
Heijenoordseweg 5
The Netherlands
6813 GG Arnhem
830 6 22503

Dwarf Athletic Association of America (DAAA)
Len Sawisch, PhD
3725 W. Holmes
Lansing, MI 48910
517-393-3116

International Blind Sports Association (IBSA)
Secreteriart c/o SHIF Idrottens Hus
S-12387 Farsta, Sweden
8-7136221 (Telephone)

International Sports Organization for the
  Disabled (ISOD)
SRD Guillermo Cabezas
Garcia de Paredos 74
Madrid 3, Spain
34-1-308-1797

National Handicapped Sports (NHS)
451 Hungerford Rd., Ste. 100
Rockville, MD 20850
301-217-0960

National Wheelchair Athletic Association
  (NWAA)
3595 E. Fountain Blvd., Ste. L-1
Colorado Springs, CO 80910
719-574-1150

Ontario Wheelchair Sport Association (OWSA)
585 Tretheway Drive
Toronto, ON
Canada M6M 4B8
416-495-4086

United States Association for Blind Athletes
  (USABA)
33 N. Institute
Brown Hall #015
Colorado Springs, CO 80903
719-630-0422

United States Cerebral Palsy Athletic Association
  (USCPAA)
500 S. Ervay, Ste. 452B
Dallas, TX 75201
214-761-0033

United States Les Autres Sports Association
  (US-LAS)
1475 W. Gray St., Ste. 165
Houston, TX 77019
713-521-3737

United States Organization for Disabled Athletes
  (USODA)
George Navarro
143 California Ave.
Uniondale, NY 11553
516-485-3701

United States Quad Rugby Association
Brad Mikkelsen
1605 Mathews St.
Ft. Collins, CO 80525
303-484-7395

United States Wheelchair Weightlifting
  Federation
39 Michael Pl.
Levittown, PA 19057
215-945-1964

Sports Medicine, Fitness, and Aerobics

Aerobics and Fitness Association of America
(AFAA)
15250 Ventura Blvd., Ste. 310
Sherman Oaks, CA 91403
800-445-5950

American College of Sports Medicine (ACSM)
401 W. Michigan Street
P.O. Box 1440
Indianapolis, IN 46206-1440
317-637-9200

American Council on Exercise (ACE)
P.O. Box 910449
San Diego, CA 92191-0449
619-535-8227

American Kinesiotherapy Association
P.O. Box 611
Dayton, OH 45409
800-326-0268

Institute for Aerobics Research
12200 Preston Rd.
Dallas, TX 75230
800-527-0362

International Dance Exercise Association (IDEA)
6190 Cornerstone Ct., East, Ste. 204
San Diego, CA 92121
800-825-3636

National Strength and Conditioning Association
P.O. Box 81410
Lincoln, NE 68501-1410
402-472-3000

Disability and Disabled Sports Publications

Able Bodies
AAHPERD
1900 Association Dr.
Reston, VA 22091
703-476-3400

Adapted Physical Activity Quarterly
Human Kinetics Publications
P.O. Box 5076
Champaign, IL 61825-5076
217-351-5076

Mainstream
2973 Beech St.
San Diego, CA 92102
617-234-3138

National Wheelchair Athletic Association
Newsletter
2107 Templeton Gap Rd., Ste. C
Colorado Springs, CO 80907
303-632-0698

Palaestra
Challenge Publications
P.O. Box 508
Macomb, IL 61455
309-833-1902

Paraplegia News and Sports 'N Spokes
PVA Publications
5201 North 19th Ave., Ste. 111
Phoenix, AZ 85015
602-224-0500

Sportsline
National Association of Sports for Cerebral Palsy
66 E. 34th St.
New York, NY 10016
212-481-6359

Fitness Equipment

Dyna-Bands
Fitness Wholesale, Inc.
3064 W. Edgerton
Silver Lake, OH 44224
800-537-5512

Equalizer Exercise Machines
911 Kings Point Rd.
Polson, MT 59860
406-883-2147
(multistation accessible exercise machines)

Freedom Machine
P.O. Box 32453
Phoenix, AZ 85064-2453
602-271-4931
(accessible weight machines)

G.E. Miller, Inc.
484 South Broadway
P.O. Box 266
Yonkers, NY 10705
800-431-2924
(arm ergometers, recumbant ergometers)

Magic In Motion, Inc.
20604 84th Ave. South
Kent, WA 98032
206-872-0722
(hand-pedaled attachment for wheelchairs)

Power Trainer
Sinties Scientific, Inc.
5616A S. 122nd East Ave.
Tulsa, OK 74145
(arm ergometer)

Saratoga Access & Fitness
6 Birch St.
Saratoga Springs, NY 12866-3834
518-587-6974
(the Saratoga Cycle)

Therabands
The Hygenic Corporation
1245 Home Avenue
Akron, OH 44310
216-633-8460

Versatrainer by Pro-Max
Bowflex of America Inc.
2200 N.E. 65th Avenue, Ste. C
Vancouver, WA 98661
800-654-3539
(accessible progressive resistance machine)

Glossary

active-assisted stretching—Assistance provided by an external force (usually a partner) to supplement active stretching by the participant

active stretching—Stretching accomplished exclusively by the efforts of the participant

acute—A condition of rapid onset and short term

aerobic—With oxygen

afferent—Pathways that conduct inward to an organ, gland, or other structure (such as the brain) and relay sensory information, as with arteries or sensory neurons

agonist—The primary contracting muscle responsible for an intended action that opposes the action of the antagonist of the muscle pair

Alzheimer's disease—A form of dementia occurring with aging marked by short-term memory impairment, hypertonia, loss of kinesthetic sense, and incoordination

amputation—The removal or absence of part or all of an appendage

amyotrophic lateral sclerosis (ALS)—Progressive atrophy of muscle due to degeneration in anterior horn cells of motor nerves

anaerobic—Without oxygen

anaerobic threshold—A level of exercise at which lactic acid concentration in the muscle begins to increase during graded exercise, signifying the level beyond which continuous aerobic exercise is limited

antagonist—A muscle capable of directly opposing the action of a prime mover or agonist in a muscle pair

aphasia—Impaired ability to speak and express thoughts (expressive aphasia) or to understand spoken or written speech (receptive aphasia)

arthritis—Joint inflammation

arthrogryposis multiplex congenita—A congenital disease that causes complete immobility in the joints of the hands and feet resulting from the formation of fibrous lesions in the joint

assistor—A muscle that contributes to an intended action

ataxia—A condition caused by injury to the cerebellum or afferent nerve tracts from skeletal muscles that causes significant movement incoordination, an impaired kinesthetic sense, and poor body balance due to loss of control over voluntary movements

athetosis—A condition caused by injury to extrapyramidal tracts in the brain and characterized by slow, nonrhythmical, random, and involuntary movements that are circular and jerky in nature; most often affecting distal segments of the upper extremities

ATP—Adenosine triphosphate; the high-energy phosphate compound produced and stored within skeletal muscle that provides the energy for muscular contraction

atrophy—Decrease in size of an organ or tissue; decrease in the diameter of muscle fibers, also referred to as "muscle wasting"

autogenic inhibition—See inverse stretch reflex

autonomic dysreflexia—A potentially life-threatening condition caused by dysfunction of the autonomic nervous system with symptoms including profuse or absent sweating, a pounding headache, skin splotching, etc.

ballistic stretching—Elongation of muscle that involves repeated bouncing, twisting, or swinging movements

bilateral—Pertaining to the same parts or similar actions on both the left and right sides of the body

biofeedback—A technique used to regulate involuntary mechanisms (such as heart rate and blood pressure) normally controlled by the autonomic nervous system

blindisms—Self-stimulatory movements such as rocking, finger waving, and hand shaking that are common to some individuals with visual impairment

bulbar polio—Viral attack upon the nuclei of the brain stem, affecting circulation and respiration

cardiac output ($\dot{Q}$)—The volume of blood pumped from the heart per minute: $\dot{Q}$ = heart rate (HR) × stroke volume (SV)

cardinal planes—Three planes of the body that divide it into left and right (sagittal plane), front and back (frontal plane), and top and bottom (transverse plane)

cardiorespiratory endurance—The ability to maintain an activity involving repeated muscular contractions of large muscle groups indefinitely

catecholamines—Substances, such as epinephrine and norepinephrine, that are released to mediate physiological responses to stress, thereby increasing heart rate, blood pressure, and blood levels of glucose and lipids

cauda equina—The collection of spinal roots descending from the lower spinal cord (T1 level) and occupying the vertebral canal below the cord

central nervous system (CNS)—One of two major branches of the nervous system that includes the brain, cranial nerves, and nerves of the spinal cord

cerebral palsy—A nonprogressive motor disorder resulting from injury to the brain before, during, or following birth that may involve motor and cognitive dysfunction

cerebrovascular accident (CVA)—Injury to the brain caused by oxygen deprivation (ischemic stroke) or hemorrhage in the brain (hemorrhagic stroke)

Charcot-Marie-Tooth disease—A hereditary disease mainly of the peripheral nerves involving progressive weakness and atrophy of distal muscles, usually beginning with the lower leg

chronic—Continual, of long duration

closed head injury—Traumatic brain injury caused by an impact to the head that causes tearing, shearing, or bruising of the soft brain tissues

collagen—Fibrous protein found in connective tissue that provides strength and resists deformation (stretching)

concentric contraction—Contraction of a skeletal muscle while it is shortening

contracture—Adaptive shortening of soft tissues crossing a joint that may or may not be reversible

coordination—Ability of muscles or different systems to work harmoniously in carrying out specific movements or actions

decubitus ulcers—See pressure sores

diabetes mellitus—A metabolic disorder resulting from insufficient production of insulin or inability to use available insulin

diastolic blood pressure—Arterial blood pressure during diastole (between heart beats)

diplegia—Paralysis in all four limbs, usually more so in the legs

disarticulation—Separation or amputation at a joint, without cutting through a bone

dynamic constant resistance—Dynamic exercise involving movement about a joint against a constant external load

dynamic variable resistance—Dynamic exercise involving movement about a joint against a variable external load

dysmelia—Amputation involving the congenital absence of a complete limb

eccentric contraction—Contraction of a skeletal muscle while it is lengthening

edema—A local, generalized condition involving accumulation of excessive amounts of fluids in body tissues

efferent—Pathways (nerves, vessels) that conduct outward or away from a part, organ, gland, or structure; motor neurons that activate or inhibit muscular actions in response to afferent sensory information relayed to the spinal cord, the brain, or both

elastin—Protein fibers of a tissue that provide extensibility

epilepsy—A condition characterized by the recurrence of seizures and convulsions

exacerbation—A period of worsening symptoms or increase in the severity of a disease

exercise hypotension—Abnormally low blood pressure during exercise

extrapyramidal tract—A functional classification of motor nerves outside the pyramidal tracts that control and coordinate postural, static, supporting, and locomotor mechanisms

fatigue, muscle—The failure of a muscle to maintain an expected force or power output

flaccid paralysis—A type of paralysis that results in complete loss of muscle tone and tendon reflexes, resulting in extreme muscle atrophy

flexibility—The ability of a muscle to elongate, enabling the joint to move through a range; extensibility

Friedreich's ataxia—A hereditary disease that causes progressive degeneration of sensory nerves in the limbs and trunk, impairing balance and coordination and causing an unsteady gait

functional range of motion—Range of motion defined by the limits imposed by disease or dysfunction; the range of motion at a joint needed to permit adequate functioning for a particular activity

gait—A manner of walking

Golgi tendon organ (GTO)—Sensory organ in tendons that detects changes in muscle tension and initiates the inverse stretch reflex

goniometer—An instrument used to measure the degrees of movement at a joint

Guillain-Barré Syndrome—A disease affecting spinal roots and peripheral nerves that causes progressive ascending weakness and paralysis from the feet to the facial muscles, impairing tendon reflexes, with recovery occurring in two thirds of affected people

hemiplegia—Paralysis on one side of the body due to damage of upper motor neurons

homeostasis—A state of dynamic equilibrium of the internal environment maintained by feedback and regulatory mechanisms among the physiologic systems of the body

hydrocephaly—"Water on the brain," an abnormal increase of cerebrospinal fluid in the skull

hyperplasia—Increase in the number of cells in a part

hyperreflexia—A condition of exaggerated reflexes

hyperthermia—Excessively high body temperature

hypertonicity—A condition of excessive tension or activity

hypertrophy—Increase in the size of tissue cells

hypoglycemia—A condition of low blood sugar (glucose)

incontinence—Inability to control bowel and bladder function

inverse stretch reflex—Action of the GTO that inhibits contraction of the agonist and initiates contraction of the antagonist (also referred to as autogenic inhibition)

ischemia—Insufficient supply of blood to a part of the body due to obstructed circulation

isokinetic—Movement of a limb at a constant angular velocity

isometric contraction—Contraction of a muscle that generates tension without limb movement

isotonic contraction—Contraction of a muscle against a constant external resistance through a movement range

ketoacidosis—Excessive acidity in body fluids due to the presence of ketone bodies, resulting from incomplete metabolism of fatty acids occurring with diabetes mellitus or other conditions of insufficient or deficient use of carbohydrates

lability—Instability; with behavior, unstable, fluctuating, or uncontrolled expression of emotions

lesion—Any pathological condition, injury, or wound in a tissue; loss of function of a part

lower motor neurons—Motor nerves of the peripheral nervous system originating in the gray matter of the spinal cord and terminating at skeletal muscles

maximal oxygen consumption ($\dot{V}O_2$max)—The greatest rate of oxygen consumption attained during exercise expressed as liters per minute (L/min) or milliliters per kilogram of body weight per minute (ml/kg/min); an indicator of overall cardiorespiratory fitness

maximal voluntary contraction (MVC)—A singular effort of maximal force by a muscle or muscle group

meninges—The three membranes covering the brain and spinal cord (dura mater, arachnoid, and pia mater)

metabolism, energy—Processes that convert chemical energy to mechanical energy to accomplish work

monoplegia—Paresis or paralysis in one muscle, limb, or body part; monoplegic cerebral palsy involves one limb, usually an arm

motor neuron—An efferent neuron having a motor function that conveys motor impulses to muscles

motor unit—A group of muscle fibers and the single efferent motor neuron that innervates them

multiple sclerosis—A chronic, neurologic disease that destroys the myelin sheath covering neurons in the CNS, possibly affecting motor function, balance, vision, speech, and cognitive function

muscle spindle—Sensory organ in muscle that detects changes in muscle length with passive elongation and responds by initiating the stretch reflex and reciprocal inhibition

muscle tone—The active resistance of muscle to passive stretch

muscular dystrophy—A collection of progressive genetic diseases causing degeneration of muscle tissue due to loss of protein in the muscle fiber and gradual replacement by fat and connective tissue

muscular endurance—A muscle's ability to repeatedly perform submaximal muscular contractions over a short period of time, measurable as the number of repetitions completed against 50% to 60% of maximum

myasthenia gravis—A progressive autoimmune disease affecting the neuromuscular junction and causing abnormal fatigue and muscular weakness in facial and neck muscles, the trunk, and extremities

myelomeningocele—Protrusion of the spinal cord and its meninges through a defect in the vertebral column; a type of spina bifida

necrosis—Tissue or cell death

one-repetition-maximum (1RM)—The amount of

force a muscle can generate during one maximal effort (a measure of muscular strength)

open head injury—Traumatic brain injury caused by a penetrating wound to the skull

osteoarthritis—A noninflammatory, degenerative joint disease caused by progressive disintegration of articular cartilage

osteogenesis imperfecta (OI)—A hereditary disease characterized by brittle bones and frequent fractures before birth (the congenital form) or occurring with the onset of walking (tarda form), with the tendency for fracture decreasing or disappearing with age

overstretch weakness—Weakness in a muscle caused by elongation for an extended period

overwork—The cumulative effects of excessive exercise stress over time causing temporary or permanent decline in muscle function

oxidation—The process of a substance combining with oxygen; process of metabolizing fuels in the presence of oxygen for the release of energy (ATP) that can be used for muscular contractions

oxygen consumption ($\dot{V}O_2$)—The rate at which the body utilizes oxygen as an indicator of the energy cost of aerobic exercise

paralysis—Loss of motor function caused by impaired neural or neuromuscular mechanisms

paraplegia—Paralysis in the lower trunk, lower extremities, or both; SCI paraplegia refers to spinal cord injury at or below the T1 level

paresis—Muscle weakness; partial or incomplete muscle paralysis

Parkinson's disease—A slowly progressive disease of the nervous system marked by resting tremor, muscular weakness, rigidity, and a shuffling gait

passive stretching—Stretching accomplished by application of an external force rather than active participation by the individual

peripheral nervous system (PNS)—One of two major branches of the nervous system that includes the nerves that emanate from the central nervous system (brain and spinal cord)

phocomelia—Congenital amputation marked by the absence of the proximal segment of a limb with the hands or feet articulating at the trunk

plasticity—The capability of being molded; the quality of muscle and connective tissue that enables it to assume a new permanent resting length after a stretch force has been applied under certain conditions

poliomyelitis—An acute, contagious viral disease that destroys or injures motor nerves, specifically anterior horn cells, in the spinal cord,

the medulla, or motor area of the cerebral cortex and cerebellum, causing paralysis, weakness, or respiratory weakness

postpolio syndrome—A condition experienced by about 25% of polio survivors decades after the initial virus has been contracted, involving joint or muscle pain, fatigue, and weakness

power—The rate at which work is performed (power = force × velocity)

pressure sores—A sore resulting from prolonged pressure on a body part that causes poor circulation and skin breakdown; decubitus ulcers

prime mover—The muscle or muscle group supplying the primary force for a specific action

primitive reflexes—Reflex actions inherent in the newborn that are normally suppressed (become integrated) during the first year of life

progressive resistive exercise—Resistive exercise training that employs progressive increases in load

proprioceptive neuromuscular facilitation (PNF)—A group of stretching techniques based on principles of neuromuscular mechanisms that involve proprioceptors in the muscles, tendons, and joints

prosthesis—An artificial substitute that replaces a missing part, such as an artificial limb

pyramidal tracts—Descending motor nerve fibers arising from cells in the motor areas of the cerebral cortex and passing through the spinal cord to anterior horn cells

quadriplegia—Paralysis of all four limbs and the trunk; SCI quadriplegia involves cord injuries above the T1 level

range of motion (ROM)—Range of movement at a joint, measurable in inches or centimeters (linear units) or degrees (angular units)

Rating of Perceived Exertion (RPE)—A scale developed by Borg (1982) to provide a qualitative measure of an individual's perception of physical exertion during exercise

reciprocal inhibition (innervation)—Reflex action of muscle pairs that causes the antagonist of a contracting muscle to relax

reflex—An involuntary response to a stimulus

reflex arc—A neural pathway between a point of stimulation and the responding organ or muscle

residual limb—The remaining segment of an amputated limb

rheumatoid arthritis—A chronic systemic disease that causes inflammation of connective tissues, stiffness, hypertrophy of cartilage, joint deformities, and pain

rigidity—Inflexibility or stiffness; increased muscle tone in extensor muscles with passive flexion as seen with some upper motor neuron diseases

spasticity—A condition caused by lesions to upper motor neurons and marked by a muscle's continuous resistance to stretch due to hypertonia (increased muscle tone) in one group of a muscle pair (often flexors) and hyperreflexia (exaggerated tendon reflexes) in response to voluntary movement

spastic paralysis—Paralysis with increased muscle tone and peripheral reflexes due to loss of control from the pyramidal system

spina bifida—A congenital defect involving the failure of one or more vertebrae (usually in the lumbar region) to completely fuse on the posterior side during fetal development, leaving a gap in the bony encasement of the spinal cord through which the cord and meninges may or may not protrude

spinal cord injury (SCI)—Injury to motor or sensory neurons that lie within the spinal cord

spinal polio—Viral attack upon the anterior horn cells of the spinal cord that affects peripheral motor nerves (most often in the legs) and causes paralysis or weakness

spinal reflex—A reflex whose center (between the afferent and efferent nerve tracts) lies in the spinal cord

stabilizer—Muscles that contract to stabilize a joint during movement at another joint

stasis—Absence of movement or flow in blood vessels

static stretching—A stretching procedure involving slow elongation of a muscle followed by maintenance of the stretched position for a predetermined period of time

steady state—An exercise rate that allows metabolic processes within the muscle to stabilize for an extended period of time

strength—The maximum force a muscle can generate during a single effort or repetition without regard to the velocity of movement

stretching—The process of elongating muscles and connective tissue for the purpose of increasing ROM and improving flexibility

stretch reflex—Reflexive contraction of a muscle in response to stretch

stroke volume (SV)—Contraction force of the heart measured as the volume of blood pumped from the heart with each heartbeat

synergist—A muscle that contracts to enhance the action of another or to rule out unintended actions

systolic blood pressure—Arterial blood pressure during systole (ventricular contraction of the heart)

tendon reflex—Deep reflex in the tendons exaggerated in diseases of upper motor neurons and diminished or lost in diseases of lower motor neurons

tenodesis—Surgical fixation of a tendon to restore lost function or power of a joint; with hand function, passive finger flexion with wrist extension that enables passive grasping by the fingers

thermoregulation—Processes in the body that attempt to regulate internal temperature

training volume—The total amount of work performed during an exercise session

tremor—An involuntary trembling of the body or limbs resulting from alternate contractions of opposing muscle groups; trembling can occur with the initiation of movement (intention tremors) or continuously (nonintentional tremors)

triplegia—Paralysis in three limbs, usually both legs and one arm

unilateral—Pertaining to parts or actions on one side of the body only

upper motor neurons—Motor neurons of the central nervous system originating in the motor cortex of the cerebrum

vasoconstriction—Narrowing of blood vessels

vasodilation—Dilation of blood vessels

ventilation ($\dot{V}_E$)—The volume of air breathed per minute; $\dot{V}_E$ = tidal volume (air breathed per breath) × breathing rate (breaths per minute)

viscoelastic—A property of a tissue that involves both its resistance to stretch and its ability to return to its resting length after being stretched

viscosity—Resistance to flow

vital capacity—Volume of air that can be expelled following a maximal inspiration

References

Adams, R.C., Daniel, A.N., McCubbin, J.A., & Rullman, L. (1982). Games, sports and exercises for the physically handicapped. Philadelphia: Lea and Febiger.

Alter, M.M. (1988). Science of stretching. Champaign, IL: Human Kinetics.

American College of Sports Medicine. (1991). Guidelines for exercise testing and prescription (4th ed.). Philadelphia: Lea & Febiger.

Americans with Disabilities Act of 1990.

Astrand, P.O., & Rodahl, K. (1977). Textbook of work physiology. New York: McGraw-Hill Book Company.

Bennett, R.L., & Knowlton, G.C. (1958). Overwork weakness in partially denervated skeletal muscle. Clinical Orthopedics, 12, 22-29.

Benson, H. (1980). The relaxation response. New York: Avon Books.

Borg, G.A. (1982). Psychophysical bases of perceived exertion. Medicine and Science in Sports and Exercise, 14, 377-381.

Carroll, M.W., Otto, R.M., & Wygand, J. (1991). The metabolic cost of two ranges of arm position height with and without hand weights during low impact aerobic dance. Research Quarterly for Exercise and Sport, 62(4), 420-423.

Chretien, R., Simard, C.P., & Dorion, A. (1985). Effects of relaxation on the peripheral chronaxie of people having multiple sclerosis. In International Federation of Adapted Physical Activity, The Fifth International Symposium on Adapted Physical Activity. Champaign, IL: Human Kinetics.

Cobble, N.D., & Maloney, F.P. (1985). Effects of exercise on neuromuscular disease. In F.P. Maloney, J.S. Burks, & S.P. Ringel (Eds.), Interdisciplinary rehabilitation of multiple sclerosis and neuromuscular disorders. Philadelphia: Lippincott.

Corbin, C.B., & Lindsey, R. (1985). Concepts of physical fitness. Dubuque, IA: Brown.

Corbin, C.B., & Noble, L. (1980). Flexibility: A major component of physical fitness. The Journal of Physical Education and Recreation, 51(6), 23-24, 57-60.

deVries, H.A. (1966). Quantitative electromyographic investigation of the spasm theory of muscle pain. American Journal of Physical Medicine, 45, 119-134.

DiRocco, P. (1986). Values for aerobic capacity of individuals with physical disabilities compared to able-bodied subjects. Unpublished data.

Edwards, R.H.T. (1986). Interaction of chemical with electromechanical factors in human skeletal muscle fatigue. Acta Physiologica Scandinavica, 128 (Suppl. 556), 149-155.

Feldman, R.M. (1985). The use of strengthening exercises in postpolio sequelae. Orthopedics, 8(7), 889-890.

Figoni, S.F. (1990). Perspectives on cardiovascular fitness and SCI. Journal of the American Paraplegia Society, 13, 63-71.

Fleck, S.J. (1988). Cardiovascular adaptations to resistance training. Medicine and Science in Sports and Exercise, 20(5), S146-151.

Fleck, S.J., & Dean, L.S. (1987). Resistance training experience and the pressor response during resistance exercise. Journal of Applied Physiology, 63, 116-120.

Fleck, S.J., & Falkel, J.E. (1986). Value of resistance training for the reduction of sports injuries. Sports Medicine, 3, 61-68.

Ford, J.R., & Duckworth, B. (1974). Physical management for the quadriplegic patient. Philadelphia: Davis.

Frustace, S.J. (1988). Poliomyelitis: Late and unusual sequelae. American Journal of Physical Medicine, 66(6), 328-336.

Gettman, L.R., & Pollock, M.L. (1981). Circuit weight training: A critical review of its physiological benefits. Physician and Sports Medicine, 9, 44-60.

Gordon, N.F. (1993a). Arthritis: Your complete exercise guide. Champaign, IL: Human Kinetics.

Gordon, N.F. (1993b). Stroke: Your complete exercise guide. Champaign, IL: Human Kinetics.

Graves, J.E., Welsch, M., & Pollock, M.L. (1991). Exercise training for muscular strength and endurance. IDEA Today, July-August, 33-40.

Grimby, G., & Einarsson, G. (1991). Post-polio

management. *Physical and Rehabilitation Medicine*, **2**(4), 189-200.

Halstead, L.S. (1990). Postpolio syndrome and exercise. In J.V. Basmajian & S.L. Wolf (Eds.), *Therapeutic exercise* (pp. 231-240). Baltimore: Williams & Wilkins.

Hegey, C., & Aceves, K. (1991). *Fitness programs for individuals with visual impairments: Tips for the exercise leader.* Unpublished report.

Holland, L.J., & Steadward, R.D. (1990, Summer). Effects of resistance and flexibility training on strength, spasticity, muscle tone, and range of motion of elite athletes with cerebral palsy. *Palaestra,* 27-31.

Hooker, S.P., Figoni, S.F., Rodgers, M.M., Glaser, R.M., Mathews, T., Suryaprasad, A.G., & Gupta, S.C. (1992). Physiological effects of electrical stimulation leg cycle exercise training in spinal cord injured persons. *Archives of Physical Medicine and Rehabilitation,* **73**, 470-476.

Houston, M.E., Froese, E.A., Valeriote, St.P., Green, H.J., & Ranney, D.A. (1983). Muscle performance, morphology and metabolic capacity during strength training and detraining: A one leg mode. *European Journal of Applied Physiology,* **51**, 25-35.

Hurley, B.F., Seals, D.R., Ehsani, A.A., Cartier, L.J., Dalsky, G.P., Hagberg, J.M., & Holloszy, J.O. (1984). Effects of high intensity strength training on cardiovascular function. *Medicine and Science in Sports and Exercise,* **16**, 483-488.

Inaba, M., Edberg, E., Montgomery, J., & Gillis, K.M. (1973). Effectiveness of functional training, active exercise, and resistive exercise for patients with hemiplegia. *Physical Therapy,* **53**(1), 28-35.

Jacobson, E. (1978). *You must relax* (5th ed.). New York: McGraw-Hill.

Jencks, B. (1977). *Your body: Biofeedback at its best.* Chicago: Nelson Hall.

Johnson, E.W., & Braddom, R. (1971). Overwork weakness in facioscapulohumeral muscular dystrophy. *Archives of Physical Medicine and Rehabilitation,* **52**, 333-336.

Johnson, M.A., Polgar, J., Weightman, D., & Appleton, D. (1973). Data on the distribution of fibre types in thirty-six human muscles: An autopsy study. *Journal of Neurological Science,* **18**, 111-129.

Kabat, H. (1965). Proprioceptive facilitation in therapeutic exercise. In S. Licht (Ed.), *Therapeutic exercise* (pp. 327-343). Baltimore: Waverly Press.

Kisner, C., & Colby, L.A. (1990). *Therapeutic exercise: Foundations and techniques.* Philadelphia: F.A. Davis.

Knapik, J.J., Mawdsley, R.H., & Ramos, M.U. (1983). Angular specificity and test mode specificity of isometric and isokinetic strength training. *Journal of Orthopedic Sports Physical Therapy,* **5**, 58-65.

Knott, M., Ionta, M.K., and Myers, B.J. (1985). *Proprioceptive neuromuscular facilitation.* New York: Harper & Row.

Knott, M., & Voss, D.E. (1968). *Proprioceptive neuromuscular facilitation: Patterns and techniques.* New York: Haeber-Harper.

Komi, P.V. (1979). Neuromuscular performance: Factors influencing force and speed production. *Scandinavian Journal of Sport Science,* **1**, 4.

MacDougall, J.D., Tuxen, D., Sale, D.G., Moroz, J.R., & Sutton, J.R. (1985). Arterial blood pressure response to heavy resistance exercise. *Journal of Applied Physiology,* **58**, 785-790.

MacLaren, D.P., Gibson, H., Parry-Billings, M., & Edwards, R.H.T. (1989). A review of metabolic and physiological factors in fatigue. In K.B. Pandolf (Ed.), *Exercise and sport science reviews* (pp. 29-66). Baltimore: Williams & Wilkins.

Mathers, L.H. (1985). *The peripheral nervous system: Structure, function, and clinical correlations.* Menlo Park, CA: Addison-Wesley.

McArdle, W.D., Katch, F.I., & Katch, V.L. (1991). *Exercise physiology: Energy, nutrition and human performance* (3rd ed.). Philadelphia: Lea & Febiger.

McAtee, R.E. (1993). *Facilitated stretching.* Champaign, IL: Human Kinetics.

McCubbin, J.A., & Shasby, G.B. (1985). Effects of isokinetic exercise on adolescents with cerebral palsy. *Adapted Physical Activity Quarterly,* **2**, 56-64.

Meyers, C.R. (1967). Effect of two isometric routines on strength, size and endurance in exercised and non-exercised arms. *Research Quarterly,* **38**, 430-440.

Milner-Brown, H.S., & Miller, R.G. (1988). Muscle strengthening through high resistance weight training in patients with neuromuscular disorders. *Archives of Physical Medicine and Rehabilitation,* **69**, 14-19.

Moritani, T., & deVries, H.A. (1979). Neural factors versus hypertrophy in time course of muscle strength gain. *American Journal of Physical Medicine and Rehabilitation,* **58**, 115-130.

Normansell, K.F. (1986). *Guidelines for exercise from a wheelchair.* (unpublished outline).

Olgiati, R., Burgunder, J.M., & Mumenthaler, M. (1988). Increased energy cost of walking in multiple sclerosis: Effects of spasticity, ataxia, and weakness. *Archives of Physical Medicine and Rehabilitation*, **69**, 846-849.

Parker, S.B., Hurley, B.F., Hanlon, D.P., & Vaccaro, P. (1989). Failure of target heart rate to accurately monitor intensity during aerobic dance. *Medicine and Science in Sports and Exercise*, **21**(2), 230-234.

Pate, R.R. (1988). The evolving definition of physical fitness. *Quest*, **40**, 174-179.

Pate, R.R., & Lonnett, M. (1988). Terminology in exercise physiology. In S.N. Blair, P. Painter, R.R. Pate, L.K. Smith, & C.B. Taylor (Eds.), *Resource manual for guidelines for exercise testing and prescription*. Philadelphia: Lea & Febiger.

Pauletto, B. (1986). Let's talk training series. 1: Sets and reps. 2: Intensity. 3: Choice and order of exercise. *National Strength & Conditioning Association Journal*, **7**(6), 67; **8**(1), 33IT; **8**(2), 71IT.

Peach, P.E. (1990). Overwork weakness with evidence of muscle damage in patients with residual paralysis from polio. *Archives of Physical Medicine and Rehabilitation*, **71**, 248-250.

Poliquin, C. (1989, July-Sept.). Theory and methodology of strength training. *Sports Coach*, 25-27.

Rosenthal, B.J., & Scheinberg, L.C. (1990). Exercise for multiple sclerosis patients. In J.V. Basmajian and S.L. Wolf (Eds.), *Therapeutic exercise* (pp. 241-250). Baltimore: Williams & Wilkins.

Rowell, L.B. (1986). *Human circulation: Regulation during physical stress*. New York: Oxford University Press.

Rutherford, O.M., & Jones, D.A. (1986). The role of learning and co-ordination in strength training. *European Journal of Applied Physiology*, **55**, 100-105.

Sale, D.G. (1988). Neural adaptation to resistance training. *Medicine and Science in Sports and Exercise*, **20**(5), S135-145.

Sapega, H.A., Quedenfield, T.C., Moyer, R.A., & Butler, R.A. (1981). Biophysical factors in range-of-motion exercise. *Physician and Sportsmedicine*, **9**, 57-65.

Shephard, R.J. (1990). *Fitness in special populations*. Champaign, IL: Human Kinetics.

Skerker, R.S. (1991). Review and update: The aerobic exercise prescription: Critical reviews. *Physical Rehabilitation Medicine*, **2**(4), 257-271.

Stone, M.H. (1988). Implications for connective tissue and bone alterations resulting from resistance exercise training. *Medicine and Science in Sports and Exercise*, **20**(5), S162-S168.

Stone, M.H., O'Bryant, H., Grahammer, J., McMillan, J., & Rozenek, R. (1982). A theoretical model of strength training. *National Strength and Conditioning Association Journal*, **4**, 4.

Surburg, P.R. (1986). New perspectives for developing range of motion and flexibility for special populations. *Adapted Physical Activity Quarterly*, **3**, 227-235.

Swash, M., & Schwartz, M.S. (1988). *Neuromuscular disease: A practical approach to diagnosis and management* (2nd ed.). New York: Springer-Verlag.

Talag, T.S. (1973). Residual muscle soreness as influenced by concentric, eccentric and static contractions. *Research Quarterly*, **44**, 458-469.

Tesch, P.A. (1988). Skeletal muscle adaptations consequent to long-term heavy resistance exercise. *Medicine and Science in Sports and Exercise*, **20**(5), S132-S134.

Tortora, G. (1986). *Principles of human anatomy*. New York: Harper and Row.

Vogel, J.A. (1988). Introduction to the symposium: Physiological responses and adaptations to resistance exercise. *Medicine and Science in Sports and Exercise*, **20**(5), S131.

Whaley, D.L., & Malott, R.W. (1971). *Elementary principles of behavior*. New York: Appleton-Century-Crofts.

Winnick, J.P. (1990). *Adapted physical education and sport*. Champaign, IL: Human Kinetics.

Yasuda, Y., & Miyamura, M. (1983). Cross-transfer effects of muscular training on blood flow in the ipsilateral and contralateral forearms. *European Journal of Applied Physiology*, **51**, 321-329.

Index

About the Editor DISCARD

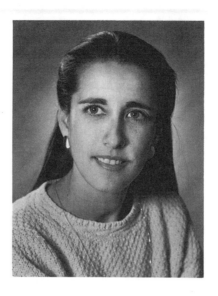

Patricia D. Miller, MA, is an exercise physiologist and consultant in exercise programs for people with disabilities. As the former director of National Handicapped Sports' "Fitness Is For Everyone[SM]" program, Miller coordinated the development of the Adaptive Fitness Instructor Certification Workshops for which this book serves as the text. These workshops have provided training for more than 350 health care, fitness, and recreation professionals throughout the country in modifying exercise routines for people with disabilities. In addition,

Miller initiated mainstream community exercise programs in 26 cities nationwide as part of a grant program funded by the U.S. Department of Education.

An avid triathlete and distance runner, Miller knows firsthand the fitness challenges faced by people with physical impairments. In 1988, she underwent surgery to implant a cardiac pacemaker, yet she continues to train for and participate in road races and triathlons.